Psychotraumatology

Key Papers and Core Concepts in Post-Traumatic Stress

The Plenum Series on Stress and Coping

Series Editor:
Donald Meichenbaum, *University of Waterloo, Waterloo, Ontario, Canada*

Current Volumes in the Series:

COMBAT STRESS REACTION
The Enduring Toll of War
Zahava Solomon

COPING WITH WAR-INDUCED STRESS
The Gulf War and the Israeli Response
Zahava Solomon

INFERTILITY
Perspectives from Stress and Coping Research
Edited by Annette L. Stanton and Christine Dunkel-Schetter

INTERNATIONAL HANDBOOK OF TRAUMATIC STRESS SYNDROMES
Edited by John P. Wilson and Beverley Raphael

PSYCHOTRAUMATOLOGY
Key Papers and Core Concepts in Post-Traumatic Stress
Edited by George S. Everly, Jr. and Jeffrey M. Lating

THE SOCIAL CONTEXT OF COPING
Edited by John Eckenrode

STRESS AND MENTAL HEALTH
Contemporary Issues and Prospects for the Future
Edited by William R. Avison and Ian H. Gotlib

THE UNNOTICED MAJORITY IN PSYCHIATRIC INPATIENT CARE
Charles A. Kiesler and Celeste G. Simpkins

WOMEN, WORK, AND HEALTH
Stress and Opportunities
Edited by Marianne Frankenhauser, Ulf Lundberg, and
Margaret Chesney

Psychotraumatology

Key Papers and Core Concepts in Post-Traumatic Stress

Edited by

George S. Everly, Jr.

International Critical Incident Stress Foundation
Ellicott City, Maryland
Union Memorial Hospital
Baltimore, Maryland
and Loyola College
Baltimore, Maryland

and

Jeffrey M. Lating

Union Memorial Hospital
Baltimore, Maryland

PLENUM PRESS • NEW YORK AND LONDON

Library of Congress Cataloging-in-Publication Data

On file

ISBN 0-306-44782-7 (Hardbound)
ISBN 0-306-44783-5 (Paperback)

A Division of Plenum Publishing Corporation
233 Spring Street, New York, N.Y. 10013

10 9 8 7 6 5 4 3 2

Printed in the United States of America

To Andrea Newman Everly, may you know only peace, happiness, and love

To George S. Everly, Sr., who has provided and continues to provide steadfast love and support

Finally, to Kathleen Webster Everly, whose strength, courage, and love were my blessings to receive

—GSE

To George and Dorothy Lating for a lifetime of unconditional love and support

To my wife Kathy, who has added special meaning to my life

—JML

Contributors

Joel Osler Brende, Regional Psychiatric Division, Central State Hospital, Milledgeville, Georgia 31061; and Department of Psychiatry, Mercer University School of Medicine, Macon, Georgia 31207

Paul Brown, Northpark Hospital Centre, Bundoora, Melbourne, Victoria, Australia

Dennis S. Charney, Department of Veterans Affairs Medical Center, West Haven, Connecticut 06516

Peter Dunn, Staff Counseling Service, State Bank Victoria, Melbourne, Victoria 3000, Australia

George S. Everly, Jr., International Critical Incident Stress Foundation, Ellicott City, Maryland 21242; Union Memorial Hospital, Baltimore, Maryland 21218; and Department of Psychology, Loyola College, Baltimore, Maryland 21210.

John A. Fairbank, Research Triangle Institute, Research Park, North Carolina 27709

Charles R. Figley, Psychosocial Stress Research Program, and the Marriage and Family Therapy Center, Florida State University, Tallahassee, Florida 32306-2024

Matthew J. Friedman, National Center for PTSD, Department of Veterans Affairs Medical and Regional Office Center, White River Junction, Vermont 05009; and Dartmouth College Medical School, Hanover, New Hampshire 03756

Judith Lewis Herman, 61 Roseland St., Somerville, Massachusetts 02143

Mardi J. Horowitz, Center for the Study of Neuroses, Langley Porter Institute, University of California, San Francisco, California 94143

A. MacNeill Horton, Jr., Psych Associates, Towson, Maryland 21204

Ronnie Janoff-Bulman, Department of Psychology, University of Massachusetts, Amherst, Massachusetts 01003

David R. Johnson, Department of Veterans Affairs Medical Center, West Haven, Connecticut 06516

Nancy B. Kaltreider, Center for the Study of Neuroses, Langley Porter Institute, University of California, San Francisco, California 94143

Terence M. Keane, Outpatient Clinics, Department of Veterans Affairs Medical Center, Boston, Massachusetts 02130

John H. Krystal, Department of Veterans Affairs Medical Center, West Haven, Connecticut 06516

Jeffrey M. Lating, Division of Psychology and Behavioral Medicine, Union Memorial Hospital, Baltimore, Maryland 21218

Monica Manton, Staff Counseling Service, State Bank Victoria, Melbourne, Victoria 3000, Australia

Jeffrey T. Mitchell, Emergency Health Services, University of Maryland, Baltimore County, Baltimore, Maryland 21228; and International Critical Incident Stress Foundation, Ellicott City, Maryland 21042

Elana Newman, National Center for PTSD, Boston Medical Center, Boston, Massachusetts 02130

Robert A. Nicholson, Department of Veterans Affairs Medical Center and University of Mississippi Medical Center, Jackson, Mississippi 39216

Frank M. Ochberg, Department of Psychiatry, Michigan State University, East Lansing, Michigan 48824

Susan Roth, Department of Psychology, Duke University, Durham, North Carolina 27706

Steven M. Southwick, Department of Veterans Affairs Medical Center, West Haven, Connecticut 06516

Alison Talbot, Staff Counseling Service, State Bank Victoria, Melbourne, Victoria 3000, Australia

Leonore C. Terr, 450 Sutter Street, San Francisco, California 94108

Onno van der Hart, Department of Clinical and Health Psychology, University of Utrecht, Utrecht, The Netherlands; and Dissociation Team, Regional Institute for Ambulatory Mental Health Care, Amsterdam South/New West, Amsterdam, The Netherlands

Bessel A. van der Kolk, Trauma Clinic, Massachusetts General Hospital and Harvard Medical School, Boston, Massachusetts 02114

Joseph Westermeyer, Department of Psychiatry, University of Minnesota Hospitals and Clinics, Minneapolis, Minnesota 55455, and Department of Psychiatry, Department of Veterans Affairs Medical Center, Minneapolis, Minnesota 55417

John P. Wilson, Department of Psychology, Cleveland State University, Cleveland, Ohio 44115

Amos Zeichner, Department of Psychology, University of Georgia, Athens, Georgia 30602

Preface

The nosological roots of post-traumatic stress disorder (PTSD) may be traced back to the American Psychiatric Association's DSM-I entry of gross stress reaction, as published in 1952. Yet the origins of the current enthusiasm with regard to post-traumatic stress can be traced back to 1980, which marked the emergence of the term *post-traumatic stress disorder* in the DSM-III. This reflected the American Psychiatric Association's acknowledgment of post-traumatic stress as a discrete, phenomenologically unique, and reliable psychopathological entity at a time in American history when such recognition had important social, political, and psychiatric implications.

Clearly, prior to DSM-I the lack of a generally accepted terminology did little to augment the disabling effects that psychological traumatization could engender. Nor did the subsequent provision of an official diagnostic label alone render substantial ameliorative qualities. Nevertheless, the post-Vietnam DSM-III recognition of PTSD did herald a dramatic increase in research and clinical discovery. The American Red Cross acknowledged the need to establish disaster mental health services, the American Psychological Association urged its members to form disaster mental health networks, and the Veterans Administration established a national study center for PTSD.

As this text is published, we stand with 15 years of temporal distance and sufficient intellectual, emotional, and political distance to reflect in a meaningful way upon the origins and current status of the field this text refers to as *psychotraumatology*. Similarly, it seems to be an appropriate point in the evolution of this field to offer this text as a scholarly—yet clinically relevant—benchmark.

Indeed, the objective being sought through the creation of this volume is not to produce an exhaustive, definitive treatise. Rather, this volume represents a unique blending of original contributions, scholarly reviews, and a selection of previously published papers that are in some way deemed to be key contributions to the psychotraumatology literature. The volume then superimposes an overarching integrative two-factor formulation of post-traumatic stress that attempts to unify and bring order to the extant information contained herein. Thus the goal of this volume is merely to tempt the reader to speculate as to the phenomenology of post-traumatic stress, with the subsequent goal of improving clinical therapeutics. Indeed, effective therapy is the corollary of phenomenology.

The text is offered as an academically challenging—yet clinically relevant—presentation for students as well as professionals in clinical psychology, psychiatry, nursing, social work, sociology, health education, and public health. In the final analysis, this volume is an effort, albeit ever so small and indirect, to lessen human suffering associated with post-traumatic stress.

George S. Everly, Jr.
Jeffrey M. Lating

Acknowledgments

I am indebted to Mark Greenberg, Ph.D., and Bessel van der Kolk, M.D., both of whom greatly stimulated my academic interests in the study of posttraumatic stress while I was at Harvard University.

I am grateful to the American Red Cross for allowing me to become part of its historic efforts to provide mental health services to victims of disaster, both locally and nationally. Special thanks go to Kay Hunley and Mike Ritter at the Central Maryland Chapter of the American Red Cross, as well as to Jane Morgan and Bev Clayton at the national headquarters.

I would like to thank Joe Chamberlin at the national headquarters of Catholic Relief Services for allowing me to gain a truly unique international perspective on humanitarian aid and disaster.

My thanks to Bertram Brown, M.D., one of mental health's senior statesmen, for his encouragement to investigate psychological trauma cross-culturally and internationally.

Finally, I am most indebted to Jeffrey T. Mitchell, Ph.D., developer of critical incident stress debriefing (CISD), for opening my career to a realm of experiences rich and unique in all the world. From him I have learned much.

GSE

I would like to thank Amos Zeichner, Ph.D., University of Georgia, and Terence M. Keane, Ph.D., Boston VA, for their scholarly contributions. I would also like to thank Stephen F. Bono, Ph.D., and Jennifer A. Haythornthwaite, Ph.D., both of whom provided helpful suggestions, encouragement, resources, and support. I would especially like to thank Kathy Niager, Ph.D., who provided the patience, tolerance, and comfort necessary for me to stay focused on my work.

JML

Finally, we would both like to thank Eliot Werner and Donald Meichenbaum, Ph.D., for their useful suggestions.

Contents

I. THE NATURE OF POST-TRAUMATIC STRESS

II. ASSESSMENT OF POST-TRAUMATIC STRESS

V. SPECIAL ISSUES IN POST-TRAUMATIC STRESS

I

The Nature of Post-Traumatic Stress

First study the science, then practice the arts.
—Leonardo da Vinci

The purpose of Part I is to examine the nature of post-traumatic stress. In doing so we will review conceptual, historical, biological, and psychological evidence as well as speculation.

The importance of pursuing such inquiry is underscored by the words of Leonardo da Vinci above. For the phenomenologist, such a discussion dedicated to foundational underpinnings may be an end unto itself. For the clinician, though, it can prove to be the basis for sound clinical practice. Indeed, the most effective clinical interventions will be those based on an understanding of the phenomenology of the disorder at hand.

Chapter 1 introduces the overarching concept of psychotraumatology as a more precise umbrella construction under which post-traumatic stress—and specifically post-traumatic stress disorder (PTSD), with its broad spectrum of factors and facets—may be studied. Chapter 1 argues for the creation of an integrative model of post-traumatic stress.

Chapter 2 underscores the importance of reviewing the past to uncover the historical roots of traumatic stress as a means of understanding extant formulations.

Chapter 3 provides the reader with a macroanalytic integrative construction of post-traumatic stress wherein PTSD is viewed as an epiphenomenon. Chapter 3 builds for the reader an integrative two-factor model wherein biological factors are inextricably intertwined with psychological factors to explain the post-traumatic stress phenomenon. This two-factor neurocognitive theme will be used as a unifying construct throughout the text.

Chapter 4 presents a detailed but useful review of major biological mechanisms at work in PTSD. In doing so, it represents a microanalysis of the first of the two constituent factors of PTSD as discussed in Chapter 3 (i.e., neurological arousal).

Chapter 5 continues the theme of microanalysis by examining some of the core dynamics undergirding psychological discord, (the second of the two constituent factors of PTSD) which is based on a violation of the victim's assumptions about the self and worldview.

Finally, Chapter 6 examines PTSD that is engendered via prolonged or repeated traumatization. This chapter on complex PTSD represents an important extension of the psychological trauma concept.

1

Psychotraumatology

GEORGE S. EVERLY, JR.

BASIC FOUNDATIONS

It has been estimated that excessive stress and its various physical manifestations account for more than 80% of all visits to health care professionals (Cummings & Vanden Bos, 1981). According to the National Council on Compensation Insurance, excessive stress accounts for about 14% of all "occupational disease" workers' compensation claims (McCarthy, 1988); the council notes that the per-claim benefit payments for stress-related disorders average roughly twice those of physical disorders. Estimates have placed the overall cost of stress on the American economy as high as $150 billion per year (Miller et al., 1988). Data such as these have caused some to consider excessive stress as a virtual plague on society that has, indeed, reached epidemic proportions. Yet the common images of workaholic executives, overpressured middle managers, and burned out nurses, doctors, teachers, or sales personnel represent only one aspect of the plague. Another aspect, one that may give no warning of its approach nor of its destructive force, is post-traumatic stress.

Descriptions of post-traumatic stress reactions date back to the 6th century B.C. within the context of warfare (Holmes, 1985), and such reactions are well documented beginning in the 17th century A.D. in response to civilian tragedy (e.g., train disasters, large fires; Trimble, 1981). Despite such recognition, though, systematic inquiry into the phenomenon of post-traumatic stress was remarkably late in coming. The origins of the current enthusiasm with regard to post-traumatic stress can be traced to the year

---

GEORGE S. EVERLY, JR. • International Critical Incident Stress Foundation, Ellicott City, Maryland 21242; Union Memorial Hospital, Baltimore, Maryland 21218; and Department of Psychology, Loyola College, Baltimore, Maryland 21210.

Psychotraumatology, edited by George S. Everly, Jr. and Jeffrey M. Lating. Plenum Press, New York, 1995.

1980, when the term *post-traumatic stress disorder* (PTSD) entered into the official psychiatric nosology (American Psychiatric Association [APA], 1980). This recognition, of at least one form of post-traumatic stress as a discrete, phenomenologically unique, and reliable psychopathological disorder heralded a dramatic proliferation of theoretical and empirical expositions into the nature and treatment of post-traumatic stress.

We now stand with sufficient intellectual, emotional, and temporal distance from the spawning of the concept of post-traumatic stress to attempt to provide order and commentary to this field, which has become a virtual clinical subspecialty. In such an effort, Everly (1992; 1993) has referred to this field as psychotraumatology.

PSYCHOTRAUMATOLOGY DEFINED

The term *psychotraumatology* is used in the present context to define or order the conduct of inquiry and the categorization of information relevant to psychological trauma. Psychotraumatology may be defined as the study of psychological trauma; more specifically, the study of the processes and factors that lie (a) antecedent to, (b) concomitant with, and (c) subsequent to psychological traumatization (Everly, 1992; 1993).

Donovan (1991) suggested that the term *traumatology* be used to unite the various endeavors within the field of traumatic stress studies. As Donovan notes, however, the term *traumatology* also denotes the branch of medicine that deals with wounds and serious injuries. Schnitt (1993) expressed concern over Donovan's choice of a term that has at least two meanings. He urged clarity of communications as this new field expands; indeed, expansion is often built upon and facilitated by clarity of communications fostered by sematic precision. In a rebuttal of sorts, Donovan (1993) argued for a term broader in scope than *traumatic stress studies,* the phrase that has been used historically to unite the field.

Clearly Schnitt's (1993) commentary offers insight to be considered. There is significant potential for ambiguity in the use of *traumatology* as a unifying term for the field of psychological trauma. Donovan (1993) argues that the term is "socially influential as well as conceptually and pragmatically useful" (p. 410). The potential ambiguity serves to diminish the promised pragmatics, but the lack of sematic precision is easily corrected. The addition of the prefix *psycho-* to the root *traumatology* appears to clarify potential ambiguities and more clearly defines the conduct at hand. Such reasoning serves as the foundation for the choice of *psychotraumatology* as the title of this volume.

Using the tripartite schema that defines psychotraumatology as the study of the process and factors that lie antecedent to, concomitant with, and subsequent to psychological traumatization, issues and variables for theoretical, controlled empirical, and clinical inquiry may be more easily identified and classified. An example is shown below:

1. Factors antecedent to psychological traumatization
   a. Personal developmental history
   b. Familial history (both of origin and procreation)
   c. Predisposing personality factors
   d. Occupational risk factors
   e. Behavioral risk factors
   f. Predisposing psychological states
   g. Psychiatric risk factors
2. Factors concomitant with psychological traumatization
   a. Traumatogenetic environmental factors
   b. Traumatogenetic interpersonal factors
   c. Traumatogenetic situational factors
   d. Traumatogenetic biological factors
   e. The psychology of traumatogenesis
   f. Biological substrates of traumatogenesis
3. Factors emerging subsequent to psychological traumatization
   a. Psychological responses to trauma
   b. Central nervous system sequelae
   c. Systemic pathophysiological sequelae
   d. Psychophysiological sequelae
   e. Behavioral sequelae
   f. Familial patterns
   g. Sociological patterns (occupational, community, national, international)

PREVALENCE: WAR-RELATED POST-TRAUMATIC STRESS

Warfare is a fertile breeding ground for post-traumatic stress. Most who have experienced the terror of human warfare would agree with General William Sherman's utterance during the American Civil War that "all war is hell." Yet this notion is not a new one. As noted earlier the adverse psychological effects of warfare were recorded as early as 600 B.C.; in the Napoleonic War 24 centuries later, General Sir Thomas Picton wrote to Lord Wellington, "My Lord, I must give up. I am grown so nervous . . . it is impossible for me to sleep at nights. I cannot possibly stand it, and I shall be forced to retire" (Holmes, 1985).

Efforts have been made throughout history to quantify the prevalence of post-traumatic stress reactions as a result of warfare. Some difficulty was encountered, however, as a result of the varying diagnostic labels that were applied prior to the advent of PTSD as a classification. For example terms like *shell shock, soldier's heart, battle fatigue, gross stress reaction,* and *traumatic neurosis* have all been employed as diagnostic labels, as will be discussed in Chapter 2. Nevertheless, some estimates do indeed exist. During the American Civil War, psychiatric casualties were estimated at between 2.3 and 3.3 per 1,000 troops. During World War I the prevalence rose to 4.0 per 1,000. Data generated from the National Vietnam Veterans' Readjustment Study (Kulka et al., 1990) reveal the lifetime prevalence of PTSD to be 30%, with 15.2% of Vietnam veterans showing a current diagnosis of PTSD.

PREVALENCE: CIVILIAN-RELATED POST-TRAUMATIC STRESS

Although society most commonly associates post-traumatic stress with warfare, it is clear that such stress can be engendered by noncombat situations as well. The revised third edition of the *Diagnostic and Statistical Manual of Mental Disorders,* (DSM-III-R) explicitly noted that PTSD may arise from the exposure to

> a psychologically distressing event that is outside the usual range of human experience. . . . The trauma may be experienced alone (e.g., rape or assault) or in the company of groups of people (e.g., military combat). Stressors . . . include natural disasters . . . accidental disasters (e.g., car accidents with serious physical injury, airplane crashes, large fires, collapse of physical structures), or deliberately caused disasters (e.g., bombing, torture, death camps). (APA, 1987, p. 248).

DSM-IV sustains the belief that PTSD may be engendered in civilian life by emphasizing the perception of threat in the diagnostic criteria (APA, 1994).

Trimble (1981) noted that post-traumatic stress was well documented subsequent to the Great Fire of London in 1666. No less a historian than Charles Dickens described, in his personal diary, his own battle with post-traumatic stress after his involvement as a passenger in a tragic rail disaster outside of London.

An epidemiological investigation conducted by Helzer et al. (1987) found the prevalence of PTSD in the general population of the United States to be about 1%, roughly equivalent to that of schizophrenia. Breslau et al. (1991) found the prevalence of PTSD to be about 9% in a cohort of young adults living in an urban setting. Norman and Getek (1988) have estimated that nearly half of all patients admitted to urban shock-trauma medical centers are likely to suffer from PTSD in addition to their physical trauma. Lastly, it is useful to note at "four in 10 Americans have been exposed to a major traumatic event before the age of 30: Of these, one in four developed post-traumatic stress disorder (PTSD)" (Davidson, 1991, p. 62). Given the events that are usually associated with post-traumatic stress, it is safe to say that it is probably underreported and underdiagnosed. Thus the prevalence of post-traumatic stress in the general population is most likely woefully underestimated.

POST-TRAUMATIC STRESS VERSUS PTSD

Using the far-reaching conceptualization of psychotraumatology suggested earlier, we see that the study of psychological trauma is far more than just the study of PTSD. For example, other than the sudden death phenomenon, post-traumatic stress represents potentially the most severe and incapacitating form of human stress known (Everly, 1989). Post-traumatic stress is directly associated with the DSM-IV Axis I diagnoses of PTSD, acute stress disorder, dissociative disorders, and brief psychotic disorder with marked stressor(s). It is likely to be similarly associated with the DSM-IV Axis II diagnosis of borderline personality disorder (Herman & van der Kolk, 1987).

It also seems clear that post-traumatic stress may be related, in varying degrees, to alcohol abuse and other forms of substance abuse via compensatory or self-medicating drives. Various mood disorders, panic disorders, phobias, family dysfunctions, various patterns of compulsivity, and various eating disorders may be related to trauma in some cases as well. Finally, post-traumatic stress may give rise to a diverse myriad of stress-related physical complaints and disorders in addition to or in concomitance with the psychiatric and behavioral disorders already enumerated. Given the perspectives just enumerated, PTSD may be viewed as an epiphenomenon arising from the more central phenomenon of post-traumatic stress.

PLAN OF THE BOOK

As just noted, the study of psychological trauma is far more than merely the study of PTSD. The purpose of this volume is to make note of the breadth of such an endeavor while also offering an opportunity for theoretical reflection and phenomenological integration. This text offers the reader a macroanalytic, conceptually integrative, global perspective within which the constructs of psychological trauma, traumatic stress, and related constructions may be amalgamated. It attempts to provide a form and structure from which traumatic stress may be better understood.

Two primary integrative efforts are offered within this volume. First, the use of the amalgamating term *psychotraumatology* is rendered as a means of more succinctly defining the field. Second, after a review of historical foundations in Chapter 2, Chapter 3 offers the reader an integrative two-factor model of post-traumatic stress that may applied in an overarching manner to integrate phenomenological, diagnostic, and treatment issues as well as technologies.

The text itself is divided into five sections. Part I is dedicated to an analysis of post-traumatic stress from conceptual, historical, biological, and psychological perspectives. It attempts to set the stage for the remainder of the text by offering the reader an integrative macroanalytic two-factor model of post-traumatic stress in Chapter 3 that may be used as a framework of reference for the various microanalytic chapters which follow. Part II addresses the assessment of post-traumatic stress; psychological, psychophysiological, and neuropsychological approaches are discussed.

Part III focuses on the treatment of post-traumatic stress. The integrative two-factor phenomenological model is once again employed to guide therapeutic strategy formulation in Chapter 10. Various microanalyses follow in the way of discussions of various post-traumatic therapeutic tactics. Part IV offers the reader a discussion of the prevention of post-traumatic stress from one highly specialized perspective. Finally, Part V addresses issues and concerns for special populations in regard to psychological trauma.

REFERENCES

American Psychiatric Association (1980). *Diagnostic and statistical manual of mental disorders* (3rd ed.). Washington, DC: Author.

American Psychiatric Association (1987). *Diagnostic and statistical manual of mental disorders* (rev. 3rd ed.). Washington, DC: Author.

American Psychiatric Association (1994). *Diagnostic and statistical manual of mental disorders* (4th ed.). Washington, D.C.: Author.

Breslau, N., Davis, G., & Andreski, P. (1991). Traumatic events and post-traumatic stress disorder in an urban population of young adults. *Archives of General Psychiatry, 48,* 216–222.

Cummings, N. A., & Vanden Bos, G. R. (1981). The twenty year Kaiser-Permanente experience with psychotherapy and medical utilization. *Health Policy Quarterly, 1,* 159–175.

Davidson, J. (1991, September). Clinical efficacy shown in pharmacologic treatment of post-traumatic stress disorder. *Psychiatric Times,* 62–63.

Donovan, D. M. (1991). Traumatology: A field whose time has come. *Journal of Traumatic Stress, 4,* 433–436.

Donovan, D. M. (1993). Traumatology: What's in a name? *Journal of Traumatic Stress, 6,* 409–412.

Everly, G. S. (1989). *A clinical guide to the treatment of the human stress response.* New York: Plenum.

Everly, G. S. (1992, February). *Psychotraumatology: A two-factor formulation of post-traumatic stress.* Paper presented to the Montreux Congress on Stress, Montreux, Switzerland.

Everly, G. S. (1993). Psychotraumatology: A two-factor formulation of post-traumatic stress. *Integrative Physiological and Behavioral Science, 28,* 270–278.

Helzer, J., Robins, L., & McEvoy, L. (1987). Post-traumatic stress disorder in the general population. *New England Journal of Medicine, 317,* 1630–1634.

Herman, J., & van der Kolk, B. (1987). Traumatic antecedents of borderline personality disorder. In B. van der Kolk (Ed.), *Psychological trauma* (pp. 111–126). Washington, DC: American Psychiatric Press.

Holmes, R. (1985). *Acts of war.* New York: Free Press.

Kulka, R., et al. (1990). *Trauma and the Vietnam war generation.* New York: Brunner Mazel.

McCarthy, M. (1988, April 7). Stress employees look for relief in workers' compensation claims. *Wall Street Journal,* 34.

Miller, A., et al. (1988, April 25). Stress on the job. *Newsweek,* pp. 40–41.

Norman, E., & Getek, D. (1988). Post-traumatic stress disorder in victims of physical trauma [Abstract]. *Proceedings of the 15th Annual National Teaching Institute of the American Association of Critical Care Nurses* (p. 671). Newport Beach, CA: American Association of Critical Care Nurses.

Schnitt, J. M. (1993). Traumatic stress studies: What's in a name? *Journal of Traumatic Stress, 6,* 405–408.

Trimble, M. (1981). *Post-traumatic neurosis.* New York: Wiley.

2

The Historical Evolution of PTSD Diagnostic Criteria

From Freud to DSM-IV

JOHN P. WILSON

INTRODUCTION

In the last quarter of this century, there has been a rapid proliferation of interest in traumatic stress syndromes, especially in post-traumatic stress disorder (PTSD) as a diagnostic category of the *Diagnostic and Statistical Manual of Mental Disorders, Third Edition-Revised* (DSM-III-R) (American Psychiatric Association, 1987). Viewed from a historical perspective, the emergence of widespread interest in PTSD by the medical and behavioral sciences as well as in legal arenas of litigation is quite understandable perhaps, expectable when examined by a retrospective look at some major events of the 20th century: two world wars, the atomic bombing of Hiroshima, scores of nationalistic and colonial wars, widespread civil violence, mass genocide, catastrophic disasters of human and natural origin, the growing awareness of domestic violence and childhood sexual abuse, technological disasters, famine, widespread diseases such as acquired immune deficiency syndrome (AIDS), and many more forms of catastrophic stress. When it is considered that hundreds of millions of human lives have been adversely effected by such traumatic events, it only stands to reason that sooner or later scientific inquiry would begin examining the multifaceted aspects of what traumatiza-

---

JOHN P. WILSON • Department of Psychology, Cleveland State University, Cleveland, Ohio 44115.

Psychotraumatology, edited by George S. Everly, Jr. and Jeffrey M. Lating. Plenum Press, New York, 1995.

tion means and its potential long-term impact to human lives of such events. Today there is a convergence of interest in PTSD. Such seemingly odd bedfellows as the neurosciences, experimental psychology, clinical psychiatry, and sociology are probing new areas of traumatic impact and discovering the complex psychobiological processes that control reaction patterns, symptom manifestation, and other aspects of coping and adaptation following a traumatic event (Wilson, 1989; Wilson & Raphael, 1993).

The psychic residue of such exposure has most commonly been approached by examining the stress response, which itself has been conceptualized in many different ways (Horowitz, 1986; Peterson, Prout & Schwarz, 1991; Trimble, 1981, 1985; Wilson, 1989). Although it is beyond the scope of this chapter to review the many theories of traumatic stress, it is worthwhile to examine seminal contributions that have had a profound influence on the evolution of the diagnostic criteria of the American Psychiatric Association (APA) for PTSD as well as other medico-legal definitions throughout the world. In particular, the contributions of Sigmund Freud will be briefly reviewed because of their importance to European and American thinking about psychic trauma and placed into a historical and cultural perspective. Freud's conceptualization of traumatic neurosis dominated thinking in the medical-psychiatric profession from about 1895 to the end of the Vietnam War era in the United States (1962–1975). This conceptualization of traumatic neurosis was basically rewritten into the DSM (APA, 1952) diagnostic criteria for gross stress reaction, the earliest diagnostic category for what was later codified as PTSD in the DSM-III-R (APA, 1987). Between DSM and DSM-II (APA, 1968) changes began to unfold that, on the one hand, are very puzzling (if not regressive) and, on the other hand, reflect the paucity of hardheaded thinking and empirical inquiry about the human consequences of victimization and traumatization. After the DSM-II, PTSD appeared in the DSM-III (APA, 1980); since then, knowledge has accumulated rapidly, and research has proliferated on a global level (Wilson, 1989; Wilson & Raphael, 1993).

FREUD'S PERSPECTIVE OF PSYCHOLOGICAL TRAUMA: 1895–1939

In 1895 Freud published *Studies in Hysteria* with Josef Breuer, which launched Freud's brilliant career. Between 1895 and 1897, Freud shifted emphasis in his thinking away from a PTSD paradigm of neurosis to a paradigm that centered around intrapsychic fantasy.

While a complete discussion of Freud's contribution to the understanding of psychic trauma is beyond the scope of this chapter, there are several issues in his work of major significance to the understanding of how the diagnostic criteria evolved in the United States and elsewhere.

To establish a broader historical framework, it should be noted that

Freud's original view of neuroses was a post-traumatic paradigm known within psychoanalytic circles as "seduction theory." In this early theoretical and clinical formulation (e.g., *Aetiology of Neuroses,* 1896), Freud stated that during childhood development there was a range of traumatic experiences and events that could be profoundly distressing to an individual (Brett, 1993). As a result of the degree of threat experienced to the ego and the subsequent anxiety, the victim typically used repression as an ego defense to remove unpleasant memories and emotions of the traumatic event from awareness. Once repression was employed, various neurotic symptoms and behaviors would appear and potentially lead the person into treatment. Moreover, Freud's early thinking about trauma also involved the concepts that children were sexual beings from birth onward and that the sexual instinct was one of the basic libidinal forces that could lead to intrapsychic conflict. This conflict could result in neurotic symptoms, neuroses or "the psychopathology" of everyday life. As many scholars have noted (Jones, 1953, p. 287–319), Freud's emphasis on sexuality as a cause of neurosis was not well received in conservative Vienna during his early years as a physician. Amidst criticism and peer pressure, he began revising seduction theory in 1897 to suggest that the memories of patients seeking treatment may only have been *fantasies* of such events, which had their origins in libidinal drives and conflicted or deprived attachments to parental figures (Masson, 1984). Freud's biographer, Ernest Jones (1953) noted this change in Freud's theories of hysteria, neuroses, and their relation to trauma. He emphasized that Freud wanted to shift emphasis away from the reality of trauma to a focus on "psychical" phenomena in which Freud thought fantasy, imagery, and thoughts were more central to analysis than actual memories of early childhood abuse. Thus, in an 1897 letter to his friend Wilhelm Fleiss, Freud revealed his abandonment of the seduction theory to a conceptual model which emphasized the role of fantasy in intrapsychic processes. This view was later stated directly, as in this passage from *The Introductory Lectures on Psychoanalysis* (1917, 1966).

> It will be a long time before [the patient] can take in our proposal that we should equate phantasy and reality and not bother to begin with whether the childhood experiences under examination are the one or the other. Yet, this is clearly the only correct attitude to adopt towards mental productions. They too possess a reality of a sort. It remains a fact that the patient has created these phantasies for himself, and this fact is of scarcely less importance for his neurosis than if he had really experienced what the phantasies contain. These phantasies possess psychical as contrasted with material reality, and we gradually learn to understand that in the world of neuroses it is psychical reality which is the decisive kind (p. 368).

Freud's shift of emphasis away from a post-traumatic seduction theory to an instinct-driven Oedipal model with focus on intrapsychic mechanisms also had the consequence of disavowing, minimizing, or recasting the role of external, event-based stressor experiences that negatively impacted on the process of psychosexual development (Masson, 1984). Further, while it is clear that Freud understood traumatic neurosis (see below), his shift away from a post-traumatic paradigm of neurosis to an Oedipal model replete with "phantasies of a physical versus a material reality" naturally led to an examination of *premorbid* psychic functioning as a determinant of mental disturbances, especially anxiety states and neuroses. As will be evident in the explicit DSM criteria for gross stress reaction (GSR), Freud's shift in paradigms also led to the formulation that traumatic impacts to the self-structure were acute and transient in nature. Thus, if there were prolonged reactions to trauma, they were not caused directly by the "material reality" of stressor events but by the premorbid traits and psychodynamics of the individual.

Sigmund Freud was no stranger to understanding trauma and its symptom constellations. In various works, he elaborated on the nature of traumatic neurosis and its mechanisms. For example, in *The Introductory Lectures on Psychoanalysis* (1917, 1966), Freud wrote as follows:

> The closest analogy to this behavior of our neurotics is afforded by illnesses which are being produced with special frequency precisely at the present time by the war—what are described as traumatic neuroses. Similar cases, of course, appeared before the war as well, after railway collisions and other alarming accidents involving fatal risks. Traumatic neuroses are not in essence the same thing as the spontaneous neuroses which we are in the habit of investigating and treating by analysis; nor have we yet succeeded in bringing them into harmony with our views, and I hope I shall be able at some time to explain to you the reason for this limitation. But in one respect we may insist that there is a complete agreement between them. The traumatic neuroses give a clear indication that a fixation to the traumatic accident lives at their root. These patients regularly repeat the traumatic situation in their dreams; where hysteriform attacks occur that admit of an analysis, we find that the attack corresponds to a complete transplanting of the patient into the traumatic situation. It is as though these patients had not yet finished with the traumatic situation, as though they were still faced by it as an immediate task which has not been dealt with; and we take this view quite seriously (pp. 274–275).

This passage is quite interesting from a historical perspective for several reasons when scrutinized by the DSM-III-R diagnostic criteria for PTSD. First, Freud recognizes that, prior to the 1917 publication date of his book, there were stressor events (e.g., World War I, railroad collisions, physical injuries, fatal risk accidents, child abuse, etc.) that generated "illnesses" with "special frequency." He acknowledges that it was not uncommon for such traumatic events to produce a "traumatic neurosis." Second, he hints at the fact that traumatic neuroses are not the same phenomena as spontaneous neuroses, yet fails to explain the difference. Third, he very clearly describes the core PTSD symptom clusters listed in the DSM-III-R 70 years before the revision of the diagnostic category. For example, (a) intrusive imagery ("patients regularly repeat the traumatic situation in their dreams"); (b) physiological hyperactivity ("hysteriform attacks occur—the attack corresponds to a complete transplanting of the patient into the traumatic situation" and (c) active reliving the event as if it was recurring ("it is as though these patients had not finished with the traumatic situation, as though they were still faced by it as an immediate task which has not been dealt with"). This last criterion implies that the traumatic event was not yet metabolized psychologically (Lindy, 1993). Further, it was active not only in the form of intrusive imagery associated with the trauma but also in attempts to ward off its impact to the ego.

While it appears that Freud was attempting to build a parsimonious psychological theory of behavior in which instinctual forces gave rise to epiphenomenal psychic reality in various states of consciousness, it is apparent that he sought to understand different types of traumatic neurosis, especially those created by warfare. For example, in 1918, at the proceedings of the fifth International Psycho-Analytical Congress held in Budapest, Hungary (later published in 1955), he wrote of traumatic neuroses in a way which illustrated his difficulty in explaining the different mechanisms that underlie "ordinary neuroses" and "war neuroses." In war neuroses, the conflict between the superego and the id is such that the neurosis is a form of compromise to the horror of warfare, states of fear, and aggression. He further elaborates on this change in ego state (i.e., peacetime ego versus war-affected ego) and notes that in war neuroses, the threat to the ego is external, in the form of annihilation or physical injury. Nevertheless, he deduces that in both traumatic neurosis and war neurosis, repression is the central psychological defense against anxiety and libidinal gratification.

> In traumatic and war neuroses, the human ego is defending itself from a danger which threatens it from without or which is embodied in a shape assumed by the ego itself. In the transference neuroses of peace, the enemy from which the ego is defending itself is actually the libido, whose demands seem to it to be menacing. In both cases, the ego is afraid of being damaged—in the latter case by the libido and in the former by external violence. It might, indeed, be said that in the case of the war neuroses, in contrast to the pure traumatic neuroses and in approximation to the transference neuroses, what is feared is nevertheless an internal enemy. The theoretical difficulties standing in the way of a unifying hypothesis of this kind do not seem insuperable: after all, we have a perfect right to describe repression, which lies at the basis of every neurosis, as a reaction to a trauma—as an elementary traumatic neurosis.

Moreover, in a continuing analysis of the etiology of traumatic neuroses, Freud rejects the theory that they are due to an organic cause (i.e., shell stock or physical concussion to brain tissue) and suggests that they are functional in nature.

> Although the war neuroses manifested themselves for the most part as motor disturbances-tremors and paralyses-and although it was plausible to suppose that such a gross impact as that produced by the concussion due to the explosion of a shell near by or to being buried by a fall of earth would lead to gross mechanical effects, observations were nevertheless made which left no doubt as to the psychical nature of the causation of these so-called war neuroses. How could this be disputed when the symptoms appeared behind the front as well, far from the horrors of war, or immediately after a return from leave? The physicians were therefore led to regard war neurotics in a similar light to the nervous subjects of peace-time.

This passage foreshadows his later (1928) thinking that trauma produces physical and psychological disequilibrium within the ego; nevertheless, he sustains the view that it is the "psychical nature of the causation" that is decisive in the determination of symptomatology.

BEYOND THE PLEASURE PRINCIPLE: TRAUMA AS DISEQUILIBRIUM

In 1928, Freud published one of his last books, *Beyond the Pleasure Principle.* Once again, he addressed the issue of traumatic neuroses and utilized the metaphor of the "protective shield of the ego" for defensive mechanisms (Brett & Ostroff, 1985). In this work, he considered traumatic events as external stressors that were strong enough to break through the "protective shield" and inflict injury or harm to the person.

> We describe as "traumatic" any excitations from outside which are powerful enough to break through the protective shield. It seems to me that the concept of trauma necessarily implies a connection of this kind with a breach in an otherwise efficacious barrier against stimuli. Such an event as an external trauma is bound to provoke a disturbance on a large scale in the functioning of the organisms energy and to set in motion every possible defensive measure. At the same time the pleasure principle is for the moment put out of action. There is no longer any possibility of preventing the mental apparatus from being flooded with large amounts of stimulus, and another problem arises instead—the problem of mastering the amounts of stimulus which broken in and of binding them, in a psychical sense, so that they can then be disposed of (p. 56–57).

In this later treatise, one can now see that Freud further elaborated the concept of trauma as involving: (1) an external stressor event which overwhelms normal ego functioning; (2) a change in the steady state of the organism (i.e., disequilibrium); (3) a reduction of ego-defensive and coping capacity; and (4) the problem of "mastery," in that other stressors can take on traumatic proportion. Thus, both the traumatic stressors and secondary ones can overwhelm the now-depleted ego defenses, thereby setting up the possibility of long term post-traumatic stress disorder and other comorbid conditions.

While it may be surprising to some that Freud seemed to grasp the essence of post-traumatic stress disorder in the early part of the 20th century, what followed his death in terms of establishing diagnostic categories to aid victims of trauma both reflects his personal contributions to the field and then a kind of intellectual vacuum in which the collective clinical wisdom about psychic traumatization seems to have gone "underground" and evaporated by the time of DSM-II (APA, 1968). What makes this so peculiar is that by 1968, the cumulative historical events involving war, civil violence, nuclear warfare, etc. produced more trauma, killing, mass destruction, and death in a delimited time frame than at any prior time in recorded history. Nevertheless, Freud's contribution to understanding PTSD-like states was in recognizing the power of trauma to change ego states and adaptive behavior. The greatest impact of his work, however, lay in the shift of conceptual paradigms from that of reality-based, stressor-event determinants of PTSD to a focus on fantasy and what he termed the "psychical reality of memory." The implications of this conceptual shift in paradigm were enormous because it made premorbid determinants a primary consideration to the exclusion of the nature, magnitude and social–historical context in which traumatization occurred.

FROM DSM-I TO DSM-IV: A RETROSPECTIVE LOOK AT THE PTSD DIAGNOSTIC CRITERIA

Sigmund Freud died in 1939 after a protracted struggle with cancer. Thirteen years after his death, the American Psychiatric Association published its first diagnostic and statistical manual, which contained a diagnostic category known as "Transient Situational Personality Disorders," which included the category (000-x81) Gross Stress Reaction. Table 1 presents the reproduction of the DSM-I for this category, which will be reviewed as it bears on the current diagnosis of PTSD.

DSM-I: Gross Stress Reaction

In the DSM-I the current diagnostic category of PTSD was formerly classified as gross stress reaction (GSR). The description of GSR clearly reflects the influence of Freud's thinking about traumatic neurosis. As Table 1 indicates, there are several criteria implied by the narrative description. First, the placement of GSR into a category of transient situational personality disorders reflects the view that such conditions are expected to be acute reactions to "unusual stress" that resolve quickly. Second, if there are prolonged or persistent reactions, an alternative diagnosis was to be considered by the clinician, and implied the possibility of a premorbid condition. In DSM-I,

Table 2.1 DSM-I (1952) Criteria for Transient Situational Personality Disorders

This general classification should be restricted to reactions which are more or less transient in character and which appear to be an acute symptom response to a situation without apparent underlying personality disturbance.

The symptoms are the immediate means used by the individual in his struggle to adjust to an overwhelming situation. In the presence of good adaptive capacity, recession of symptoms generally occurs when the situational stress diminishes. Persistent failure to resolve will indicate a more severe underlying disturbance and will be classified elsewhere.

000-x80 Transient Situational Personality Disturbance

Transient situational disorders which cannot be given a more definite diagnosis in the group, because of their fluidity, or because of the limitation of time permitted for their study, may be included in this general category. This category is designed also for the use of record librarians and statisticians dealing with incomplete diagnoses.

000-x81 Gross Stress Reaction

Under conditions of great or unusual stress, a normal personality may utilize established patterns of reaction to deal with overwhelming fear. The patterns of such reactions differ from those of neurosis or psychosis chiefly with respect to clinical history, reversibility of reaction, and its transient character. When promptly and adequately treated, the condition may clear rapidly. It is also possible that the condition may progress to one of the neurotic reactions. If the reaction persists, this term is to be regarded as a temporary diagnosis to be used only until a more definitive diagnosis is established.

This diagnosis is justified only in situations in which the individual has been exposed to severe physical demands or extreme emotional stress, such as in combat or in civilian catastrophe (fire, earthquake, explosion, etc.). In many instances this diagnosis applies to previously more or less "normal" persons who have experienced intolerable stress.

The particular stress involved will be specified as (1) combat or (2) civilian catastrophe.

these alternatives included psychosis, neurosis (e.g., anxiety neurosis), and character disorders. Third, the criteria also notes that "when promptly treated, the condition may clear rapidly." This statement apparently reflected an assumption that rapid intervention facilitates recovery from the impact of the stressful event, no matter how great the degree of victimization.

The DSM-I (1952) category of GSR had features which in many ways parallel the later DSM-III (APA, 1980) criteria for PTSD, such as the recognition that in "conditions of great or unusual stress" a normal person may manifest stress-related behaviors in response to "intolerable stress." Hence, a recognizable stressor could generate reactions and symptoms, but only for the duration of the stressful event, since it was presumed that "recession of symptoms generally occurs when the situational stress diminishes." It is here that we see the Freudian influence that a traumatic neurosis is caused by a "penetration of the protective shield of the ego" due to an excess influx of excitation in the mental apparatus within a short period of time. Thus, while a traumatic neurosis (i.e., GSR) may be produced, it was presumed to diminish once the event terminated. Thus, the persistence of traumatic reactions could only be due to underlying psychopathology, which became more apparent because the ego now lacked the capacity to defend itself against premorbid and repressed infantile conflicts. Stated more basically, this view of GSR implies that trauma may aggravate repressed, latent, or pre-existing intrapsychic conflicts, but that the persistence of reactions is not primarily caused by the traumatic event. Thus, while the stress might be great, it also may weaken ego defenses in such a way that other emotional problems become manifest as well.

DSM-II: Adjustment Reaction of Adult Life

Table 2 summarizes the diagnostic criteria for PTSD as found in the DSM-II (1968). GSR was into category (DSM 307.3) Adjustment Reaction of Adult Life, and provided three short (and inadequate) illustrations. However, the asterisks by the diagnostic category name told the user of the manual to look in the appendices for additional examples of stressful life events and listed such things as car accidents, railway accidents, boat accidents, airplane accidents, and more, ad nauseum, in a highly compartmentalized and obsessive-compulsive style. However, what is interesting about these examples is that the DSM-II committee clearly recognized that there were stressor events that contained a possible physical threat of injury or death, or were psychologically associated with states of fear and anxiety. However, given such extensive codification of external stressor events, one must question why the committee did not go further in determining how these types of events relate specifically to adjustment reactions.

It is puzzling that in the 16-year interval between the publication of DSM and DSM-II, there were more traumatic events worldwide that were the focus of both national and international attention: the Korean and Vietnam Wars; colonial wars and revolutions; the assassination of John F. Kennedy; civil violence in Northern Ireland; wars in the Middle East; major natural disasters in many parts of the world; and recognition of the prevalence of childhood sexual abuse. These events and those that preceded in

Table 2.2 DSM-II (1968) Criteria for Adjustment Reaction of Adult Life

307.3 Adjustment Reaction of Adult Life

EXAMPLE: Resentment with depressive tone associated with an unwanted pregnancy and manifested by hostile complaints and suicidal gestures.

EXAMPLE: Fear associated with military combat and manifested by trembling, running, and hiding.

EXAMPLE: A Ganser syndrome associated with death sentence and manifested by incorrect but approximate answers to questions.

the period from 1900–1952 were being investigated, researched, and published in medical and scientific journals, such as A. Kardiner's book *Traumatic Neurosis of War* (1941, 1959) and Lifton's landmark 1967 book on Hiroshima, *Death in Life*. And yet the DSM-II equivalent of PTSD contained a mere three examples of "adjustment reaction to adult life": (1) an unwanted pregnancy accompanied by depression and hostility, (2) a frightened soldier in combat, and (3) a prisoner facing execution in a death penalty case.

The simplicity and inadequacy of these examples makes one wonder why there was not a more adequate and complete delineation of the various types of trauma, their common effects on psychological functioning, and the known clinical features associated with stressful life experiences. At one level, it is apparent that the committee who drew up the revised DSM-II category of PTSD implicitly understood that certain types of events were more likely than others to be associated with difficulties in adjustment. And yet it was apparent, as suggested earlier, that Freud understood, 70 years before DSM-III-R, the core system clusters of PTSD that are currently accepted by most professionals who work with traumatized clients. While it is beyond the purpose of this chapter, a retrospective analysis and reconstruction of how the DSM-II (307.3) diagnostic criteria came into being in the form they did, in light of the extensive extant literature *at that time* on various trauma populations, would be interesting and important to understand.

DSM-III: PTSD

Table 3 presents the DSM-III (APA, 1980) diagnostic criteria for PTSD. Twelve years after DSM-II, PTSD emerged as a separate diagnostic entity and was placed among the anxiety disorders, presumably because anxiety, emotional distress, and physical disequilibrium were among the primary affective reactions associated with traumatization. Further, to receive a diagnosis of PTSD, the individual had to manifest *at least* four symptoms (e.g., intrusive recollections) from three clusters of symptoms (i.e., 12 total symptoms), which include reexperiencing the trauma, numbing and detachment responses, and changes in personality that were not present before the trauma (e.g. sleep disturbance, survival guilt). As with the other mental disorders listed in DSM-III, the PTSD diagnostic considerations were constructed as an algorithm for differential diagnosis and were not meant to be exhaustive of all possible symptoms a survivor might possess. Moreover, a careful look at the PTSD diagnostic criteria reflects what Freud (1917) had earlier observed, namely, that the impact of trauma is systemic and influences emotional expressiveness, cognitive processes, motivation and goal striving, intrapersonal and object relations, physiological functioning, and ego states.

The DSM-III also made a number of advances over the DSM and DSM-II in that the narrative description of the disorder contained in the manual explained PTSD syndrome dynamics and made other observations that were

Table 2.3 DSM-III (1980) Criteria for Post-Traumatic Stress Disorder

A. Existence of a recognizable stressor that would evoke significant symptoms of distress in almost everyone.
B. Reexperiencing of the trauma as evidenced by at least one of the following:
  (1) Recurrent and intrusive recollections of the event
  (2) Recurrent dreams of the event
  (3) Sudden acting or feeling as if the traumatic event were reoccurring, because of an association with an environmental or ideational stimulus
C. Numbing of responsiveness to or reduced involvement with the external world, beginning some time after the trauma, as shown by at least one of the following:
  (1) Markedly diminished interest in one or more significant activities
  (2) Feeling of detachment or estrangement from others
  (3) Constricted affect
D. At least two of the following symptoms that were not present before the trauma:
  (1) Hyperalertness or exaggerated startle response
  (2) Sleep disturbance
  (3) Guilt about surviving when others have not, or about behavior required for survival
  (4) Memory impairment or trouble concentrating
  (5) Avoidance of activities that arouse recollection of the traumatic event
  (6) Intensification of symptoms by exposure to events that symbolize or resemble the traumatic event

not previously elucidated, such as the role of dissociative process (e.g., "flashbacks," forms of reenactment) in post-traumatic attempts at coping and processing the trauma. Moreover, the prime criterion of diagnostic consideration was "the existence of a recognizable stressor that would evoke significant symptoms of distress in almost everyone."

Clearly, this statement is of etiological significance since it implies that the *magnitude of the stressor* is sufficient to generate traumatic reactions in almost everyone, which, in turn, might develop into a pathological state. In this regard, it is possible to see how researchers such as Lifton (1988) indicated that, to a large extent, PTSD can be thought of as the normal human reaction to abnormally stressful life events. In this perspective, the reactions and symptoms of the syndrome are expectable, predictable, and normative. However, the psychopathology of traumatic reactions is discerned when the presence of the symptoms persists and exerts an adverse effect on adaptive functioning. Thus, there is not only a continuum of symptom severity but also a continuum of pathological impact on psychosocial functioning. Further, the concept of a continuum of symptom severity and pathological impact implies that there are variables and processes that moderate both manifestations. Most typically, researchers have postulated that personal variables (e.g., personality traits) or environmental factors (e.g., level of perceived social support) influence the specific patterns of PTSD expression (Wilson, 1989).

While it is possible to engage in an extended discussion of the historical importance of PTSD as a separate diagnostic entity in the DSM-III (APA, 1980), a few points should be mentioned at this juncture. First, the nomenclature of the disorder was important. The words "post-traumatic" mean "after injury" and indicate that there is a change in state of well-being which is associated with various reaction patterns and symptom formations. Second, although PTSD was initially a controversial diagnostic category in some medical–legal circles, the net effect to date has been to stimulate more research programs and promote clarification in terms of differential diagnosis and the understanding comorbid conditions (Davidson & Foa, 1993; Wilson & Raphael, 1993). Third, the existence of PTSD also helped to validate and legitimate the suffering of those victimized by stressful life events. Similarly, the availability of PTSD as a diagnostic category for consideration also helped to avoid misdiagnosis and, by implication, possible mistreatment. Fourth, the existence of PTSD as an officially recognized mental disorder enabled it to be used in legal considerations for such things as securing disability payments and pensions, compensation for injury, or as a form of legal defense in criminal litigation. Fifth, the rapid proliferation of clinical and research studies with different populations of trauma victims (e.g., childhood abuse victims, rape victims, war veterans, disaster survivors, etc.), led to new questions and refinements in understanding the complexity of stress response syndromes. Today, this process is in full momentum, and such new publications as *International Handbook of Traumatic Stress Syndromes* (Wilson & Raphael, 1993) reflect the emerging international collaboration in studies of disaster, trauma, and victimization. Finally, interest in PTSD generated during the 1980s has brought forth new revisions in the criteria that are evident in the DSM-III-R and the DSM-IV (Davidson & Foa, 1993).

DSM-III-R: PTSD, Revised

In 1987, the committee of the APA decided to revise the diagnostic criteria for PTSD.[1] These revisions reflected a knowledge based on research and clinical work with victims of trauma. The total number of diagnostic symptoms was expanded to 17, and to receive a clinical diagnosis, the client had to manifest six symptoms from the 3 major clusters: reexperiencing the traumatic event (DSM-III-R-B criteria), avoidance and numbing reactions associated with the traumatic event that were *not present before it* (DSM-III-R-C criteria), and symptoms of increased physiological arousal that *were not present before the trauma* (DSM-III-R-D criteria). Additionally, the criteria also stated that the duration of the disturbance (i.e., symptoms or reactions) had to be at least one month. If the onset and offset of the reactions was less than a month, the condition was to be regarded as a normal pattern of stress response that was not pathological in nature.

The changes made in the DMS-III-R diagnostic criteria were more than simply additional symptoms added to a list. The revision also attempted to

[1]The author was a member of the DSM-III-R committee on PTSD.

clarify language, meaning, and specificity of reactions to trauma. The DSM-III-R criteria for PTSD are listed in Table 2.4.

Definition of Trauma. In DSM-III (1980) the "A" criteria for PTSD was a generic definition of stressors associated with post-trauma symptom development. As investigators evaluated impacts of different stressful events, it became less clear what was meant by the 1980 ("A" criterion) phrase, "a

Table 2.4 DSM-III-R (1987) Criteria for Post-Traumatic Stress Disorder

A. The person has experienced an event that is outside the range of usual human experience that would be markedly distressing to almost anyone, e.g., serious threat to one's life or physical integrity; serious threat or harm to one's children, spouse, or other close relatives and friends; sudden destruction of one's home or community; or seeing another person who has recently been, or is being, seriously injured or killed as the result of an accident or physical violence.

B. The traumatic event is persistently reexperienced in at least one of the following ways:
   (1) Recurrent and intrusive distressing recollections of the event (in young children, repetitive play in which themes or aspects of the trauma are expressed)
   (2) Recurrent distressing dreams of the event
   (3) Sudden acting or feeling as if the traumatic event were recurring (includes a sense of reliving the experience, illusions, hallucinations, and dissociative [flashback] episodes, even those that occur upon awakening or when intoxicated)
   (4) Intense psychological distress at exposure to events that symbolize or resemble an aspect of the traumatic event, including anniversaries of the trauma

C. Persistent avoidance of stimuli associated with the trauma or numbing of general responsiveness (not present before the trauma), as indicated by at least three of the following:
   (1) Efforts to avoid thoughts or feelings associated with the trauma
   (2) Efforts to avoid activities or situations that arouse recollections of the trauma
   (3) Inability to recall an important aspect of the trauma (psychogenic amnesia)
   (4) Markedly diminished interest in significant activities (in young children, loss of recently acquired developmental skills such as toilet training or language skills)
   (5) Feeling of detachment or estrangement from others
   (6) Restricted range of affect, e.g., unable to have loving feelings
   (7) Sense of a foreshortened future, e.g., does not expect to have a career, marriage, or children, or a long life

D. Persistent symptoms of increased arousal (not present before the trauma), as indicated by at least two of the following:
   (1) Difficulty falling or staying asleep
   (2) Irritability or outbursts of anger
   (3) Difficulty concentrating
   (4) Hypervigilance
   (5) Exaggerated startle response
   (6) Physiologic reactivity upon exposure to events that symbolize or resemble an aspect of the traumatic event (e.g., a woman who was raped in an elevator breaks out in a sweat when entering any elevator)

E. Duration of the disturbance (symptoms in B, C, and D) of at least one month

Specify delayed onset if the onset of symptoms was at least six months after the trauma.

recognizable stressor that would evoke significant symptoms of distress in almost everyone." As noted earlier, the problem that there is a stress–threshold continuum. A recognizable stressor to one person may not be so to another. Thus, the DSM-III-R "A" criterion attempted to clarify that the stressors associated with the onset of PTSD were external events outside the usual range of daily hassles that would be "markedly distressing to almost everyone." This criteria is then followed by examples of (1) physical life threat, (2) psychological threat to well-being, (3) physical *or* psychological threat to the well-being of significant others, (4) witnessing of horrific trauma, or (5) involvement in a disaster of natural or human-induced origin. In essence, the revised (1987) "A" criteria indicated that the stressors associated with the onset of PTSD are generally at the extreme end of the stress continuum and that the more severe and life-threatening the event is, the higher the probability is that it will produce traumatic consequences such as PTSD.

Reenactment and Reliving Trauma. The 1987 revision also sought to clarify the various ways that traumatic events can be reexperienced. First, the explicit "B" criteria noted that the traumatic event is persistently reexperienced. Second, reexperiencing trauma as a part of PTSD is different than remembering trauma. The visual imagery and emotional distress in PTSD is *intrusive, unbidden, involuntary,* and *unexpected* (Horowitz, 1986). Third, the different ways individuals relive trauma were also more finely detailed in the 1987 revision and included (1) nightmares of the traumatic event, (2) daytime intrusive imagery and effect of the trauma (e.g., emotional "flooding") (3) suddenly acting or feeling that the traumatic event might reoccur, (4) dissociative states in which the traumatic is reexperienced or acted out in behavior (i.e., symbolically or as repetition of the earlier event), (5) hallucinations that are trauma-based, (6) increased distress upon exposure to events or stimuli that either symbolize or resemble the original trauma, (7) anniversary reactions during the course of the year, and (8) repetitive play activities in children that are an expression of preoccupation with the traumatic event. Thus, the revised "B" criteria in DSM-III-R indicated 8 possible forms of reexperiencing a traumatic event, 5 more than the 1980 revision.

Avoidance, Numbing, Detachment, Emotional Constriction, and Amnesia. It should come as no surprise that if there were more ways discovered in which people relive a traumatic event, there would be a corresponding number of ways to avoid its impact or to numb or diminish painful emotions associated with memories of the trauma. The 1987 revision described 7 categories of avoidance symptoms and included the following: (1) avoidance of thoughts, feelings, situations and activities either associated with the trauma or likely to stimulate recollections, (2) psychogenic amnesia, (3) regression or developmental arrestation, (4) loss of interest or meaning in previously enjoyed activities, (5) detachment, estrangement and isolation from others, (6) loss of emotional expressiveness and capacity for love, sexuality, intimacy, and friendship, and (7) changed beliefs about personal well-being in the future.

In summary, the avoidance and numbing criteria can be thought of, in an overly simplistic sense, as characterizing self–other object relations. There is intrapersonal constriction, numbing, denial, and splitting. Similarly, there is interpersonal detachment, distancing, withdrawal, and avoidance. In terms of ego function there may be cognitive constriction, loss of memory, meaning, purpose, and qualities of self structure.

Physiological Hyperarousal: Psychobiological Manifestations. Among the more significant major changes in the DSM-III-R was the reorientation of the "D" diagnostic category. In the 1980 version, the symptom cluster was concerned with changes in personality and behavior that were not present before the traumatic event. In the 1987 revision, the category directly concerned states of increased physiological arousal, underscoring recent advances in the psychobiology of PTSD (Friedman, 1993; Wilson, 1989). Further, whereas there still remained 6 symptoms within the "D" category, survivor guilt, memory impairment, and hyperalertness had been deleted from the DSM-III edition and replaced with irritability or outbursts of anger, hypervigilance, and physiologic reactivity upon exposure to stimuli that activated memories of the traumatic event. Thus, the revised "D" category for "persistent systems of increased arousal" was added to the other two categories to form an interrelated symptom triad: (1) intrusive states of reexperiencing the traumatic event, (2) avoidance and numbing reactions; and (3) disequilibrium states as expressions of changes in nervous system activity (van der Kolk, 1993; van der Kolk, Krystal & Greenberg, 1984; van der Kolk & van der Hart, 1989).

DSM-IV

The DSM-IV was published in May, 1994. Table 2.5 contains the diagnostic criteria for DSM-IV and reflects minor changes from the previous revision in 1987. However, one noteworthy change is in the definition of the traumatic event, which has a two-pronged criteria indicating that the person must have experienced or witnessed a life-threatening event and responded to it with fear, horror, or helplessness. But with the rate at which new discoveries are being made in the study of traumatic stress syndromes, there are considerations for the future that must be addressed more thoughtfully and systematically. Let us consider a few of them.

Is PTSD an environmentally caused disorder? If the answer is an unequivocal yes, should PTSD then be classified separately in the diagnostic manual? Pynoos and Nader (1993) have suggested separate diagnostic criteria for childhood PTSD. Similarly, Terr (1991) has identified Type I and Type II childhood stressor events with differential consequences for PTSD manifestations and character changes. Ochberg (1988, 1993) has also suggested that victims of torture, terrorism and degradation may experience a victimization disorder which overlaps with PTSD but has different psychic consequences. Braun (1993) has also suggested that PTSD and dissociative disorders may have a common psychological pathway to symptom formation.

Table 2.5 DSM-IV (1994) Diagnostic Criteria for Post-Traumatic Stress Disorder

A. The person has been exposed to a traumatic event in which both of the following were present:
   (1) Event or events that involved actual or threatened death or serious injury, or a threat to the physical integrity of self or others
   (2) The person's response involved intense fear, helplessness, or horror. **Note:** In children, this may be expressed instead by disorganized or agitated behavior.

B. The traumatic event is persistently reexperienced in one (or more) of the following ways:
   (1) Recurrent and intrusive distressing recollections of the event, including images, thoughts, or perceptions. **Note:** In young children, repetitive play may occur in which themes or aspects of the trauma are expressed
   (2) Recurrent distressing dreams of the event. **Note:** In children, there may be frightening dreams without recognizable content
   (3) Acting or feeling as if the traumatic event were recurring (includes a sense of reliving the experience, illusions, hallucinations, and dissociative flashback episodes, including those that occur on awakening or when intoxicated). **Note:** In young children, trauma-specific reenactment may occur
   (4) Intense psychological distress at exposure to internal or external cues that symbolize or resemble an aspect of the traumatic event
   (5) Physiological reactivity on exposure to internal or external cues that symbolize or resemble an aspect of the traumatic event

C. Persistent avoidance of stimuli associated with the trauma and numbing of general responsiveness (not present before the trauma), as indicated by three (or more) of the following:
   (1) Efforts to avoid thoughts, feelings, or conversations associated with the trauma
   (2) Efforts to avoid activities, places, or people that arouse recollections of the trauma
   (3) Inability to recall an important aspect of the trauma
   (4) Markedly diminished interest or participation in significant activities
   (5) Feeling of detachment or estrangement from others
   (6) Restricted range of affect (e.g. unable to have loving feelings)
   (7) Sense of a foreshortened future (e.g., does not expect to have a career, marriage, children, or a normal life span)

D. Persistent symptoms of increased arousal (not present before the trauma), as indicated by two (or more) of the following:
   (1) Difficulty falling or staying asleep
   (2) Irritability or outbursts of anger
   (3) Difficulty concentrating
   (4) Hypervigilance
   (5) Exaggerated startle response

E. Duration of the disturbance (symptoms in Criteria B, C, and D) is more than 1 month.

F. The disturbance causes clinically significant distress or impairment in social occupational, or other important areas of functioning.

Specify if:
Acute: if duration of symptoms is less than 3 months
Chronic: if duration of symptoms is 3 months or more

Specify if:
With Delayed Onset: if onset of symptoms is at least 6 months after the stressor

There are several other phenomena associated with trauma and disaster that require much more research and evaluation. For example, Laibow and Laue (1993), Wilson (1990) and Vyner (1987) have described anomalous traumatic experiences, such as exposure to invisible toxic contaminants that have unique properties such as difficulties discerning the nature of the stressors or their long term consequences to physical and emotional wellbeing. In technological disasters, those affected often manifest states of chronic uncertainty, anxiety, obsessive behavior, hypervigilance and somatoform processes (Vyner, 1987). Are such reactions a form of PTSD? Are there subclinical levels of PTSD as well? Moreover, how do we understand the acute or persistent effects of dysfunctional families, civil chaos and violence, unstable cultural systems, or similar events that impact adversely on the well-being of victims? Do the persistent effects of unstable, chaotic, threatening, (e.g., civil violence, gang warfare,) and inconsistent environments eventually begin to function in a manner similar to a discrete, major catastrophic life events? If so, are these patterns of adaptation a subtype of PTSD?

These and other questions await future research and clinical insights. What seems clear at this point in the continuing evolution of PTSD diagnostic criteria is that the inquiry probed by Freud, expanded by others in the wake of unprecented historical 20th-century events of cataclysmic proportion, and pursued vigorously by scholars worldwide at the dawn of the 21st century, is nothing less than a willingness to address the psychic impact of traumatic injury and thereby seek solutions to healing and the restoration of humaneness.

REFERENCES

American Psychiatric Association (1952). *Diagnostic and statistical manual of mental disorders.* Washington, DC: Author.

American Psychiatric Association (1968). *Diagnostic and statistical manual of mental disorders,* 2nd Edition. Washington, DC: Author.

American Psychiatric Association (1980). *Diagnostic and statistical manual of mental disorders,* 3rd Edition. Washington, DC: Author.

American Psychiatric Association (1994). *Diagnostic and statistical manual of mental disorders,* 4th Edition. Washington, DC: Author.

American Psychiatric Association (1993). *DSM-IV draft criteria.* Washington, DC: Author.

Braun, B. (1993). Multiple personality disorder and post traumatic stress disorder: Similarities and differences. In J. P. Wilson and B. Raphael (Eds.), *International handbook of traumatic stress syndromes.* New York: Plenum.

Brett, B. (1993). Psychoanalytic contributions to a theory of traumatic stress. In J. P. Wilson and B. Raphael (Eds.), *International handbook of traumatic stress syndromes.* New York: Plenum.

Brett, B & Ostroff, R. (1985). Imagery and post-traumatic stress disorder: An overview. *American Journal of Psychiatry, 142,* 417–424.

Davidson, J. R. T. & Foa, E. (Eds.), *Post-Traumatic stress disorder: DSM-IV and beyond.* Washington, DC: American Psychiatric Press.

Friedman, M. (1993). Psychobiology and pharmacological approaches to treatment. In J. P. Wilson and B. Raphael (Eds.), *International handbook of traumatic stress syndromes.* New York: Plenum.

Freud, S. (1928). *Beyond the pleasure principle.* New York: Liveright (1956).

Freud, S. (1955). Introduction to psychoanalysis and the war neuroses. In J. Strachey (Ed.

and Trans.), *The standard edition of the complete psychological works of Sigmund Freud* (vol. 17, pp. 166–211). London: Hogarth. (Original work published 1918.)
Freud, S. (1917, 1966). *Introductory lectures on psychoanalysis.* New York: Liveright.
Freud, S. & Breuer, J. (1895, 1956) *Studies in hysteria.* London: Hogarth Press.
Horowitz, M. J. (1986). *Stress response syndromes* (2nd Ed.). Northvale, NJ: Jason Aronson.
Jones, E. (1953). *The life and work of Sigmund Freud,* Vol. 1. New York: Basic Books.
Kardiner, A. (1941). *The traumatic memories of war.* New York: Hoeber.
Kardiner, A. (1959). Traumatic memories of war. In Arieti (Ed.). *American handbook of psychiatry.* New York: Basic Books.
Laibow, R. & Laue, S. (1993). Posttraumatic stress disorder and anomalous trauma. In J. P. Wilson and B. Raphael (Eds.), *International Handbook of traumatic stress syndromes.* New York: Plenum.
Lifton, R. J. (1967). *Death in life: Survivors of Hiroshima.* New York: Simon & Schuster.
Lifton, R. J. (1988). Understanding the traumatized self: Imagery, symbolization, and transformation. In J. P. Wilson, Z. Harel, & B. Kahana (Eds.), *Human adaptation to extreme stress: From the Holocaust to Vietnam.* New York: Plenum.
Lindy, J. D. (1993). Focal psychoanalytic therapy. In J. P. Wilson and B. Raphael (Eds.), *International handbook of traumatic stress syndromes.* New York: Plenum.
Maslow, A. H. (1970). *Motivation and personality.* New York: Harper & Row.
Masson, J. (1984). *The assault on truth.* New York: Farrar, Straus and Giroux.
Ochberg, F. (1988). *Post-traumatic therapy and victims of violence.* New York: Brunner/Mazel.
Ochberg, F. (1983). Post-traumatic therapy. J. P. Wilson and B. Raphael (Eds.), *International Handbook of traumatic stress sydrome.* New York: Plenum.
Peterson, K. C., Prout, M. F., & Schwarz, R. A. (1991). *Post-traumatic stress disorder.* New York: Plenum.
Putnam, F. W. (1989). *Diagnosis and treatment of multiple personality disorder.* New York: Guilford.
Pynoos, R., & Nader, K. (1993). Issues in the treatment of posttraumatic stress in children and adolescents. In J. P. Wilson and B. Raphael (Eds.), *International handbook of traumatic stress syndromes.* New York: Plenum.
Terr, L. (1991). Childhood trauma: An outline and overview. *American Journal of Psychiatry, 148,*(1), 10–20.
Terr, L. C. (1985). Children traumatized in small groups. In S. Eth and R. S. Pynoos (Eds.), *Post-traumatic stress disorder in children.* Washington, DC: American Psychiatric Press.
Trimble, M. R. (1981). *Post-traumatic neurosis.* Chicester: Wiley.
Trimble, M. R. (1985). Post-traumatic stress disorder: History of a concept. In C. R. Figley (Ed.), *Trauma and its wake: The study and treatment of post-traumatic stress disorder* (pp. 5–14). New York: Brunner/Mazel.
van der Kolk, B., & van der Hart, O. (1989). Pierre Janet and the breakdown of adaptation in psychological trauma. *American Journal of Psychiatry,* 146:(12),1530–1540.
van der Kolk, B. A., Krystal, H., & Greenberg, M. S. (1984). Post-traumatic stress disorder as a biological based disorder: Implications of the animal model of inescapable shock. In B. A. van der Kolk (Ed.), *Post-traumatic stress disorder: Psychological and biological sequelae.* Washington, DC: American Psychiatric Press.
van der Kolk, B. (1993). Biological basis of trauma. In J. P. Wilson and B. Raphael (Eds.), *International handbook of traumatic stress syndromes.* New York: Plenum.
Vyner, H. (1987). *Invisible trauma: The psychosocial effects of invisible environmental contaminants.* Lexington, MA: D. C. Heath.
Wilson, J. P. (1989). *Trauma, transformation, and healing.* New York: Brunner/Mazel.
Wilson, J. P., Harel, Z. & Kahana, B. (Eds.) (1988). *Human adaptation to extreme stress: From the Holocaust to Vietnam.* New York: Plenum.
Wilson, J. P. (1990). PTSD and Experienced Anomalous Trauma. Similarities in reported UFO abductions and exposure to toxic contaminants. *Journal to UFO Studies, 2,* 1–19.
Wilson, J. P. & Raphael, B. (1993). *International handbook of traumatic stress syndromes.* New York: Plenum.
Wilson, J. P. (in press). The need for an integrative theory of PTSD. In M. B. Williams (Ed.), *The handbook of posttraumatic therapies.* New York: Praeger.

3

An Integrative Two-Factor Model of Post-Traumatic Stress

GEORGE S. EVERLY, JR.

There is nothing so practical as a good theory.
—KURT LEWIN

As noted earlier, Part I of this text is dedicated to analyzing traumatic stress from conceptual, historical, biological, and psychological perspectives. The preceding chapters have addressed the broader issues. Chapter 1 introduced psychotraumatology as an overarching concept within which to examine traumatic stress and its related phenomena, and Chapter 2 provided a detailed historical perspective on traumatic stress. The purpose of this chapter is to provide the reader with a conceptually integrative model of the post-traumatic stress phenomenon. The primary goal of such a phenomenological model is not to provide an exhaustive microanalysis, but rather to offer one possible overarching integrative perspective on the biological and psychological constituents of post-traumatic stress. This perspective will serve as an engendering foundation or point of integration for the more exhaustive and detailed microanalyses that will follow in subsequent chapters. Further, an integrative model may provide a framework within which to capture the "heterogeneity" of PTSD (Kolb, 1989). Such a conceptual amalgamation

GEORGE S. EVERLY, JR. • International Critical Incident Stress Foundation, Ellicott City, Maryland 21042; Union Memorial Hospital, Baltimore, Maryland 21218; and Department of Psychology, Loyola College, Baltimore, Maryland 21210.

Psychotraumatology, edited by George S. Everly, Jr. and Jeffrey M. Lating. Plenum Press, New York, 1995.

is likely to have clinical as well as heuristic value; it will also be used as a unifying theme in the remaining text.

AN INTEGRATIVE TWO-FACTOR NEUROCOGNITIVE MODEL

In what may be the most significant of the earlier conceptually integrating treatises, Kardiner (1941) viewed post-traumatic stress as a "physioneurosis." This term eloquently embodies the exquisite intertwinings of psychological and biological substrates that represent the essence of traumatic stress. Although Freud (1920) seemed to appreciate that the traumatic stress process was somehow a blending of psychological and biological processes, Kardiner appears to be the first to delineate specifically how these two domains were inextricably integrated to create the post-traumatic stress phenomenon.

Almost 40 years after Kardiner's psychophysiological appreciation of post-traumatic stress, the American Psychiatric Association (APA, 1980) operationalized post-traumatic stress disorder (PTSD) as a form of anxiety disorder, blending more primitive physiological components with higher-order cognitive and affective processes. The APA criteria (APA, 1980, 1987, 1994) conceptualized PTSD within three symptom clusters temporally subsequent to the sine qua non of the diagnosis—exposure to a psychologically overwhelming stressor outside the usual realm of human experience (i.e., a traumatic event.) The three symptom clusters are (1) intrusive psychological reexperiencing of the traumatic event; (2) psychological numbing to, or reduced involvement with, the external environment; and (3) autonomic nervous system hyperreactivity and/or hyperfunction (although we now understand that the physiological arousal is not limited to the autonomic nervous system).

Based upon a review of the efforts of Lazarus (Lazarus & Folkman, 1984), Wilson (1989), and Everly (1989) to construct meaningful models of human stress, this chapter attempts to bring some phenomenological order to the DSM criteria for PTSD. The model offered in Figure 3.1 is an integrative model that blends the three DSM symptom clusters into one psychophysiological construct.

An analysis of Figure 3.1 reveals several significant factors worth noting. First, immediately subsequent to the traumatic event, an individual may suffer what is most typically an acute hypothalamically mediated "shock" or numbing reaction. Neural mechanisms most likely account for this reaction as opposed to endocrine pathways. Second, the figure places great pivotal emphasis on the cognitive interpretation the individual places upon the traumatic event. This concept preceded contemporary writers

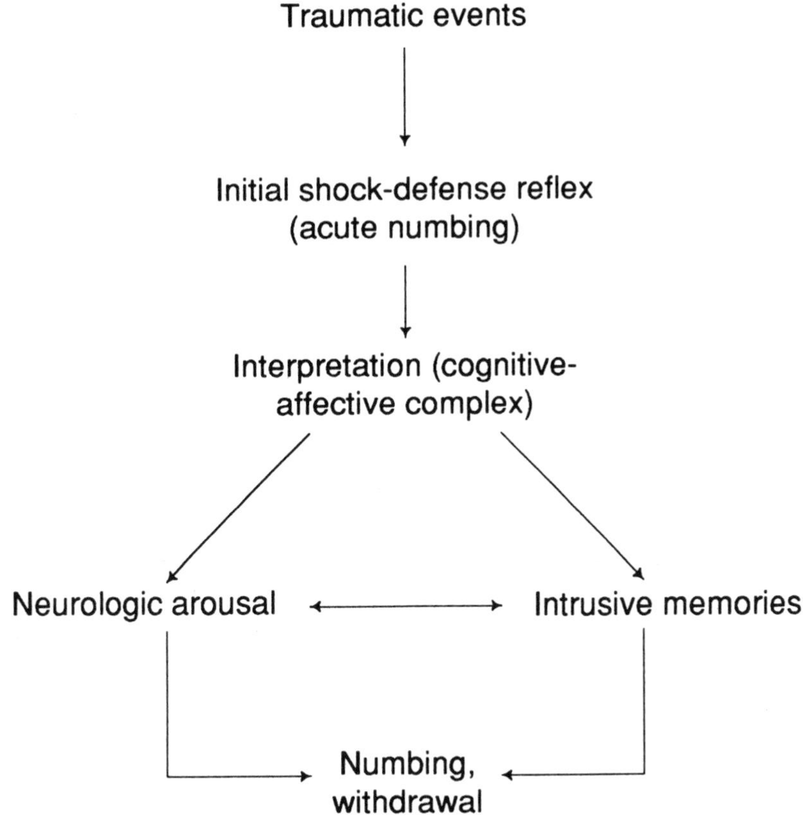

Figure 3.1 A model of post-traumatic stress disorder

and may be traced to the work of pioneering psychotraumatologist Pierre Janet. Janet argues that it is the cognitive appraisal of the traumatic event in combination with the resultant emotion that ultimately determines the intensity of the traumatic stressor's overall impact upon psychological functioning and, in the final analysis, whether the overall reaction is pathological. Third, based upon an integration of high-intensity reflexive neurological and appraisal processes, the core two-factor "neurocognitive" phenomenology of PTSD, consistent with DSM-IV criteria (APA, 1994), is seen to emerge in the form of (1) *neurological arousal* and (2) *intrusive cognitive recollections* of the traumatic event. Finally, the model in Figure 3.1 can be seen to express the bias that chronic numbing (hormonally mediated as opposed to neurally mediated), avoidance, and withdrawal behaviors reside phenomenologically subsequent and reactive to the two primary core constituents just enumerated.

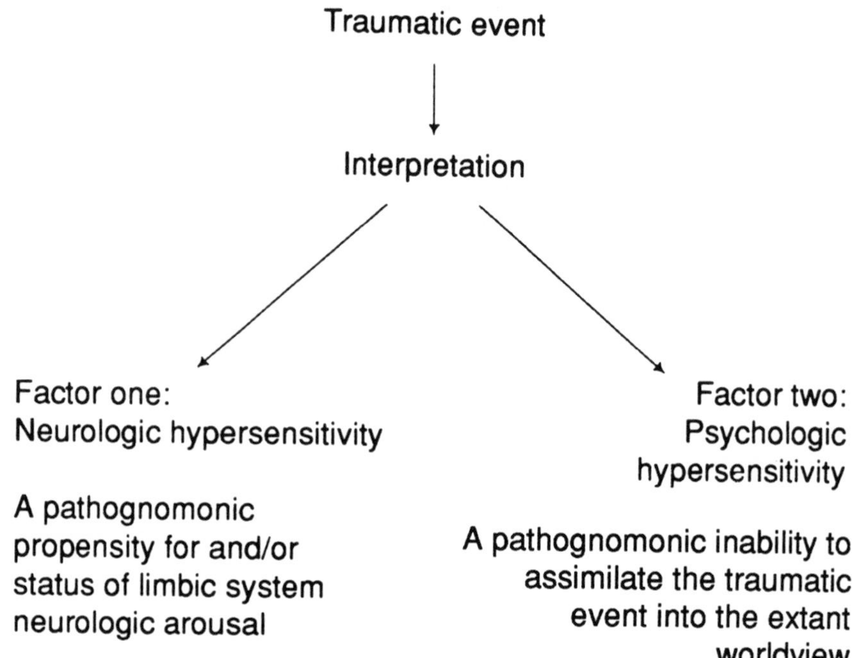

Figure 3.2 A two-factor formulation of post-traumatic stress

To summarize, viewing the model of PTSD in Figure 3.1 as an epiphenomenological construction, a two-factor "neurocognitive" primary process model is revealed (see Figure 3.2). The factors are as follows:

1. A *neurological hypersensitivity* yielding a pathognomonic propensity for and/or status of *neurologic arousal* (Everly, 1990; van der Kolk, 1988) existing within the limbic circuity and its neural effectors (e.g., amygdaloid and hippocampal cells; Everly, 1993a, b).
2. A *psychological hypersensitivity* in the form of intrusive cognitive recollection of some uniquely meaningful aspect of the psychotraumatogenetic process. This psychological hypersensitivity may be viewed as some form of violation or contradiction of the individual's worldview (or Weltanschauung) regarding safety, security, or overall sense of self and the subsequent inability to assimilate the traumatic event in the individual's idiosyncratic worldview (Bowlby, 1969; Everly, 1993a; Janoff-Bulman, 1992; Lifton, 1988; Peterson, Prout, & Schwarz, 1991; Wilson, 1989). This two-factor model will be used as a unifying theme in the rest of the text.

POST-TRAUMATIC STRESS AS A SPECTRUM DISORDER

Some authors (Everly, 1989; Wilson, 1989) have suggested that extreme stress and trauma may engender a wide variety of symptoms not limited to the DSM criteria. Kolb (1989) has even discussed the "heterogeneity" of PTSD symptoms.

It seems clear that post-traumatic stress represents a form of spectrum disorder. Brown and Fromm (1986) have discussed the notion of a "complicated" variant of PTSD within the context of a continuum of severity. It may be that as the intensity of traumatization increases, there is a qualitative change in symptoms as well as an increase in their quantitative intensity. This concept can be visually captured by converting the binary two-factor formulation described earlier into two intersecting dimensions (see Figure 3.3).

As the figure depicts, the two factors that have been posited to represent the core elements of post-traumatic stress can be conceived of not as static nosological monoliths but as dimensional dynamic phenomenological

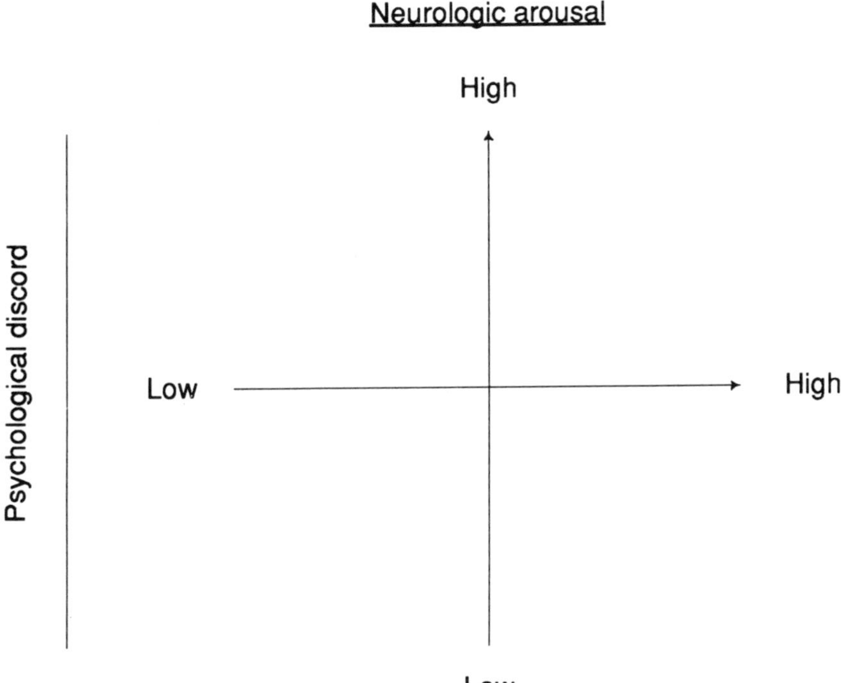

Figure 3.3 Post-traumatic stress as a spectrum disorder

constituents that exist on continua. This dimensional representation allows us to appreciate the dynamism of symptoms, the notion of remission and exacerbation, and the concept of recovery. More in-depth analysis of Figure 3.3 may also allow the clinician to consider psychopharmacological vis-à-vis psychotherapeutic interventions depending upon where the patient's symptoms may be plotted to the two-factor dimensions. In effect, diagnostically the phenemonology of each individual case of post-traumatic stress may be clinically conceptualized by noting the intensity of the arousal symptoms on the arousal dimension; similarly, the degree of psychological incongruence/discord created by the traumatic stressor may be noted on the psychological-discord dimension.

FACTOR ONE: NEUROLOGICAL HYPERSENSITIVITY

In the previous section, it was posited that post-traumatic stress disorder possessed a two-factor neurocognitive phenomenological core: (1) pathognomonic hypersensitivity for and/or status of arousal, and (2) intrusive recollective ideation relevant to some traumatic event (in effect, a psychological hypersensitivity based upon a contradiction to one's worldview). Let us examine each of these two factors in detail.

As noted earlier, Kardiner (1941) conceptualized post-traumatic syndromes as variants on a theme of "physioneurosis." This term is the reflection of the notion that post-traumatic syndromes reflect an inextricable combination of biological and psychological phenomena. Kardiner recognized five consistent clinical features of post-trauma syndromes:

1. Exaggerated startle reflex and irritability
2. Atypical dream experiences
3. A propensity for explosive and aggressive reactions
4. Psychic fixation upon the trauma
5. Constriction of personality functioning.

A review of Kardiner's criteria, as well as DSM criteria (Everly, 1990), reveals that the core physiology of post-traumatic stress is the physiology of arousal of the central nervous system (CNS), the autonomic nervous systems, and various neuroendocrine effector mechanisms. Consistent with Kardiner's perspective, van der Kolk (1988), views PTSD as a pathological inability to modulate arousal.

It then appears as if the patient suffering from a post-traumatic syndrome exhibits a pathognomonic status of CNS neurological hypersensitivity and hyperfunction. This hyperfunction may be characterized by hypertonus, reactive hyperphasic amplitude, or both (Everly, 1990). Ernst Gellhorn was the first to describe the conceptual underpinnings of CNS neurological hypersensitivity clearly via his construct of "ergotropic tuning."

Gellhorn described this hypothalamically based process as the neurophysiological basis for affective lability, autonomic nervous system hyperfunction, anxiety, stress response syndromes, and related emotional disorders (Gellhorn, 1965, 1967; Gellhorn & Loofbourrow, 1963): "The sensitization of autonomic centers has been designated 'tuning' and we speak of sympathetic tuning and parasympathetic tuning . . . and refers merely to the 'sensitization' or 'facilitation' of a particular centers of the brain" (Gellhorn & Loofbourrow, 1963, p. 91).

The term *ergotropic* tuning was chosen by Gellhorn to describe a preferential pattern of sympathetic nervous system responsiveness. Such a neurological status could then serve as the basis for a host of psychiatric disorders (Gellhorn, 1965; Weil, 1974). Etiologically, Gellhorn (1965) states, "in the waking state the ergotropic division of the autonomic is dominant and responds primarily to environmental stimuli. If these stimuli are very strong or follow each other at short intervals, the tone and reactivity of the sympathetic system increases" (pp. 494–495). This sympathetic hyperfunction, according to Gellhorn, then serves as the basis for the psychiatric sequelae observed in stress response syndromes. The pattern may be sustained by continuously reverberating circuits in the emotional centers of the limbic brain (Weil, 1974) and/or by a positive feedback loop involving the skeletal musculature. Gellhorn (1965) has noted that affective discharge from the limbic brain sends neural impulses in two simultaneous directions: to neocortical targets, and to the skeletal musculature via pyramidal and extrapyramidal projections. The neocortical centers then send impulses back to the limbic areas, thus sustaining affective arousal. At the same time, proprioceptive impulses from the skeletal musculature ascend via the reticular system and further stimulate limbic and neocortical targets. This complex positive feedback loop serves to sustain and intensify ergotropic tone (Gellhorn, 1965, 1967).

John Weil (1974) developed a model similar to that constructed by Gellhorn. In fact, Weil makes brief reference to the work of Gellhorn in his construction of a neurophysiological model of emotional behavior. Weil agrees with Gellhorn that the activation thresholds of the limbic system can be altered. More specifically, Weil noted that the neurological activation thresholds of the limbic system and its efferent mechanisms can be lowered enough to render the limbic system hypersensitive. This process he calls "charging of the arousal system." Similar to Gellhorn, Weil notes that the arousal system can be charged (i.e., rendered hypersensitive), through high-intensity and/or chronically repetitive stimulation. The behavioral result of a "charged" limbic arousal system, according to Weil, would be affective lability, anxiety-related dysfunction, and stress-related somatic discord.

Robert Post (1985, 1986; Post & Ballenger, 1981) has proposed that extreme stress may serve to stimulate limbic structures, resulting in a condition whereby the neurological tissues themselves become hypersensitive to subsequent excitation. Drawing on the classic experiments of Goddard (Goddard et al., 1969) on "kindling," which demonstrated that intense or protracted stimulation of limbic nuclei could create permanent changes in the structure and function of the limbic systems, Post chose the term *behavioral sensitization* to reflect the condition where limbic neurons could become hypersensitive based upon exposure to psychosocially related stimuli. This hypersensitivity, Post notes, is considered to be reversible. He has implicated such a behavioral sensitization phenomenon as being involved in various affective mood disorders and other psychopathological conditions.

More recently, Post (1992) has boldly postulated that psychosocial stressors may possess the ability to create a form of neurological sensitization that can encode itself at the level of gene expression. More specifically, the biochemical concomitants of exposure to a stressor (or repeated stressor exposure) may be able to induce the proto-oncogene c-fos to alter gene expression by binding at DNA sites and inducing mRNAs for other substances. Post (1992) notes that transcription factors such as c-fos and c-jun "may provide the basis for a spatiotemporal cascade of events that result in more enduring neurotransmitter, receptor and peptide changes that might provide the . . . basis for long-term synaptic adaptations and memory that could last indefinitely" (p. 1002). He adds, "It is now apparent that a variety of neurochemical systems can induce c-fos" (p. 1002). Among the factors that can induce c-fos are activation of noradrenergic (alpha-1 and beta), dopaminergic (D1), glutamanergic (NMDA), and opiate receptors (see Post, 1992).

Thus we see that the patient suffering from post-traumatic stress is one who is best thought of as neurologically sensitized (i.e., possessing a neurological hypersensitivity or lowered functional threshold for neurologic hyperexcitation). There exist several mechanisms potentially responsible for this posited neurological hypersensitivity:

1. An augmentation of available excitatory neurotransmitters, such as norepinephrine (Davidson & Baum, 1987; Murburs, McFall, & Veith, 1990; Krystal et al., 1989); dopamine (Kalivas & Duffy, 1989); and glutamate (McGeer & McGeer, 1988; Palkovits, Lang, Patthy, & Elekes, 1986)
2. A functional decrease in inhibitory neurochemicals, such as gamma aminobutyric acid (GABA) (Biggio, 1983; Drugan et al., 1989; Gray, 1982; Krnjevic, 1983; van Gelder, 1986)
3. changes in neuronal structural and intraneuronal function that bias the neuron toward a status of or tendency for hyperexcitability, such as an augmentation of excitatory postsynaptic receptors and/or a decrease in inhibitory receptors (see Biggio, 1990; Gray, 1982; Joy, 1985; Nutt, 1989; Perry, Southwick, & Giller, 1990; Post & Ballenger, 1981; Post & Kopanda, 1976).

Given this chronic and potentially intense activation of subcortical CNS excitatory mechanisms, one wonders what the implications may be for what Hans Selye (1976) called "wear and tear" upon the organism. Let us take a closer look at the implications for excessively chronic or intense arousal.

EXCITATORY TOXICITY AND NEURAL DAMPENING

It is now well documented that excessively intense stimulation of CNS mechanisms can actually be toxic to neural substrates. This phenomenon is known as *excitatory toxicity* (McGeer & McGeer, 1988; Olney, 1978). First articulated by Olney and his colleagues, the phenomenon represents a metabolic cascade originating in the form of a massive release of excitatory neurotransmitters—especially glutamate, but perhaps including norepinephrine, dopamine, and others. In high concentrations, these neurotransmitters may become "excitotoxins" capable of damaging or destroying the very neural substrates they serve.

McGeer and McGeer (1988) note that the flood of excitotoxins overstimulate the excitatory receptors on the postsynaptic membranes, especially N-methyl-D-aspartate (NMDA) receptors.

The stimulation of receptor sites causes an opening of calcium ion channels in the affected neurons. A massive influx of positively charged calcium ions results; potassium ions appear to be pushed out of the neuron. This ion influx causes an increase in anaerobic glycolysis as the ion pumps within the neurons attempt to clear the excess ions and prevent a neural bloating phenomenon. Anaerobic glycolysis, protracted because of continued overstimulation, results in a buildup of lactic acid. The buildup in lactic acid may lead to a lowering of the cells' pH level, and acidosis may follow. Ultimately neural cell death occurs if the process is not interrupted (i.e., unless overstimulation is reduced).

Neural excitatory toxicity within hippocampal, septal, and corpus callosum cells may explain some aspects of memory and concentration dysfunctions (Everly & Horton, 1989), intractable aggressive behavior, diminished social or family interaction or bonding, and diminished affiliative behavior, as well as post-trauma alexithymia (Henry, 1993) or even what may be a myriad of attention-deficit-related disorders. The elegant research of Sapolsky and his colleagues (Sapolsky, Uno, Rebert, & Finch, 1990) has demonstrated that high levels of glucocorticoids in the primate brain may cause neural lesions, especially in the area of the hippocampus. This may explain the concentration and memory encoding problems noted by Everly and Horton (1989), as well as other cognitive deficits that may be related to PTSD.

Finally, research by van der Kolk and his colleagues (van der Kolk, Greenberg, Boyd, & Krystal, 1985; van der Kolk, Greenberg, Orr, & Pitman, 1989) argues convincingly for the involvement of some form of CNS opioid-mediated stress-induced analgesia in PTSD. This analgesia appears to be acutely reversible by naloxone, but as it appears naturalistically it would prove to be extremely chronic in nature.

NEUROENDOCRINOLOGY AND ENDOCRINOLOGY

The characteristic overarousal of PTSD is not limited to the CNS; evidence of the overarousal phenomenon can be seen in peripheral or "downstream" mechanisms as well. It is generally accepted that a core constituent of PTSD is the elevation of circulating catecholamine levels (Davidson & Baum, 1986; Mason et al., 1986), which may be evidence of augmentation of the sympatho-adrenal-medullary neuroendocrine axis (Everly, 1989).

There is conflicting evidence, however, surrounding the activity of the hypothalamic-anterior pituitary-adrenal cortical (HPAC), axis. Andrew Baum and his colleagues investigating the Three Mile Island nuclear accident (Davidson & Baum, 1986; Schaeffer & Baum, 1984) found significantly elevated levels of cortisol in those affected by the disaster. Rahe et al. (1990) also found plasma and salivary cortisol highly elevated in the American hostages freed from captivity in Iran. Pitman and Orr (1990), as well as Smith et al. (1989), found similar results with varied populations. Mason and his colleagues (Mason et al., 1986), though, have consistently found evidence of lowered cortisol in combination with elevated catecholamine activity. The work of van der Kolk and his colleagues, noted earlier, would support the conclusion that an augmentation within the HPAC axis, does indeed exist. Finally, Mason et al. (1990) assessed activity of the gonadotropic axis by measuring serum testosterone in patients diagnosed with PTSD. Evidence indicated that the PTSD patients had consistently higher testosterone levels than other patient groups.

The above noted findings are generally consistent with the global formulations of Everly (1989) with regard to generalized human stress. These suggest that post-traumatic stress disorder may represent an extreme variation on the age-old theme of human stress *arousal.*

FACTOR TWO: PSYCHOLOGICAL HYPERSENSITIVITY

This chapter has posited the existence of a two-factor phenomenological core undergirding post-traumatic stress disorder (PTSD). Factor one, described earlier, exists as a neurological hypersensitivity. Factor two, as examined within this section, will be revealed to be a *psychological hypersensitivity.* It may be thought of as the traumatic event leaving in its wake a violation or contradiction of some aspect of the trauma victim's worldview (or Weltanschauung) as it pertains to (1) safety or security or (2) some important aspect of self-perception. In many respects, the essence of the trauma from a psychological perspective *is* the violation of the worldview, combined with the person's inability to assimilate the traumatic event into a personal view of self and/or the world. Let us take a closer look at this notion.

Weltanschauung

Developmentalists and existentialists appear to agree that human beings are engaged in a never-ending struggle to make sense out of the world around them. As Pennebaker and Susman (1988) noted: Most living organisms seek to learn about contingencies of rewards and punishments in their environments. Humans are unique, however, in wanting to understand themselves as well as the world around them. Striving for understanding of the environment and self, then, serves as a fundamental human motive. . . . The issue of understanding the world is particularly relevant to our confronting upsetting or traumatic experiences. (p. 327)

It was William James who in 1868 reportedly first used, in English text, the German word *Weltanschauung* (*welt-* meaning "world"; *anschauung-* meaning "perspective") to refer to an overarching assumption or philosophy about life. Although *Weltansicht* more literally means "worldview," it was *Weltanschauung* that gained more popular usage as the term used to refer to a philosophical perspective/assumption about the world. The term *Weltanschauung* can now be found as an essential aspect of the study of rhetoric, where it is believed important to analyze the worldview of the listener in order to better encode a rhetorical message in concert with the listener's existing set of assumptions, expectations, and the like. Aristotle believed that such conformity was useful in establishing ethos (credibility).

Events that are parallel or in concert to the Weltanschauung may be viewed as ego syntonic for the person experiencing those events. Events that are discordant or contradictory to the Weltanschauung may be viewed as ego dystonic, threatening, or stressful.

Two essential aspects to the overarching Weltanschauung are those aspects that deal specifically with (1) safety and security and (2) a sense of self. It may be argued that the primary reason that humans search for meaning and understanding in their world is to provide a sense of safety and security as well as a meaningful role or sense of self.

John Bowlby

Developmentalist John Bowlby places extreme importance upon an individual's need to create working models of the environment (called the *environmental model*) and of one's self (i.e., one's own skills, resources, etc., called the *organismic model*). The achievement of any predetermined life goal, including safety and security, requires a functional environmental model continually interacting with an organismic model.

> To be useful both working models must be kept up-to-date. As a rule this requires only a continuous feeding in of small modifications, usually a process so gradual that it is hardly noticeable. Occasionally, however, some major change in environment or organism occurs. . . . At those times radical changes of model are called for. Clinical evidence suggests that the necessary revisions of model are not always easy to achieve. Usually, they are completed but only slowly, often they are done imperfectly, and sometimes done not at all. (Bowlby, 1969, p. 82)

This description of Bowlby's terminology describes, in somewhat different terminology, the essence of psychological trauma: the contradiction of extant environmental or organismic (self-perception) Weltanschauung, and the often laborious road to reintegration and recovery.

Robert J. Lifton

Robert J. Lifton has written eloquently about survivors of trauma. From the Holocaust and Hiroshima to Vietnam and Buffalo Creek, he has meticulously studied victimization and survival. From these efforts, he has formulated 10 principles germane to the study of psychological trauma:

1. The importance of the concept of death to the study of psychological trauma.
2. The concept of being a survivor: "Survival is an achievement" (Lifton, 1988, p. 8).
3. The role of human connectedness in survivors. Trauma engenders a discontinuity; recovery entails becoming reconnected. Dissociation may be seen as a natural human response to extreme stress. The vulnerability for dissociation is present in all humans in varying degrees.
4. PTSD is a "normal adaptive process of reaction to an abnormal situation" (Lifton, 1988, p. 9).
5. Survivor guilt is a common post-traumatic reaction for the perception of having failed to halt the traumatic event and/or the failure to help others.
6. Emotional vitality is the conflict between intense feelings associated with the trauma and reactive psychic numbing.
7. Psychic numbing in its extreme form is dissociation and represents a discontinuity of the self.
8. The search for meaning is intimately involved in psychological trauma. According to Lifton (1988), "without addressing this idea of meaning . . . we cannot understand post-traumatic stress disorder" (p. 10).
9. Inherent in psychological trauma is the concept of moral dilemma.

10. Psychological traumatization and recovery involves issues of the transformation of the self.

Lifton concludes that survivors of trauma retain an indelible image of the trauma because of a continuing struggle to master and assimilate the traumatic event into some meaningful context.

Abraham Maslow

In 1954 Abraham Maslow proposed a theory of human motivation that was a blending of the functionalist tradition of James with the holism of Wertheimer and the dynamicism of Freud, Alder, and Jung. Maslow (1970) referred to his theory as a holistic-dynamic theory; it was based upon a hierarchy of human needs (see Figure 3.4). At the absolute foundation of all motivation was the need to satisfy basic physiological needs (e.g., food, water); second only to this drive was the need for safety. Safety was defined by

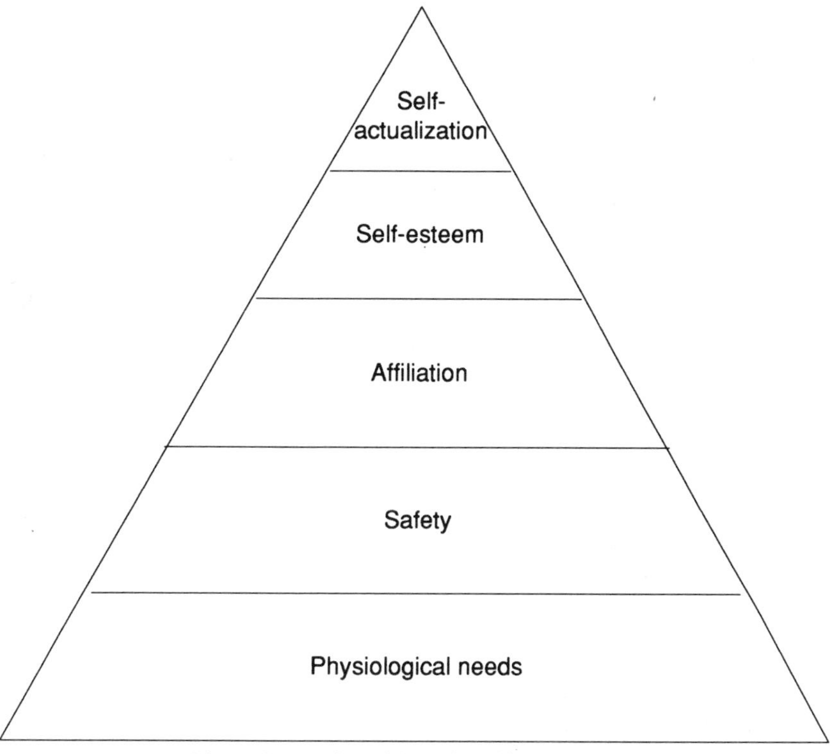

Figure 3.4 Maslow's hierarchy of human needs

Maslow as having security, freedom from fear, the need for structure and order, stability, and protection.

Maslow's hierarchy of needs was completed by the addition of the need to belong and be loved, the need for self-esteem, and finally self-actualization. Maslow makes the point that one cannot progress up the hierarchy until one has satisfied the need beneath it. Sometimes individuals "get stuck" and spend a lifetime pursuing a rudimentary need.

Trauma is the antithesis of order, protection, and security. It may also represent a devastation to one's self-perception. No matter which higher-order Maslovian need level one has attained prior to being traumatized, trauma automatically drops one back to a quest for the lower-order need for safety. Trauma represents a contradiction to the quest for safety and autonomy and stifles any further personality growth until the safety need is once again satisfied.

Trauma also serves to violate or contradict directly the aspect of the Weltanschauung that addresses safety, security, and self. The trauma represents a piece of the puzzle of life that cannot be easily explained or integrated. It is so extreme that it serves to challenge the foundations of the entire Weltanschauung. The post-traumatic world appears chaotic, malevolent, threatening, and insecure. Maslow (1970) explains that once challenged or contradicted, the need for safety becomes a consuming quest fixating the person at this rudimentary level of human existence—perhaps for a lifetime. Horowitz (1976) notes that until the trauma is resolved (i.e., integrated into the worldview), the person becomes engaged in a reiterative cognitive process called the "completion tendency": an intrusive cascade of recollections of the traumatic event with the intent of seeking resolution or integration.

Viktor Frankl

Existentialist Viktor Frankl (1959) argues that the failure to find meaning and a sense of responsibility in one's life lies at the root of psychopathology. Frankl quotes Nietzsche, who said, "He who has a why to live can bear with almost any how." Yet as Frankl explains in his treatise on logo therapy, he who loses the why to live may lose the how as well. "Man's search for meaning is the primary force in his life and not a 'secondary rationalization' of instinctual drives. This meaning is unique and specific in that it must and can be fulfilled by him alone," notes Frankl (1959, p. 99). Thus the striving to find meaning is the primary motivational force in humanity, according to Frankl.

Trauma challenges previously constructed assumptions, meanings, and understandings regarding the world and oneself. Indeed, trauma may violate or contradict both the meaning and the sense of responsibility that one may have previously found in life—hence its devastating impact. Yet Frankl is also quick to quote Nietzsche's famous motto "That which does not kill me, makes me stronger," a seemingly robust optimism for recovery from trauma.

In summarizing the psychological hypersensitivity that undergirds post-traumatic stress disorder, we see that from the perspectives of developmentalist John Bowlby, psychotraumatologist Robert J. Lifton, social and personality psychologist Abraham Maslow, and existential psychiatrist Viktor Frankl that human beings need (and therefore create) a sense of meaning, understanding, and safety regarding the world around them and the role they personally play in that world. This goal is achieved through the use of working models, assumptions about the world and oneself, and other explanatory processes. The aggregation of these psychological processes we refer to as the Weltanschauung, or worldview, regarding both the world per se and the sense of self. Psychological traumatization serves to contradict or shatter the very foundations of what makes the world safe and secure, and/or the very nature of how one perceives oneself.

A NEUROBIOLOGICAL MODEL OF PTSD

In this section I shall take the basic model of PTSD in Figure 3.1 and provide a neurobiological adaptation of that model in an attempt to underscore important neurobiological foundations. Figure 3.5 may then be considered a neurobiological model of PTSD.

As noted earlier, the sine qua non of PTSD is exposure to some traumatic event. Sokolov (1963) has argued that upon exposure to some high-intensity stimulus, typical orienting mechanisms are bypassed and the hypothalamically mediated defense reflex is initiated.

According to van der Kolk et al. (1989)—and as Janet noted, it is the intensity of the cognitive-affective reaction that determines whether an event will cause post-traumatic psychopathology. Authors such as Lazarus and Folkman (1984), Wilson (1989), and Everly (1989) argue that cognitive appraisal/interpretation is the key deterministic aspect of this complex. Arnold (1984) has elegantly mapped the neuroanatomy of cognitive appraisal through the dense neural connections of the cingulate-prefrontal labyrinth.

Everly (1993, a,b) has argued that the core phenomenology of PTSD is the integrated neurological arousal and intrusive memories of the trauma. The amygdala not only controls the sympathetic defense mechanism (Roldan et al., 1974), including the classic fight-or-flight response, but also encodes emotional memories (LeDoux et al., 1989). Emotional memories encoded via the amygdaloid appear to be "impervious to extinction and forgetting processes" (LeDoux et al., 1989). Though the amygdala plays an important role in memory, so does the hippocampus. Gloor (1986) has reported that the hippocampus plays a major role in memory and fear reac-

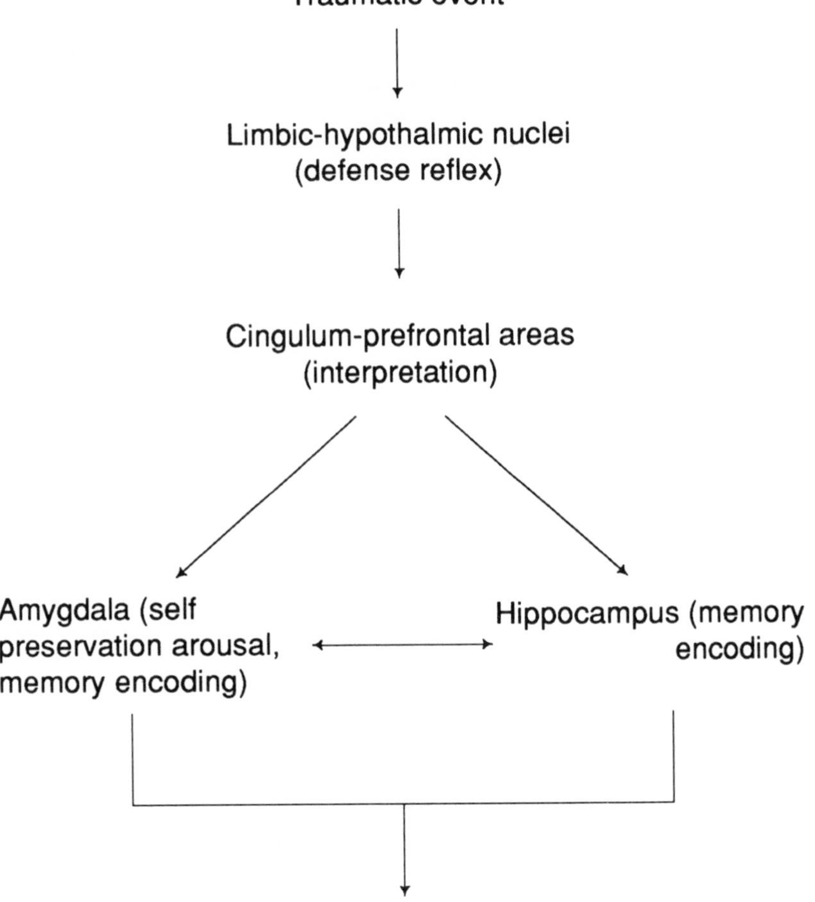

1. Sympatho-adrenal medullary augmentation (increased catecholamines)

2. Gonadatropin alteration (increased testosterone in males possible progesterone and/or estrogen dysfunction in females)

3. Potential hypothalmic anterior pituitary adrenal cortical augmentation (increased cortisol; increased endogenous opioids)

Figure 3.5 Neurobiology of post-traumatic stress disorder

tions; it is thought to be capable of engendering flashbacks, fear, worry, and even guilt reactions.

Thus the functional combination of the amygdala and the hippocampus serves to undergird the core two factors of PTSD (neurological arousal and intrusive cognitive processes). When viewed as a functional symbiosis, it may be suggested that PTSD represents a form of self-preservation mechanism. Figure 3.5 can be seen to extend Figure 3.1 by adding "downstream" efferent physiological processes—namely, the sympatho-adrenal-medullary, gonadotropic, and hypothalamic anterior pituitary adrenal cortical mechanisms (see Everly, 1989, for a review), as reviewed previously.

POST-TRAUMATIC STRESS AND DISORDERS OF AROUSAL

Everly (1989, 1990) first proposed that PTSD be considered within the phenomenological context of a "disorder of arousal." This nosological genre was first proposed and formulated by Everly and Benson (1989) and is reflective of the notion that all stress-related disorders, including PTSD, are manifestations of and variations on a theme of pathognomonic neurological hypersensitivity—in effect, a lowered threshold for psychophysiological excitation within the limbic system and its numerous efferent pathways.

The implications for manifest medical and psychophysiological disorders related to PTSD are great. Everly and Benson (1989), Post (1986), and Doane (1986) have argued that hypersensitivity within the limbic system and its effector systems can cause a multitude of psychiatric and somatic physical disorders. Based on a review of extant literature, Everly (1989) has posited a host of physical illnesses that could be predicated upon a pathogenesis of overarousal. Table 3.1 and Table 3.2 provide such a list of physical and psychiatric disorders that may be a consequence of the overarousal associated with PTSD and the broader construct of post-traumatic stress. Obviously not all traumatized individuals will develop physical symptoms of such

Table 3.1 Psychiatric Disorders Possibly Related to Arousal

1. Anxiety disorders (post-traumatic stress disorder, panic disorders, and diffuse generalized anxiety disorders)
2. Adjustment disorders (with anxious mood and with mixed emotional features)
3. Various primary and secondary affective disorders (especially fast cycling bipolar disorders and secondary reactive depression)
4. Addictive disorders (cocaine, amphetamine, nicotine)
5. Temporal lobe disorders
6. Acute atypical psychotic decompensation
7. Alcohol withdrawal (subsequent to 6 or more years alcoholism)
8. Dissociative disorders
9. Personality disorders

Table 3.2 Somatic Disorders Possibly Related to Arousal

1. Hypertension
2. Stress-related ventricular fibrillation
3. Nonischemic myofibrillar degeneration
4. Stress-related coronary artery disease
5. Migraine headaches
6. Raynaud's disease
7. Muscle contraction headaches
8. Non-head-related muscle contraction dysfunctions
9. Peptic ulcer
10. Irritable bowel syndrome

a wide array as in Table 3.2, nor will all traumatized individuals develop any physical symptoms at all. Table 3.2 is merely provided as a guide to sensitize the reader that post-traumatic stress and somatic discord could coexist in some individuals.

SUMMARY

Within this chapter, a unifying model of PTSD has been proposed. In effect, it has been suggested that PTSD is an epiphenomenon undergirded by a core two-factor phenomenology consisting of (1) subcortical neurological hypersensitivity and (2) psychological hypersensitivity. This notion was depicted in Figures 3.1, 3.2, and 3.3. The two-factor concept will be used as a unifying theme in the remainder of this text.

The neurobiology of PTSD was posited to be a combination of amygdalar-hippocampus neural networks with numerous and varied efferent projections. This concept was depicted in Figure 3.5. Finally, to summarize visually the above concepts and the possible symptom manifestations subsequent to trauma, Figure 3.6 is presented here as the last logical extension of Figure 3.1. It depicts the various symptom manifestation of post-traumatic stress.

The purpose of this chapter was to provide the reader with a unifying macroanalytic model of PTSD and post-traumatic stress. The remaining chapters within Part I will provide more detailed microanalyses of the biological and psychological aspects of post-traumatic stress. Southwick and his colleagues (Chapter 4) present a detailed but useful review of neurobiological literature, and Janoff-Bulman (Chapter 5) examines in greater detail the concept of how trauma affects assumptions about the world (i.e., worldviews). Finally, in Chapter 6 Herman extends the concept of PTSD to reflect its unique nature when engendered via prolonged or repeated traumatization.

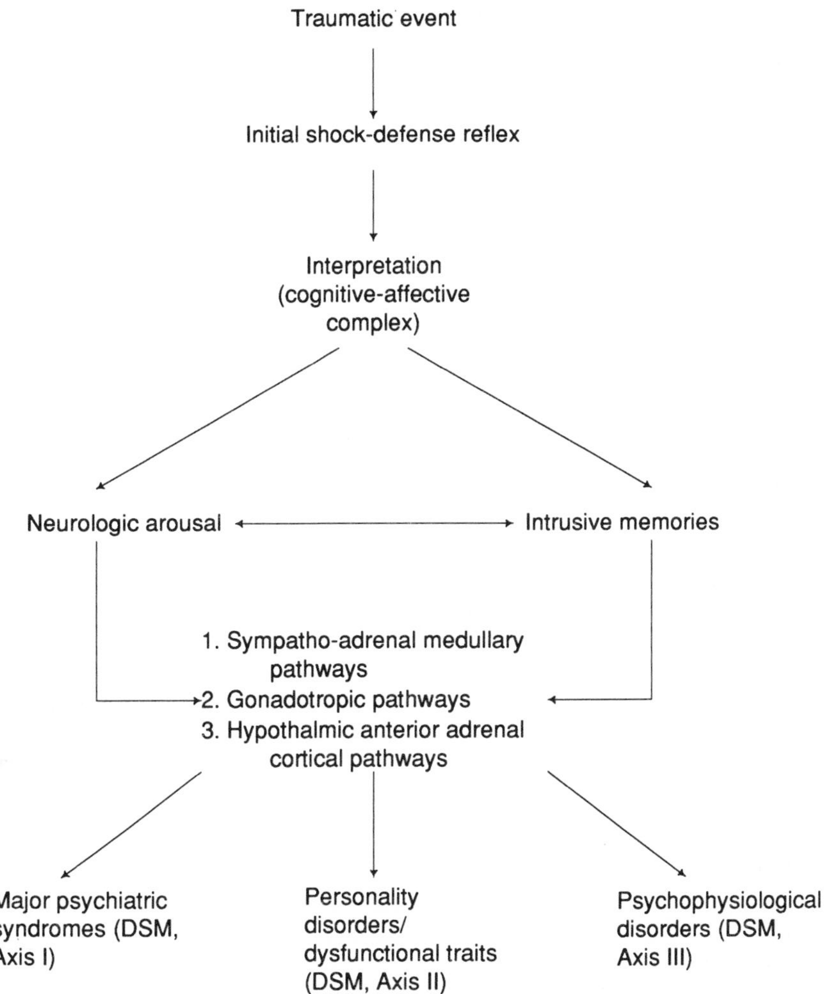

Figure 3.6 A summary of the post-traumatic stress process

REFERENCES

American Psychiatric Association (1980). *Diagnostic and statistical manual of mental disorders* (3rd ed.). Washington, DC: Author.

American Psychiatric Association. (1987). *Diagnostic and statistical manual of mental disorders* (3rd ed. rev.). Washington, DC: Author.

American Psychiatric Association (1994). *Diagnostic and statistical manual of mental disorders* (4th ed.) Washington, DC: Author.

Arnold, M. (1984). *Memory and the brain.* Hillsdale, NJ: Erlbaum.
Benson, H. (1975). *The relaxation response.* New York: Morrow.
Biggio, G. (1983). The action of stress, beta carbornes, diazepam, Ro15-1788 on GABA receptors in the rat brain. In G. Biggio & E. Costa (Eds.), *Benzodiazephine recognition and site ligands* (pp. 105–119). New York: Raven.
Brown, D. P., and Fromm, E. (1987). *Hypnosis and behavioral medicine.* Hillsdale, NJ: Erlbaum.
Bowlby, J. (1969). *Attachment and loss, vol. I: Attachment.* New York: Basic Books.
Breslau, N., Davis, G., & Andreski, P. (1991). Traumatic events and post-traumatic stress disorder in an urban population of young adults. *Archives of General Psychiatry, 48,* 216–222.
Davidson, L., & Baum, A. (1986). Chronic stress and post-traumatic stress disorders. *Journal of Consulting and Clinical Psychology, 54,* 303–308.
Doane, B. (1986). Clinical psychiatry and physiodynamics of the limbic system. In B. Doane & K. Livingston (Eds.), *The limbic system* (pp. 285–315). New York: Raven.
Drugan, R. C., Murrow, A. L., Weizman, R., et al. (1989). Stress-induced behavioral depression associated with a decrease in GABA receptor-mediated chloride ion influx and brain benzodiazepine receptor occupancy. *Brain Research, 487,* 45–51.
Everly, G. S. (1989). *A clinical guide to the treatment of the human stress response.* New York: Plenum.
Everly, G. S. (1990). Post-traumatic stress disorder as a "disorder of arousal." *Psychology and Health: An International Journal, 4,* 135–145.
Everly, G. S. (1993a). Neurophysiological considerations in the treatment of PTSD: A neurocognitive perspective. In J. Wilson & B. Raphael (Eds.), *International handbook of traumatic stress syndromes* (pp. 795–801). New York: Plenum.
Everly, G. S. (1993b). Psychotraumatology: A two-factor formulation of post-traumatic stress. *Journal of Integrative Physiological and Behavioral Science, 28,* 270–278.
Everly, G., & Benson, H. (1989). Disorders of arousal. *International Journal of Psychosomatics, 36,* 15–22.
Everly, G. S., & Horton, A. M. (1989). Neuropsychology of PTSD. *Perceptual and Motor Skills, 68,* 807–810.
Frankl, V. (1959). *Man's search for meaning.* Boston: Beacon.
Freud, S. (1959). Beyond the pleasure principle. In J. Strachey (Ed. and Trans.), *The standard edition of the complete psychological works of Sigmund Freud* (Vol. 18). London: Hogarth. (Original work published 1920).
Gellhorn, E. (1965). Neurophysiological bases of anxiety. *Perspectives in Biology and Medicine, 8,* 488–515.
Gellhorn, E. (1967). *Principles of autonomic-somatic integration.* Minneapolis: University Minnesota Press.
Gellhorn, E., & Loofbourrow, G. (1963). *Emotions and emotional disorders.* New York: Harper and Row.
Gloor, P. (1986). Role of the human limbic system in perception, memory, and affect. In B. Doane & K. Livingston (Eds.) *The limbic system* (pp. 159–169). New York: Raven.
Goddard, G., McIntyre, D., & Leech, C. (1969). A permanent change in brain function resulting from daily electrical stimulation. *Experimental Neurology, 25,* 295–330.
Gray, J. (1982). *The neuropsychology of anxiety.* New York: Oxford.
Henry, J. P. (1993, February). *Alexithymia and PTSD.* Paper presented to the Fifth Montreux Congress on Stress, Montreux, Switzerland.
Horowitz, M. (1976). *Stress response syndromes.* New York: Jason Aronson.
Janoff-Bulman, R. (1992). *Shattered assumptions.* New York: Free Press.
Joy, R. (1985). The effects of neurotoxicants on kindling and kindled seizures. *Fundamental and Applied Toxicology, 5,* 41–65.
Kalivas, P. W., & Duffy, P. (1989). Similar effects of cocaine and stress on mesocorticolimbic dopamine neurotransmission in the rat. *Biological Psychiatry, 25,* 913–928.
Kardiner, A. (1941). *The traumatic neuroses of war.* New York: Hoeber.
Kolb, L. C. (1989). Letter to the editor. *American Journal of Psychiatry, 146,* 811–812.

Krnjevic, K. (1983). GABA-mediated inhibitory mechanisms in relation to epileptic discharges, In H. Jasper & N. van Gelde (Eds.), *Basic mechanisms of neuronal hyperexcitability* (pp. 249–263). New York: Liss.

Krystal, J. H., Kosten, T. R., Southwick, S., et al. (1989). Neurobiological aspects of PTSD. *Behavior Therapy, 20,* 177–198.

Lazarus, R., and Folkman, S. (1984). *Stress, appraisal, and coping.* New York: Springer.

LeDoux, J. E., Romanski, L. M., & Xagoraris, A. E. (1980). Indelibility of subcortical emotional memories. *Journal of Cognitive Neuroscience, 1,* 238–243.

Lifton, R. J. (1988). Understanding the traumatized self. In J. P. Wilson, Z. Harel, & B. Kahana (Eds.), *Human adaptation to extreme stress* (pp. 7–31). New York: Plenum.

Maslow, A. H. (1970). *Motivation and personality.* New York: Harper & Row.

Mason, J. W., Giller, E. C., Kosten, T., & Wahby, V. (1990). Serum testosterone levels in post-traumatic stress disorder inpatients. *Journal of Traumatic Stress, 3,* 444–457.

Mason, J. W., et al. (1986). Urinary free cortisol in PTSD. *Journal of Nervous and Mental Disorders, 174,* 145–149.

McGeer, E., & McGeer, P. (1988). Excitotoxins and animal models of disease. In C. Galli, L. Manzo, & P. Spencer (Eds.), *Recent advances in nervous system toxicology* (pp. 107–131). New York: Plenum.

Murburs, M., McFall, M., & Veith, R. (1990). Catecholamines stress and PTSD. In E. Giller (Ed.), *Biological assessment and treatment of Post-Traumatic Stress Disorder* (pp. 29–64). Washington, DC: American Psychiatric Press.

Nutt, D. (1989). Altered central a-2 adrenoreceptor sensitivity in panic disorder. *Archives of General Psychiatry, 46,* 165–169.

Olney, J. W. (1978). Neurotoxicity of excitatory amino acids. In E. McGeer, J. Olney, & P. McGeer (Eds.), *Kainic acid as a tool in neurobiology* (pp. 95–122). New York: Raven.

Palkovits, M., Lang, T., Patthy, A., & Elekes, L. (1986). Distribution and stress-induced increase of glutamate and aspartate levels in discrete brain nuclei of rats. *Brain Research, 373,* 252–257.

Pennebaker, J., & Susman, J. (1988). Disclosure of trauma and psychosomatic processes. *Social Science and Medicine 26,* 327–332.

Perry, B. D., Southwick, S. M., & Giller, E. L. (1990). Adrenergic receptor regulation in post-traumatic stress disorder. In E. Giller (Ed.), *Biological assessment and treatment of post-traumatic stress disorder* (pp. 87–114). Washington, DC: American Psychiatric Press.

Peterson, P., Prout, M., & Schwarz, R. (1991). *Post-traumatic stress disorder.* New York: Plenum.

Pitman, R. K., & Orr, S. P. (1990). Twenty-four hour urinary cortisol and catecholamine excretion in combat-related post-traumatic stress disorder. *Biological Psychiatry, 27,* 245–247.

Pittman, R. K., van der Kolk, B., Orr, S. P., & Greenberg, M. (1990). Naloxone-reversible analgeric response to combat-related stimuli in post-traumatic stress disorder. *Archives of General Psychiatry, 47,* 541–544.

Post, R. (1985). Stress, sensitization, kindling, and conditioning. *Behavioral and Brain Sciences, 8,* 372–373.

Post, R. (1986). Does limbic system dysfunction play a role in affective illness? In B. Doane & K. Livingston (Eds.), *The limbic system.* New York: Raven.

Post, R. (1992). Transduction of psychosocial stress into the neurobiology of recurrent affective disorder. *American Journal of Psychiatry, 149,* 999–1010.

Post, R., & Ballenger, J. (1981). Kindling models for progressive development of psychopathology. In H. Van Pragg (Ed.), *Handbook of biological psychiatry* (pp. 609–651). New York: Marcel Dekker.

Post, R., & Kopanada, R. (1976). Cocaine, kindling and psychosis. *American Journal of Psychiatry, 133,* 627–634.

Rahe, R., et al. (1990). Psychological and physiological assessments on American hostages freed from captivity in Iran. *Psychosomatic Medicine 52,* 1–16.

Roldan, E., Alvarez-Pelaez, P., & deMolina, F. (1974). Electrographic study of the amygdaloid defense response. *Physiology and Behavior, 13,* 779–787.

Saplosky, R. M., Krey, L., & McEwen, B. (1984). Stress down regulates corticosterone receptors in a site specific manner in the brain. *Endocrinology, 114,* 287–292.

Sapolsky, R., Uno, H., Rebert, C. & Finch, C. (1990). Hippocampal damage associated with prolonged glucocorticoid exposure in primates. *Journal of Neuroscience, 10,* 2897–2902.

Schaeffer, M. A., & Baum, A. (1984). Adrenal cortical response to stress at Three Mile Island. *Psychosomatic Medicine 46,* 227–237.

Seyle, H. (1976). *The stress of life.* New York: McGraw-Hill.

Smith, M., Davidson, J., Ritchie, J., et al. (1989). The cortico-tropin hormone test in patients with post-traumatic stress disorder. *Biological Psychiatry 26,* 349–355.

Sokolov, Y. N. (1988). *Perception and the conditioned reflex.* New York: Macmillan.

van der Kolk, B. (1988). The trauma spectrum. *Journal of Traumatic Stress, 1,* 273–290.

van der Kolk, B., Greenberg, M., Boyd, H., & Krystal, J. (1985). Inescapable shock, neurotransmitters, and addiction to trauma. *Biological Psychiatry 20,* 314–325.

van der Kolk, B., Greenberg, M., Orr, S., & Pittman, R. K. (1989). Endogenous opioids, stress-induced analgesia, and post-traumatic stress disorder. *Psychopharmacology Bulletin, 25,* 417–421.

van Gelder, N. M. (1986). The hyperexcited brain: Glutamic acid release and failure of inhibition. In R. Schwarcz & Y. Ben-Ari (Eds.), *Excitatory amino acids and epilepsy* (pp. 331–347). New York: Plenum Press.

Weil, J. (1974). *A neurophysiological model of emotional and intentional behavior.* Springfield, IL: Thomas.

Wilson, J. P. (1989). *Trauma, transformation, and healing.* New York: Brunner/Mazel.

4

Neurobiology of Post-Traumatic Stress Disorder

STEVEN M. SOUTHWICK, JOHN H. KRYSTAL, DAVID R. JOHNSON, and DENNIS S. CHARNEY

In the general population, post-traumatic stress disorder (PTSD) has a 1% lifetime prevalence (Helzer et al., 1987). Estimates among war veterans are much higher, with 15% of Vietnam veterans currently meeting criteria for PTSD and 30% meeting lifetime criteria. Since their tour in Vietnam, another 20% of veterans have suffered from partial PTSD, having at least some symptoms disruptive of normal social functioning (Kulka et al., 1990).

The criteria for PTSD include exposure to a stressor beyond the range of normal human experience, with subsequent symptoms of reexperiencing, avoidance, and hyperarousal. Traumatic stressors include a wide range of experiences (e.g., natural disasters, violent crimes, accidents, and war). When PTSD lasts for longer than 6 months, it is classified as chronic and is often accompanied by symptoms of anxiety, depression, and compromised work and social functioning.

In this chapter we primarily focus on psychopharmacological treatment and neurobiological consequences of severe psychological trauma. We review both preclinical and clinical studies relevant to the proposition that PTSD appears to be associated with a significant disturbance of multiple neurobiological systems. At the conclusion of the chapter, an attempt will be

---

STEVEN M. SOUTHWICK, JOHN H. KRYSTAL, DAVID R. JOHNSON, and DENNIS S. CHARNEY • Department of Veterans Affairs Medical Center, West Haven, Connecticut 06516. Reprinted by permission from A. Tasman and M. B. Riba (Eds.), *American Psychiatric Press Review of Psychiatry, Vol. 11*. Washington, D.C., American Psychiatric Press, 1992, pp. 347–367.

Psychotraumatology, edited by George S. Everly, Jr. and Jeffrey M. Lating. Plenum Press, New York, 1995.

made to synthesize much of the data to put forth a more comprehensive theory of the pathophysiology of PTSD. In addition, potential therapeutic implications are discussed.

PSYCHOPHARMACOLOGICAL TREATMENT

Until recently, there have been surprisingly few reports of somatic treatments for the suspected neurobiological symptoms of PTSD. During World War II, amobarbital sodium and thiopental sodium were used in the treatment of acute "combat exhaustion" and "war neurosis" (Kolb, 1985), largely for purposes of abreaction and sedation. Another more extreme treatment designed to decrease sympathetic nervous system activation involved bilateral denervation of adrenal glands in war veterans with "neurocirculatory asthenia" (Crile, 1940; Krystal et al., 1989). More recently, clinicians and researchers have employed a wide variety of psychopharmacological agents to treat the acute and chronic symptoms of traumatic stress. None of these agents, however, has been successful in treating the full spectrum of symptoms associated with PTSD. Rather, most reports note the improvement of particular symptom clusters within the DSM-III-R (American Psychiatric Association, 1987) diagnosis of PTSD or within frequently occurring adjunctive symptom clusters, such as depression or explosive impulsivity.

The most commonly investigated psychopharmacological agents have been the antidepressants. Antidepressants are a logical treatment choice because of the high frequency of depressive and panic symptoms in patients with PTSD. The efficacy of antidepressants in the treatment of major depression and panic disorder is well established; thus far the literature contains four case reports (Hogben & Cornfield, 1981; Levenson et al., 1982; Shen & Park, 1983; Walker, 1982), seven open trials (Birkheimer et al., 1985; Bleich et al., 1986; J. Davidson et al., 1987; Falcon et al., 1985; Kauffman et al., 1987; Lerer et al., 1987; Milanes et al., 1984), and four double-blind, placebo-controlled trials (J. Davidson et al., 1990b; Kosten et al., 1991; Reist et al., 1989; Shestatzky et al., 1988) using antidepressants for PTSD. One open trial has addressed acute PTSD; the other have studied chronic PTSD. Subjects in most studies have been combat veterans (J. Davidson et al., 1990a).

To date, studies of antidepressant use in PTSD have primarily focused on the monoamine oxidase inhibitors and tricyclic antidepressants. Initially considerable excitement about the efficacy of phenelzine for PTSD followed a very encouraging case report by Hogben and Cornfield (1981). The authors reported on five combat veterans with traumatic war neurosis; although these patients had previously failed treatment trials of psychotherapy, antipsychotics, and tricyclic antidepressants, each showed a dramatic response to phenelzine, with a marked decrease in nightmares, flashbacks, startle reactions, and aggressive violent outbursts. The authors described phenelzine as possibly "curative." Subsequent reports of phenelzine, however, have been less enthusiastic. Although phenelzine was found to be of significant overall benefit in an open trial by J. Davidson et al. (1987) and in a double-blind, placebo-controlled trial by Kosten et al. (1991), it was found to have minimal treatment efficacy in an open trial by Lerer et al. (1987) and in a placebo-controlled trial by Shestatzky et al. (1988; Davidson et al., 1990a). In general, most tricyclic antidepressant treatment trials in PTSD have reported moderate global improvement. For example, the placebo-controlled trials by J. Davidson et al. (1990b) and Kosten et al. (1991) found tricyclics to be superior to placebo. The best-studied tricyclics have been imipramine and amitriptyline.

Although studies of antidepressant use in PTSD have differed with respect to such methodological issues as assessment, dosage, and length of treatment, most reports have noted significant improvement in the reexperiencing symptom cluster. In a quantitative review that pooled data from all published antidepressant treatment trials in PTSD, both phenelzine and imipramine were found to be effective for the treatment of reexperiencing symptoms but not for avoidance, hyperarousal, depressive, or panic symptoms (Southwick et al., 1994). The finding that depressive and panic symptoms did not respond to antidepressants needs further clarification, because most of the studies did not thoroughly assess for the presence of DSM-III (American Psychiatric Association [APA], 1980) or DSM-III-R major depressive disorder or panic disorder.

Other medications that have been used to treat PTSD also appear to decrease some symptoms but not others (Friedman, 1988). For example, autonomic reactivity reportedly diminishes with both clonidine and propranolol; impulsivity and explosiveness respond to both of these agents as well as to lithium, carbamazepine, and neuroleptics. Although neuroleptics are at times used to treat severe impulsivity, such use is controversial. Lithium may be especially useful for mood lability. Benzodiazepines, among the most frequently prescribed medications for PTSD, appear most effective for an anxiety-related symptoms rather than the core symptoms of PTSD. Their use may be limited by their abuse potential and by the tendency for acute withdrawal to increase PTSD-specific symptoms. Finally, avoidance symptoms appear to be resistant to all psychopharmacological interventions, with the possible exception of fluoxetine and amitriptyline (J. Davidson et al., 1990b; McDougle et al., 1991).

PTSD AS A MULTISYSTEM DISORDER

The fact that various symptoms and symptom clusters in patients with PTSD respond to different psychopharmacological agents with separate modes of action suggests that PTSD, from a neurobiological perspective, may represent a multisystem disorder. For example, if PTSD was caused purely by dysregulation of the noradrenergic system, clonidine would be expected to treat successfully the syndrome as a whole. As noted earlier, however, clonidine is believed to be only partially helpful for a limited number of PTSD symptoms. Similarly, if PTSD was related purely to excessive dopamine function, one might expect neuroleptics to treat the syndrome more successfully. Likewise, fluoxetine would be the only treatment needed if PTSD was solely related to a deficiency in 5-hydroxytryptamine (5-HT) neuronal activity.

A review of the preclinical and clinical neurobiological stress literature relevant to PTSD supports the notion that multiple neurochemical systems are markedly altered in animals and humans who have undergone traumatic stress. Of the enormous number of published preclinical stress studies, this review focuses on those related to the neurochemical and behavioral effects of uncontrollable stress. Uncontrollable stress (where the animal lacks control over stress presentation, intensity, and duration) is a useful animal model of PTSD because the behavioral sequelae so closely resemble symptoms seen in humans with PTSD; furthermore, stressors that result in PTSD are generally uncontrollable in nature. Our review of the relevant clinical neurobiological literature reports primarily on veterans of war, because the vast majority of investigations have studied this population.

BEHAVIORAL EFFECTS OF UNCONTROLLABLE STRESS

When laboratory animals are exposed to aversive events that are out of their control (e.g., electric shock, loud noise, or submersion in cold water), they experience profound disturbances in behavior. Initially there is an alarm response, followed by deficits in learning, reduced exploratory behavior, abnormal sleep patterns, and somatic dysfunction (including reduced feeding, weight loss, suppressed immunological function, increased gastric ulceration, and analgesia; Anisman, 1984).

Both the inability to control and the inability to predict the stressor appear to be critical variables in the development of these behavioral and somatic responses (Maier et al., 1986; Tsuda et al., 1989). Although the underlying molecular mechanisms by which uncontrollable stress exerts such profound behavioral effects are currently not known, recent studies in learning and memory suggest that long-term potentiation and behavioral sensitization may be important.

Long-Term Potentiation

Brief but intense electrical stimulation of an afferent pathway can lead to long-term potentiation, which is a long-lasting increase in synaptic responsivity to subsequent electrical stimulation. Because of its long-term course, hippocampal locus, and correlation with behavioral learning, long-term potentiation has been proposed as a putative mechanism involved in learning and memory (Teyler & DiScenna, 1987). In animals exposed to uncontrollable stress, several investigators have found that hippocampal long-term potentiation memory and behavioral learning are impaired (Shors et al., 1989). When control is introduced, partial reversal of the impairment may result. The above findings have led some to hypothesize that uncontrollable stress causes impairment in hippocampal long-term potentiation, which then results in long-standing deficits in memory and behavioral learning.

Evidence for long-term potentiation has been found not only in the hippocampus but also in the lateral and basolateral nucleus of the amygdala (Clugnet & LeDoux, 1990). Experiments pairing an acoustic stimulus with a foot shock (Chapman et al., 1990) have shown that projections from the medial geniculate body to the amygdala may mediate the formation of traumatic memories. It also has been suggested that emotional memories established via thalamoamygdala pathways may be relatively indelible (LeDoux et al., 1989). These findings raise the possibility that dysfunctional amygdala long-term potentiation may be related not only to the learning abnormalities associated with uncontrollable stress but also to the encoding, storage, and retrieval of traumatic memories.

Behavioral Sensitization

After exposure to uncontrollable threatening or noxious stimuli, animals may exhibit increased behavioral responses to a wide variety of stimuli (both threatening and nonthreatening). The development of sensitization may be strongly related to the memories imprinted by the original stress and by the hormonal and neurochemical brain systems activated by the traumatic experience (Antelman, 1988). It has been suggested that the memory traces themselves are associated with a form of sensitization (Squire, 1986) and that the intensity of a particular traumatic memory may result from the degree to which key neurochemical systems have been activated by the trauma (McGaugh, 1989). Stress-induced sensitization may also partly account for the increased startle response seen in PTSD (Davis 1986, 1989; Hitchcock et al., 1989). Both dopamine and norepinephrine systems have been implicated in the behavioral sensitization that occurs following repeated stress (Kalivas et al., 1990; Nisenbaum et al., 1991).

NEUROCHEMICAL EFFECTS OF UNCONTROLLABLE STRESS AND THE SPECTRUM OF PTSD SYMPTOMS

Profound alterations in multiple neurotransmitter systems are caused by uncontrollable stress. In both the preclinical and clinical literature, the neurochemical systems that have been most studied include noradrenergic,

Table 4.1 Preclinical Evidence for Neurobiological Dysfunction in Post-Traumatic Stress Disorder

Neurochemical System	Functional Alteration Produced by Uncontrollable Stress	Acute Adaptive Behavioral Responses
Noradrenergic	Increased regional norepinephrine turnover in limbic and cortical areas Increased responsiveness of locus coeruleus neurons	Anxiety, fear, autonomic hyperarousal, fight or flight readiness, encoding of traumatic memories, facilitation of sensory-motor responses
Dopaminergic	Increased dopamine release in frontal cortex and nucleus accumbens Activation of mesocortical dopamine neurons	Hypervigilance
Opiate	Increased endogenous opiate release in periaqueductal gray Decreased density of mu opiate receptors in cerebral cortex	Analgesia, emotional blunting, encoding of traumatic memories
Benzodiazepine	Decreased density of benzodiazepine receptors in hippocampus and cerebral cortex Reduced GABA-dependent chloride flux	Fear, hyperarousal
Hypothalamic-pituitary-adrenal axis	Elevated glucocorticoid levels at the level of the hippocampus	Metabolic activation, learned behavioral responses

Note: GABA = gamma-aminobutyric acid.

dopaminergic, endogenous opiate, gamma-aminobutyric acid (GABA), benzodiazepine, serotonergic, and hypothalamic-pituitary-adrenal (HPA) axis systems (Tables 4.1 and 4.2).

Noradrenergic Neuronal Function

Uncontrollable stress is associated with an elevated sense of fear and anxiety. In the brain, fear and anxiety may be mediated in part by increased activity of the locus coeruleus, resulting in increased synaptic norepinephrine in limbic and cortical regions innervated by the locus coeruleus. Although many types of stressful stimuli produce marked regional (e.g., hypothalamus, hippocampus, amygdala) increases in brain noradrenergic function, uncontrollable stress appears to cause greater increases than controllable stress (Gavin, 1985). In fact, when animals have mastered a coping

Table 4.2 Clinical Evidence for Neurobiological Dysfunction in Post-Traumatic Stress Disorder

Neurobiological dysfunction	Potential clinical evidence	Correlates	Reference
Autonomic reactivity	Increased resting heart rate	Hyperresponsivity to stress, increased cardiovascular morbidity	Orr (1990)
	Increased resting systolic blood pressure		
	Increased heart rate in response to visual and auditory reminders of trauma		
Adrenergic and noradrenergic function	Increased 24-hour urinary epinephrine and norepinephrine	Chronic anxiety, fear, impulsivity, anger	Kosten et al. (1987)
	Increased plasma epinephrine in response to combat-related stressful stimuli	Persistent hypervigilance	McFall et al. (1990)
	Decreased platelet alpha$_2$-adrenergic receptor number	Reactivation of traumatic memories	Perry et al. (1987)
	Increased internalization of platelet alpha$_2$-adrenergic receptors in response to in-vitro agonist stimulation	Chronic hyperarousal	Perry et al. (1990)
	Increased behavioral and MHPG responses to yohimbine		Southwick et al. (1991)
Hypothalamic-pituitary-adrenal axis function	Increased, dec 24-hour urinary cortisol	Possible difficulties in learning and memory	Pitman & Orr (1990) Yehuda et al. (1990)
	Increased lymphocyte glucocorticoid receptor number		Yehuda et al. (1991a)
	Decreased ACTH response to CRH		Smith et al. (1989)
	Increased sensitivity to dexamethasone		Yehuda et al. (1991b)
Endogenous opiate function	Increased stress-induced analgesia reversed by naloxone	Chronic "numbing" and blunting of emotional responses	Pitman et al. (1990) van der Kolk et al. (1989)

Note: MHPG = 3-methoxy-4-hydroxyphenylglycol. ACTH = adrenocorticotropic hormone. CRH = corticotropin-releasing hormone.

task to reduce stress effectively, increased norepinephrine turnover generally does not occur (Tsuda & Tanaka, 1985).

A number of investigations have shown that uncontrollable (but not controllable) stress produces increased responsivity of locus coeruleus neurons to excitatory stimulation. This locus coeruleus hyperactivity may result from the development of alpha$_2$ adrenergic autoreceptor subsensitivity (Simson & Weiss, 1988a, b). In addition, stress-induced increase in norepinephrine turnover is associated with a decrease in postsynaptic beta-receptor number (Torda et al., 1984).

Sensitization and Noradrenergic Function. Altered noradrenergic function may be associated with behavioral sensitization to repeated stress. When animals are exposed to repeated stressors, tyrosine hydroxylase, dopamine beta-hydroxylase activity, and synaptic levels of norepinephrine metabolites increase (Irwin et al., 1986b; Kramarcy et al., 1984; Melia et al., 1991). These findings suggest that repetitive stress can cause a compensatory increase in the synthesis of norepinephrine. Thus, when repeatedly shocked animals are reexposed to limited shock, they respond with a degree of norepinephrine release that is more appropriate for much higher levels of shock.

Environmental stimuli previously paired with uncontrollable shock may also lead to sensitization or fear conditioning of noradrenergic neuronal systems. Neutral stimuli that have been paired with inescapable shock produce increases in brain norepinephrine metabolism and behavioral deficits similar to that elicited by the original shock (Cassens et al., 1981). Neurophysiological studies in freely moving cats indicate that pairing a neutral stimulus with an aversive one (which increases locus coeruleus firing) results in the neutral stimulus acquiring the same property (Rasmussen et al., 1986).

Clinical Studies. For years, investigators have speculated about the relationship between symptoms of severe stress and the sympathetic nervous system in traumatized humans. Meakins and Wilson (1918) found shell-shocked veterans to have greater increases in heart rate and respiratory rate than healthy controls when exposed to sulfuric flames and the sounds of gunfire. Exaggerated psychophysiological arousal responses were noted in war veterans when they were administered intravenous epinephrine (Fraser & Wilson, 1918). Since the 1980s there have been a series of well-designed psychophysiological studies that have consistently documented heightened sympathetic nervous system arousal in combat veterans with PTSD (Orr, 1990). Compared with healthy controls, veterans with PTSD tend to have a higher mean resting heart rate and systolic blood pressure, and they tend to show greater increases in heart rate when exposed to visual and auditory combat-related stimuli in the laboratory. This same degree of hyperreactivity has not been found in combat veterans without PTSD or in combat veterans with anxiety disorders other than PTSD. Taken together, the psychophysiological studies suggest that some individuals are more susceptible to sympathetic nervous system dysregulation than others, and that neither combat alone nor the presence of anxiety disorders other than PTSD is sufficient to explain postwar physiological hyperactivity. Additionally, it has been shown that not all stressful stimuli evoke hyperactive responses in traumatized combat veterans; hyperactive responses seem relatively specific to combat-related stressful stimuli, suggesting that noradrenergic reactivity in patients with PTSD may be conditioned or sensitized to specific traumatic stimuli (Orr, 1990).

Investigations of neuroendocrine and peripheral catecholamine receptor systems have also provided evidence for a dysregulation of sympathetic nervous system activity in PTSD. Kosten et al. (1987) found that 24-hour urine norepinephrine excretion was higher in combat veterans with PTSD than in patients with schizophrenia or major depression. Further, throughout the course of hospitalization, norepinephrine excretion in the PTSD group remained markedly elevated in comparison to values reported for other subjects. In a study of alpha$_2$-adrenergic receptors, Perry et al. (1987) found 40% fewer receptors in a group of patients with PTSD compared with control subjects who were not psychiatrically ill. A decreased receptor number most likely reflects adaptive "down-regulation" in response to chronically elevated levels of circulating endogenous catecholamines. In addition, using an in-vitro model of intact platelets, high concentrations of epinephrine caused a more rapid and extensive loss of receptor protein from the platelet membrane, probably because a more rapid internalization process (Perry et al., 1990).

In the first study to evaluate psychophysiologic reactivity and peripheral catecholamines simultaneously in combat veterans with PTSD, McFall et al. (1990) found a parallel rise in blood pressure, heart rate, subjective distress, and plasma epinephrine during and after a combat film, suggesting that elevations of circulating catecholamines are related to hyperreactive physiological responses. In residents living within 5 miles of the Three Mile Island nuclear power plant (south of Harrisburg, Pennsylvania), similar elevations in resting heart rate, blood pressure, and urinary norepinephrine have been reported (Davidson & Baum, 1990).

Although most studies of neurobiological function in PTSD have employed peripheral measures of catecholamine metabolism, preliminary evidence for central catecholamine dysregulation comes from a recent investigation using intravenous yohimbine as a probe of central and peripheral noradrenergic function. Although yohimbine affects multiple neurotransmitter systems, in panic disorder it has been proposed that yohimbine induces panic attacks by increasing noradrenergic function through a blockage of alpha$_2$-adrenergic receptors (Charney et al., 1987). As predicted from preclinical studies, intravenous yohimbine induced enhanced behavioral, biochemical, and cardiovascular responses in combat veterans with PTSD compared with control subjects who were not psychiatrically ill (Southwick et al., 1991). Approximately 60% of patients with PTSD had yohimbine-induced panic attacks; approximately 40% had flashbacks. In contrast, yohimbine rarely induces panic attacks in patients with schizophrenia, major depression, obsessive-compulsive disorder, or generalized anxiety disorder, or in healthy control subjects (Charney et al., 1990a). The 60% rate of yohimbine-induced panic attacks, however, closely resembles the rate seen in patients with pure panic disorder (Charney et al., 1987), suggesting that PTSD and panic disorder share a common neurobiological abnormality related to the noradrenergic system. Comorbid panic disorder could not solely account for panic attacks in PTSD, because panic attacks were experienced by patients both with and without comorbid panic disorder.

Uncontrollable Stress and Dopaminergic Neuronal Function

The prefrontal cortex is the primary brain dopamine system involved in the stress response. Biochemical and electrophysiological studies have shown that stress preferentially activates and increases the filing rate of mesocortical neurons compared with mesolimbic and strata dopamine areas (Dunn, 1988; Roth et al., 1988). Increases in dopamine metabolism in the frontal cortex also have been noted in association with environmental cues that have been paired with a stressor (Herman et al., 1982). A number of chemically distinct afferent systems seem to play a role in stress-induced activation of mesocortical dopamine, including substance P, N-methyl-D-aspartate (NMDA), and opiates (Dunn, 1988).

Chronic stress and repeated cocaine exposure may have similar effects on dopamine neuronal function. Both appear to increase mesocortical dopamine transmission in response to acute stress. Further, locomotor responses to cocaine and amphetamine increase after daily exposure to stress (Antelman et al., 1980; Kalivas & Duffy, 1989; Maclennan & Maier, 1983; Robinson, et al., 1985).

Clinical Studies. Because enhanced dopamine function has been related to psychosis in schizophrenia, it is possible that symptoms of stress-induced psychosis are also related to dopamine neuronal hyperactivity. Trauma-related psychosis in Nazi concentration camp survivors, Vietnam veterans, and Cambodian refugees has been described in case reports and small descriptive studies (Kinzie & Boehnlein, 1989; Mueser & Butler, 1987; Nemeth, 1960). These reports are difficult to interpret because of the possibility that these individuals may have developed psychotic disorders in the absence of trauma, as well as the complexity of distinguishing dissociative and psychotic symptoms. Hypervigilance and paranoia have also been reported in traumatized individuals; in fact, these symptoms are frequently seen in combat veterans with PTSD.

Uncontrollable Stress and Endogenous Opiate System Function

Uncontrollable stress stimulates a release of endogenous opiates, causing substantial and significant hypoalgesia (Hemingway & Reigle, 1987).

Further, in rats previously exposed to uncontrollable shock, reexposure with less intense shock reproduces the same degree of hypoalgesia, suggesting that sensitization occurs. This hypoalgesia is likely to be mediated by stress-induced release of endogenous opiates, because opiate peptides are elevated after acute uncontrolled shock (Maier, 1986). Uncontrollable (but not controllable), shock decreases the density of mu opiate receptors, and stress-induced analgesia is blocked by naltrexone (Stuckey et al., 1989).

The actual induction of behavioral deficits resulting from uncontrollable stress may also in part be mediated by endogenous opiates. Hippocampal long-term potentiation and behavioral deficits do not develop when naltrexone is given prior to uncontrollable shock (Hemingway & Reigle, 1987).

Clinical Studies. Naloxone has been shown to reverse stress-induced analgesia in both nontraumatized and traumatized human populations. After noxious foot shock (Hemingway & Reigle, 1987) and during uncontrollable problem-solving tasks (Bandura et al., 1988) in nontraumatized humans, stress-induced analgesia can be reversed by naloxone. Similarly, naloxone reverses the analgesia induced by stressful combat films in Vietnam veterans with PTSD (Pitman et al., 1990). These findings suggest that stress-induced analgesia in PTSD is, at least in part, opiate mediated. These findings are consistent with the observation that soldiers in World War II required lower doses of narcotics than did civilians with less severe injuries (Beecher, 1946).

It has been hypothesized that compulsive reexposure to traumatic events (or "addition to trauma") is related to increases in endogenous opiates during episodes of reexposure to the trauma or reminders of the trauma (van der Kolk et al., 1989). Psychophysiological laboratory studies, however, have failed to support this hypothesis; combat films in veterans with PTSD evoked numbing or blunting of emotional responses as opposed to euphoria or emotional feelings of calm and control (Pitman et al., 1990). This association between psychic numbing and opiate-mediated stress-induced analgesia is supported by studies of self-mutilation in traumatized psychiatric patients (Richardson & Zaleski, 1983).

Uncontrollable Stress and Benzodiazepine Receptor Function

Decreases in GABA receptor-mediated chloride ion flux, depolarization-induced hippocampal release of GABA, and brain benzodiazepine receptor occupancy have all been associated with behavioral deficits induced by uncontrollable shock (Drugan et al., 1989). Uncontrollable stress causes a decrease in benzodiazepine receptor binding in cerebral cortex, hippocampus, and striatum, and a reduction of the density of low-affinity $GABA_A$ receptors and chloride efflux and uptake in cerebral cortex (Concas et al., 1988a; Drugan et al., 1989; Schwartz et al., 1987). Additionally, foot shock stress and anxiogenic beta-carbolines increase [^{35}S]TBPS (*t*-butylbicyclophosphomethionate) binding in rat cerebral cortex (Concas et al., 1988b). These findings suggest that the behavioral effects of uncontrollable stress are associated with a functional alteration of the benzodiazepine GABA chloride ionophore complex.

Lorazepam and chlordiazepoxide, both benzodiazepines, prevent the development of the behavioral deficits and analgesia induced by uncontrollable stress (Drugan et al., 1985). The benzodiazepine receptor inverse agonist β-carboline FG-7142 (N-methyl-β-carboline-3-carboxamide), in contrast, produces behavioral deficits very similar to those seen in uncontrollable shock. Pretreatment with a benzodiazepine receptor antagonist, Ro 15-788, prevents the effects of FG-7142 (Drugan et al., 1985).

The effects of uncontrollable stress in the benzodiazepine system may in part be related to alterations in norepinephrine, dopamine, and endogenous steroid systems. For example, benzodiazepines reduce locus coeruleus activity, as well as stress-induced increases in norepinephrine turnover (Ida et al., 1985; Redmond, 1987). Benzodiazepines also decrease stress-induced increases in prefrontal dopamine activity. Additionally, it is now known that several endogenous steroids are potent modulators of the $GABA_A$ benzodiazepine chloride ionophore receptor complex (Majewska et al., 1986).

Clinical Studies. Although there have been no specific studies to date relating the symptoms of PTSD to dysfunction of the benzodiazepine GABA system, there is extensive preclinical and accumulating clinical evidence implicating the benzodiazepine GABA receptor in the pathophysiology of human anxiety and general fear states. For example, FG-7142, a benzodiazepine receptor inverse agonist, causes severe anxiety and panic attacks in healthy subjects (Dorow et al., 1983). Similarly flumazenil, a benzodiazepine receptor antagonist, induces panic attacks in some patients with panic disorder but not in healthy subjects, suggesting that the sensitivity of benzodiazepine receptors to inverse agonists may be increased (Nutt et al., 1990; Woods et al., 1991). The use of benzodiazepine inverse agonists and antagonists in patients with PTSD and the measurement of behavioral and cerebral metabolic effects of these drugs using positron-emission tomography (PET) and single-photon-emission computed tomography (SPECT) imaging techniques will provide for a better understanding of the role of the benzodiazepine GABA system in symptom formation.

Uncontrollable Stress and Serotonergic Neuronal Function

Inescapable shock, but not escapable shock, decreases serotonin levels in the lateral septum and cortex (Petty & Sherman, 1983). In contrast, immobilization stress increases brain 5-HT turnover and 5-hydroxyindoleacetic acid (5-HIAA) concentrations (Keneth & Joseph, 1981). Supporting the finding that inescapable shock reduces serotonin levels is the fact that serotonin antagonists (methysergide and parachlorophenylalanine [PCPA]) can cause behavioral effects that resemble those seen in inescapable shock

(Morgan et al., 1975). Additionally, when serotonin agonists (parachloroamphetamine [PCA], 5-HT$_{1A}$ agonists) are administered before inescapable shock, the subsequent behavior deficits can be prevented (Giral et al., 1988).

Establishing the precise role of serotonin in the behavioral effects of uncontrollable stress is complicated by the fact that noradrenergic and serotonergic neuronal systems interact with and regulate one another in the brain. For example, 5-HT$_2$ binding sites are elevated in rat cortex as a result of acute stress and immobilization. This effect is dependent on the integrity of the brain noradrenergic system, however, and not the 5-HT system (Torda et al., 1990). Clearly, further preclinical investigations will be needed to delineate the precise role of the serotonin system in uncontrollable stress.

Clinical Studies. The role of serotonin function of human forms of anxiety, fear, and stress is not well understood. A partial serotonin agonist with complex interactions at the 5-HT receptor, m-chlorophenylpiperazine (mCPP), has been shown to have anxiogenic properties in healthy subjects and in patients with panic disorder, supporting a role for serotonergic neurons in the pathophysiology of anxiety (Charney et al., 1990b; Soubrie, 1986). Although the precise 5-HT receptor type and most affected by mCPP is not fully delineated, recent evidence suggests an important role for the 5-HT$_{1c}$ receptor (Seibyl et al., 1991). The effects of mCPP in patients with PTSD are currently being investigated.

Serotonin may play an important role in the regulation of mood, aggression, impulsivity, and compulsive behavior. These affects and behaviors are commonly seen in traumatized individuals, suggesting that dysfunction of serotonergic neurons may play a role in symptom formation in PTSD. The use of fluoxetine for the treatment of a variety of symptoms of PTSD is currently under investigation. Preliminary data appear encouraging, with possible efficacy for avoidance symptoms as well as reexperiencing symptoms (McDougle et al., 1991).

Uncontrollable Stress and HPA Axis Function

In laboratory animals, adrenocorticotropic hormone (ACTH) and cortisol levels are increased by acute stress of many types (McEwen, et al., 1986). It has been shown that high glucocorticoid levels decrease hippocampal but not other brain glucocorticoid receptors, resulting in increased corticosterone secretion and feedback resistance. With uncontrolled stress (but not controllable stress), this feedback resistance results in nonsuppression of cortisol in response to dexamethasone. With the resolution of acute stress, glucocorticoid levels again decrease, receptor number increases, and feedback sensitivity normalizes (Sapolsky & Plotsky, 1990).

Both adaptation and sensitization of glucocorticoid activity have been reported in response to chronic stress. Some investigators have reported that adaptation to chronic stress may occur, with resultant decreases in plasma ACTH and cortisol levels (Kant et al., 1985). Other investigators have reported an increased cortisol secretion following chronic stress as well as augmented cortisol responses to a subsequent stressor, particularly in animals with prior histories of stress (Irwin et al., 1986a).

It is unclear exactly how the effects of uncontrollable stress on the HPA axis affect behavior. There is some evidence to suggest that elevated glucocorticoid levels may result in learning deficits through neurotoxic effects on hippocampal neurons. In a study of vervet monkeys, marked and preferential hippocampal degeneration was noted in deceased animals after sustained social stress (Uno et al., 1989). In a second investigation with vervet monkeys, glucocorticoid administration resulted in very similar damage to the hippocampus (Sapolsky et al., 1990). Other evidence for a relationship between uncontrollable stress, alteration in the HPA axis, and behavior comes from adrenalectomy experiments. In general, adrenalectomy and resultant decreased corticosteroid levels increase the frequency of behavioral and learning deficits caused by uncontrollable stress. These deficits may be reversed by corticosteroid administration (Edwards et al., 1990). It appears, then, that a certain amount of glucocorticoid activity is necessary for learning and adaptation, but that too much activity may result in neurotoxicity.

Just as serotonergic and noradrenergic systems appear to have regulatory effects on one another in the brain, glucocorticoids and biogenic amines also appear to have modulating effects on one another (McEwen, 1987). For example, norepinephrine stimulates corticotropin-releasing hormone (CRH) secretion from the hypothalamus (Calogero et al., 1988); stress-induced glucocorticoid elevation may mediate the ability of stress to reduce norepinephrine-stimulated cyclic AMP in the hippocampus and cortex. Because CRH and corticosterone (Avanzino et al., 1987; Valentino et al., 1983) each activate locus coeruleus neurons, it is possible that under conditions of stress the CRH systems and noradrenergic systems mutually reinforce one another.

Clinical Studies. Under conditions of acute stress, both norepinephrine and cortisol secretion increase. Norepinephrine prepares the organism for action; cortisol generally serves a metabolic preservation function. In studying chronic stress, however, Mason et al. (1988) found low cortisol levels in the presence of elevated norepinephrine, suggesting a dissociation between the pituitary-adrenal-cortical axis and the sympathetic-adrenal-medullary system. This unusual discordance between norepinephrine and cortisol has been used as a means to discriminate chronic combat-related PTSD from other psychiatric diagnoses.

The data on urinary cortisol in chronically stressed combat veterans have been conflicting. One group reported an increased level (Pitman &

Orr, 1990); a second group found unusually low cortisol levels in comparison with healthy control subjects and subjects with other psychiatric diagnoses (Yehuda et al., 1990). Earlier work with animals suggested that the underlying mechanism of low cortisol is not one of pituitary-adrenal-cortical system exhaustion, but rather most likely involves a central suppressive or inhibitory mechanism (Yehuda et al., 1991c).

In a conclusion consistent with these data, combat veterans with PTSD have been found to have a greater number of lymphocyte glucocorticoid receptors compared with healthy control subjects (Yehuda et al., 1991a). Glucocorticoids appear to play a role in the regulation of glucocorticoid receptor number in a variety of tissues, with decreased cortisol levels resulting in a compensatory increase in number of receptors and increased cortisol levels in a decreased number of receptors.

Also consistent with low cortisol levels is the finding that some patients with PTSD may be overly sensitive to the ability of dexamethasone to suppress cortisol (Yehuda et al., 1991b). In other words, the HPA axis, most likely at the level of the hypothalamus or pituitary, may hyperrespond to dexamethasone. The resultant heightened negative feedback could be the result of an increased number or sensitivity of hypothalamic-pituitary glucocorticoid receptors. Heightened negative feedback to glucocorticoids might also explain the finding by Smith et al. (1989) of a blunted ACTH response to CRF in patients without abnormally high circulating cortisol levels.

COMMENT

Acute Neurobiological Responses to Severe Trauma

Under conditions of acute and severe psychological trauma, the organism mobilizes multiple neurobiological systems for the purpose of survival. Thus noradrenergic, benzodiazepine, opiate, dopaminergic, serotonergic, and HPA axis systems may all be activated simultaneously. These systems appear to interact functionally with one another as the organism attempts to cope with impending danger. In addition to the simultaneous functional alteration of different neurochemical systems during acute stress, several brain structures—most notably the amygdala, hippocampus, locus coeruleus, and prefrontal cortex—also appear to become activated. For example, activation of the locus coeruleus produces an increase in norepinephrine release at locus coeruleus projection sites, including the amygdala, hippocampus, and cerebral cortex. As reviewed above, these structures are markedly affected by uncontrollable stress, are functionally and neuroanatomically interrelated, and may mediate many of the symptoms of PTSD.

The simultaneous alterations of numerous brain neurochemical systems and structures during acute traumatic stress likely represent adaptive responses critical for survival. Endogenous norepinephrine, benzodiazepine, and dopamine appear to mediate fear, autonomic hyperarousal, and hypervigilance, each of which facilitates appropriate behavioral reactions to threat. Norepinephrine additionally appears to influence numerous somatic functions, including blood pressure, heart rate, and blood clotting. The metabolic activation necessary for sustained physical demands and tissue repair appears to be influenced by trauma-induced cortisol hypersecretion. Secretion of endogenous opiates reduces pain sensitivity of men wounded in battle; this reduction may be critical for survival. Finally, the encoding of traumatic memories that will facilitate appropriate response to future danger may be facilitated by norepinephrine and opiate systems.

Chronic Neurobiological Sequelae

Although initially beneficial, neurobiological responses to trauma may have long-term negative consequences that are related to many of the chronic symptoms of PTSD. For example, the dysregulation of noradrenergic neurons may result in a system that is persistently hyperresponsive to stress, particularly stress that is in some way related to the original trauma. Symptoms of chronic hyperarousal and anxiety may result. Preclinical studies demonstrating stress-induced alpha$_2$-autoreceptor dysfunction and stressor desensitization of noradrenergic neurons support this notion.

Noradrenergic system hyperactivity may also be related to the reexperiencing symptoms of PTSD. During the original trauma, when encoding of memories takes place, the individual is in a state of heightened noradrenergic activity. It is quite possible that this physiological state of hyperarousal becomes associated with the original trauma and by itself has the capacity to evoke traumatic memories and flashbacks. It is well known that traumatic memories can be reactivated decades after the original trauma by stressful life events completely unrelated to the original stressor. Preclinical studies invite the speculation that traumatic memories can be evoked by stress-induced activation of the locus coeruleus with increased norepinephrine release and stimulation of noradrenergic receptors in brain regions such as the amygdala and hippocampus. Recent clinical studies with yohimbine support this notion.

Patients with chronic PTSD frequently exhibit increased anger, hostility, impulsivity, and dysphoria. These symptoms may be related to abnormalities in either norepinephrine, 5-HT, or both. Further experience with selective norepinephrine and selective 5-HT pharmacological agents should clarify the relationship between specific neurotransmitter systems and particular symptoms of PTSD. Another potentially important long-term consequence of the acute response to trauma involves persistent difficulties in learning and memory, possibly as a result of glucocorticoid-induced hippocampal damage.

The high rates of substance abuse in combat veterans with PTSD may also be related to the noradrenergic system. Alcohol, opiates, and benzodiazepines are commonly considered the preferred substances of abuse among traumatized combat veterans. Each of these drugs decreases the firing rate of the locus coeruleus and decreases norepinephrine release and turnover in various brain loci. The use of these drugs by a traumatized veteran might then represent an attempt to compensate for dysregulation of catecholamine or endogenous opiate systems. Conversely, amphetamines and cocaine, which increase dopamine function, may actually increase symptoms of hyperarousal and paranoia.

Implications for Therapeutics of PTSD

PTSD can be a devastating disorder with a wide array of symptoms, including the core clusters of reexperiencing, avoidance, and hyperarousal as well as such adjunctive symptoms as paranoia, anger, impulsivity, compulsivity, depression, and panic attacks. As a disorder, it can be chronic in nature and difficult to treat. Until recently, the disorder largely has been understood from a psychological, social, and behavioral standpoint. Psychosocial treatments in PTSD rely on abreaction, desensitization, insight, cognitive restructuring, and social support (Beck, 1976; Bernstein & Borkovec, 1973; Bowen & Lambert, 1986; Brende & Parson, 1985; Brown & Fromm, 1986; Catherall, 1986; Crasilneck & Hall, 1985; Figley, 1985; Flannery, 1987; Freud, 1914/1958; Horowitz, 1986; Johnson, 1987; Lindy, 1986; Lyons & Keane, 1989; Shatan, 1973). Of these approaches, only abreactive and desensitization techniques attempt to eliminate the source of ongoing PTSD symptoms. The others focus on reducing the ill effects of trauma and increasing the individual's capacity to cope with the condition. Collectively, these psychosocial treatments have brought much relief to victims of trauma; unfortunately, however, they have had limited effectiveness in fully treating the core symptoms of PTSD. As suggested by the above review, many of the core symptoms may reflect underlying neurobiological disturbances and, as such, are more likely to respond to treatments specifically targeted at these disturbances.

To improve treatment response in patients with PTSD, many more carefully designed cognitive, physiological, behavioral, and neurobiological studies are needed. Neurotransmitter and neuropeptide functions must be comprehensively assessed shortly after (and at intervals following) different types of severe stress. The spectrum of stress-induced clinical symptoms also needs to be related to the function of identified neurochemical systems and brain regions. Important tools for investigating some of these relationships include magnetic resonance imaging, PET, and SPECT. Family and genetic studies will also be important for determining premorbid vulnerability.

With a better understanding of the psychobiology of traumatic stress, it may be possible to develop more effective and specific treatment approaches for PTSD. At present, because no one therapeutic modality has emerged as the treatment of choice, patients seem to benefit most from a combination of therapies. For example, although antidepressants may be effective for reexperiencing symptoms, concurrent behavioral therapy or traditional psychodynamic psychotherapy can be used to manage other symptoms, such as avoidance and guilt. Even after more is known about the pathophysiology of PTSD, it seems unlikely that any one pharmacological agent will be sufficient to treat the entire spectrum of symptoms seen in PTSD, because so many neurochemical systems are involved.

REFERENCES

American Psychiatric Association. (1980). *Diagnostic and statistical manual of mental disorders* (3rd ed.). Washington, DC: Author.

American Psychiatric Association. (1987). *Diagnostic and statistical manual of mental disorders* (rev. 3rd ed.). Washington, DC: Author.

Anisman, H. (1984). Vulnerability to depression: Contribution of stress. In R. M. Post & J. C. Ballenger (Eds.), *Neurobiology of mood disorders* (pp. 407–431). Baltimore, MD: Williams & Wilkins.

Antelman, S. M. (1988). Time dependent sensitization as the cornerstone for a new approach to pharmacotherapy: Drugs as foreign or stressful stimuli. *Drug Development Research, 14,* 1–30.

Antelman, S. M., Eichler, A. J., Black, C. A., et al. (1980). Interchangeability of stress and amphetamine in sensitization. *Science, 207,* 329–331.

Avanzino, G. L., Ermirio, R., Cogo, C. E., et al. (1987). Effect of corticosterone on neurones of the locus coeruleus in the rat. *Neuroscience Letter, 80,* 85–88.

Bandura, A., Cioffi, D., Taylor, C. B., et al. (1988). Perceived self-efficacy in coping with cognitive stressors and opioid activation. *Journal of Personality and Social Psychology, 55,* 479–488.

Beck, A. (1976). *Cognitive therapy and the emotional disorders.* New York: New American Library.

Beecher, H. K. (1946). Pain in men wounded in battle. *Annals of Surgery, 123,* 96–105.

Bernstein, D. A., & Borkovec, T. D. (1973). *Progressive muscle relaxation training.* Champaign, IL: Research Press.

Birkheimer, L. J., DeVane, C. L., & Muniz, C. E. (1985). Posttraumatic stress disorder: Characteristics and pharmacological response in the veteran population. *Comprehensive Psychiatry, 24,* 304–310.

Bleich, A., Seigel, B., Garb, R., et al. (1986). Post-traumatic stress disorder following combat exposure: Clinical features and psychopharmacological treatment. *British Journal of Psychiatry, 149,* 365–369.

Bowen, G. R., & Lambert, J. A. (1986). Systematic desensitization therapy with PTSD cases. In C. R. Figley (Ed.), *Trauma and its wake* (Vol. 2, pp. 280–291). New York: Brunner/Mazel.

Brende, J. O., & Parson, E. R. (1985). *Vietnam veterans: The road to recovery.* New York: Plenum.

Brown, D., & Fromm, E. (1986). *Hypnotherapy and hypnoanalysis.* Hillsdale, NJ: Erlbaum.

Calogero, A. E., Gallucci, W. T., Chrousos, G. P., et al. (1988). Catecholamine effects upon rat hypothalamic corticotropin-releasing hormone secretion *in vivo. Journal of Clinical Investigation, 82,* 839–846.

Cassens, G., Kuruc, A., & Roffman, M., et al. (1981). Alterations in brain norepinephrine metabolism and behavior induced by environmental stimuli previously paired with inescapable shock. *Behavioral Brain Research, 2,* 387–407.

Catherall, D. (1986). The support system and amelioration of PTSD in Vietnam veterans. *Psychotherapy, 23,* 472–482.

Chapman, P. F., Kairiss, E. W., Keenan, C. L., et al. (1990). Long-term synaptic potentiation in the amygdala. *Synapse, 6,* 271–278.

Charney, D. S., Woods, S. W., Goodman, W. K., et al. (1987). Neurobiological mechanisms of panic anxiety: Biochemical and behavioral correlates of yohimbine-induced panic attacks. *American Journal of Psychiatry, 144,* 1030–1036.

Charney, D. S., Woods, S. W., Price, L. H., et al. (1990a). Noradrenergic dysregulation in panic disorder. In J. C. Ballenger (Ed.), *Neurobiology of panic disorder* (pp. 91–105). New York: Wiley Liss.

Charney, D. S., Woods, S. W., Krystal, J. H., et al. (1990b). Serotonin function and human anxiety disorders. In P. M. Whitaker-Azmitia & S. J. Peroutka (Eds.), *The neuropharmacology of serotonin* (pp. 104–113). New York: New York Academy of Sciences.

Clugnet, M. C., & LeDoux, J. E. (1990). Synaptic plasticity in fear conditioning circuits: Induction of LTP in the lateral nucleus of the amygdala by stimulation of the medial geniculate body. *Journal of Neuroscience, 10,* 2818–2824.

Concas, A., Serra, M., Atsiggiu, T., et al. (1988b). Footshock stress and anxiogenic β-carbolines increase t[^{35}S]butylbicyclo-phosphorothionate binding in the rat cerebral cortex, an effect opposite to anxiolytics and γ-aminobutyric acid mimetics. *Journal of Neurochemistry, 51,* 1868–1876.

Concas, A., Serra, M., Corda, M. G., et al. (1988a). Change of 365-TBPS binding induced by stress and GABAergic drugs. In G. Biggio & E. Costa (Eds), *CA-channels and their modulation by neurotransmitters and drugs* (pp. 121–136). New York: Raven.

Crasilneck, H. B., & Hall, J. A. (1985). *Clinical hypnosis.* Orlando, FL: Grune & Stratton.

Crile, G. (1940). Results of 152 denervations of the adrenal glands in the treatment of neurocirculatory asthenia. *Military Surgeon, 87,* 509–513.

Davidson, J., Walker, J. I., & Kilts, C. (1987). A pilot study of phenelzine in the treatment of post-traumatic stress disorder. *British Journal of Psychiatry, 150,* 252–255.

Davidson, J. R. T., Kudler, H. S., & Smith, R. D. (1990a). Assessment and pharmacotherapy of posttraumatic stress disorder. In E. L. Giller, Jr. (Ed.), *Biological assessment and treatment of posttraumatic stress disorder* (pp. 203–233). Washington, DC: American Psychiatric Press.

Davidson, J. R. T., Kudler, H., Smith, R., et al. (1990b). Treatment of post-traumatic stress disorder with amitriptyline and placebo. *Archives of General Psychiatry, 47,* 259–266.

Davidson, L. M., & Baum, A. (1990). Chronic stress and post traumatic stress disorders. *Journal of Consulting and Clinical Psychology, 27,* 1165–1175.

Davis, M. (1986). Pharmacological and anatomical analysis of fear conditioning using the fear potentiated startle paradigm. *Behavioral Neuroscience, 100,* 814–824.

Davis, M. (1989). Sensitization of the acoustic startle reflex by footshock. *Behavioral Neuroscience, 103,* 495–503.

Dorow, R., Horowski, R., & Paschelke, G. (1983). Severe anxiety induced by FG7142, a beta carboline ligand for benzodiazepine receptors. *Lancet, 1,* 98–99.

Drugan, R. C., Ryan, S. M., Minor, T. R., et al. (1981). Librium prevents the analgesia and shuttlebox escape deficit typically observed following inescapable shock. *Pharmacology, Biochemistry, and Behavior, 21,* 749–754.

Drugan, R. C., Maier, S. F., Skolnick, P., et al. (1985). An anxiogenic benzodiazepine receptor ligand induces learned helplessness. *European Journal of Pharmacology, 113,* 453–457.

Drugan, R. C., Morrow, A. L., Weizman, R., et al. (1989). Stress-induced behavioral depression in the rat is associated with a decrease in GABA receptor-mediated chloride ion flux and brain benzodiazepine receptor occupancy. *Brain Research, 487,* 45–51.

Dunn, A. J. (1988). Stress-related activation of cerebral dopaminergic system. *Annals of the New York Academy of Science, 537,* 188–205.

Edwards, E., Harkins, K., Wright, G., et al. (1990). Effects of bilateral adrenalectomy on the induction of learned helplessness. *Behavioral Neuropsychopharmacology, 3,* 109–114.

Falcon, S., Ryan, C., Chamberlain, K., et al. (1985). Tricyclics: Possible treatment for posttraumatic stress disorder. *Journal of Clinical Psychiatry, 46,* 385–338.

Figley, C. R. (1985). Traumatic stress: The role of family and social support systems. In C. R. Figley (Ed.), *Trauma and its wake* (pp. 39–54). New York: Brunner/Mazel.

Flannery, R. B. (1987). From victim to survivor: A stress management approach in the treatment of learned helplessness. In B. A. van der Kolk (Ed.), *Psychological trauma* (pp. 217–232). Washington, DC: American Psychiatric Press.

Fraser, F., & Wilson, B. M. (1918). The sympathetic nervous system and the "irritable heart of soldiers." *British Medical Journal, 2,* 27–29.

Freud, S. (1958). Remembering, repeating, and working through (further recommendations on the technique of psychoanalysis II). In J. Strachey (Ed. and Trans.), *The standard edition of the complete psychological works of Sigmund Freud* (Vol. 12, pp. 145–156). London: Hogarth Press. (Original work published 1914)

Friedman, M. J. (1988). Toward a rational pharmacotherapy for post traumatic stress disorder: An interim report. *American Journal of Psychiatry, 145,* 281–285.

Gavin, G. B. (1985). Stress and brain noradrenaline: A review. *Behavioral Neuroscience Review, 9,* 233–243.

Giral, P., Martin, P., Soubrie, P., et al. (1988). Reversal of helpless behavior in rats by putative 5-HT1A agonists. *Biological Psychiatry, 23,* 237–242.

Helzer, J. E., Robins, L. N., & McEvoy, L. (1987). Post-traumatic stress disorder in the general population: Findings of the Epidemiologic Catchment Area survey. *New England Journal of Medicine, 317,* 1630–1634.

Hemingway, R. B., & Reigle, T. G. (1987). The involvement of endogenous opiate systems in learned helplessness and stress induced analgesia. *Psychopharmacology, 93,* 353–357.

Herman, J. P., Guilloneau, P. P., Dantzer, R., et al. (1982). Differential effects of inescapable footshocks and of stimuli previously paired with inescapable footshocks on DA turnover in cortical and limbic areas of the rat. *Science, 23,* 1549–1556.

Hitchcock, J. M., Sananes, C. B., & Davis, M. (1989). Sensitization of the startle reflex by footshock: Blockage by lesions of the central nucleus of the amygdala or its efferent pathway to the brainstem. *Behavioral Neuroscience, 103,* 509–518.

Hogben, G. L., & Cornfield, R. B. (1981). Treatment of traumatic war neurosis with phenelzine. *Archives of General Psychiatry, 38,* 440–445.

Horowitz, M. (1986). *Stress response syndromes.* London: Jason Aronson.

Ida, Y., Tanaka, M., Tsuda, A., et al. (1985). Attenuating effect of diazepam on stress-induced increases in noradrenaline turnover in specific brain regions of rats: Antagonism by Ro 15-1788. *Life Science, 37,* 2491–2498.

Irwin, J., Ahluwalia, P., & Anisman, H. (1986b). Sensitization of norepinephrine activity following acute and chronic footshock. *Brain Research, 379,* 98–103.

Irwin, J., Ahluwalia, P., Zacharko, R. M., et al. (1986a). Central norepinephrine and plasma corticosterone following acute and chronic stressors: Influence of social isolation and handling. *Pharmacology, Biochemistry, and Behavior, 24,* 1154–1154.

Johnson, D. (1987). The role of the creative arts therapies in the diagnosis and treatment of psychological trauma. *Arts in Psychotherapy, 14,* 7–14.

Kalivas, P. W., & Duffy, P. (1989). Similar effects of daily cocaine and stress on mesocorticolimbic dopamine neurotransmission in the rat. *Biological Psychiatry, 25,* 913–928.

Kalivas, P. W., Duffy, P., Abhold, R., et al. (1990). Sensitization of mesolimbic dopamine neurons by neuropeptides and stress. In P. W. Kalivas & C. D. Barnes (Eds.), *Sensitization in the nervous system* (pp. 119–124). Caldwell, NJ: Telford.

Kant, G. J., Eggleston, T., Landman-Roberts, L., et al. (1985). Habituation to repeated stress is stressor specific. *Pharmacology, Biochemistry, and Behavior, 22,* 631–634.

Kauffman, C. D., Reist, C., Djenderedjian, A., et al. (1987). Biological markers of affective disorders and posttraumatic stress disorder: A pilot study with desipramine. *Journal of Clinical Psychiatry, 48,* 366–367.

Keneth, G. A., & Joseph, M. H. (1981). The functional importance of increased brain tryptophan in serotonergic response to restraint stress. *Neuropharmacology, 20,* 39–43.

Kinzie, J. D., & Boehnlein, J. J. (1989). Post-traumatic psychosis among Cambodian refugees. *Journal of Traumatic Stress, 2,* 185–198.

Kolb, L. C. (1985). The place of narcosynthesis in the treatment of chronic and delayed stress reactions of war. In S. M. Sonnenberg, A. S. Blank, & J. A. Talbott (Eds.), *The trauma of war: Stress and recovery in Vietnam veterans.* Washington, DC: American Psychiatric Press.

Kosten, T. R., Mason, J. W., Giller, E. L., et al. (1987). Sustained urinary norepinephrine and epinephrine elevation in post-traumatic stress disorder. *Psychoneuroendocrinology, 12,* 13–20.

Kosten, T. R., Frank, J. B., Dan, E., et al. (1991). Pharmacotherapy for posttraumatic stress disorder using phenelzine or imipramine. *Journal of Nervous and Mental Disease, 179,* 366–370.

Kramarcy, N. R., Delanoy, R. L., & Dunn, A. J. (1984). Footshock treatment activates catecholamine synthesis in slices of mouse brain region. *Brain Research, 290,* 311–319.

Krystal, J. H., Kosten, T. R., Southwick, S. M., et al. (1989). Neurobiological aspects of PTSD: Review of clinical and preclinical studies. *Behavior Therapy, 20,* 177–198.

Kulka, R. A., Schlenger, W. E., Fairbank, J. A., et al. (1990). The National Vietnam Veterans Readjustment Study: Table of findings and appendices. *Trauma and the Vietnam War generation.* New York: Brunner/Mazel.

LeDoux, J. E., Romanski, L., & Xagoraris, A. (1989). Indelibility of subcortical emotional memories. *Journal of Cognitive Neuroscience, 1,* 238–243.

Lerer, B., Bleich, A., & Kotler, M. (1987). Posttraumatic stress disorder in Israeli combat veterans. *Archives of General Psychiatry, 44,* 976–981.

Levenson, H., Lanman, R., & Rankin, M. (1982). Posttraumatic war neurosis and phenelzine. *Archives of General Psychiatry, 39,* 1345.

Lindy, J. D. D. (1986). An outline for the psychoanalytic psychotherapy of post-traumatic stress disorder. In C. R. Figley (Ed.), *Trauma and its wake* (Vol. 2, pp. 195–210). New York: Brunner/Mazel.

Lyons, J. A., & Keane, T. M. (1989). Implosive therapy for the treatment of combat-related PTSD. *Journal of Traumatic Stress, 2,* 137–152.

Maclennan, A. J., & Maier, S. F. (1983). Coping and stress induced potentiation of stimulant stereotype in the rat. *Science, 219,* 1091–1093.

Maier, S. F. (1986). Stressor controllability and stress induced analgesia. *Annals of the New York Academy of Science, 467,* 55–72.

Maier, S. F., Ryan, S. M. Barksdale, C. M., et al. (1986). Stressor controllability and the pituitary-adrenal system. *Behavioral Neuroscience, 100,* 669–674.

Majewska, M. D., Harrison, N. I., Schwartz, R. D., et al. (1986). Steroid metabolites are barbiturate-like modulators of the GABA receptor. *Science, 232,* 1004–1007.

Mason, J. W., Giller, E. L., Kostin, T. R., et al. (1988). Elevation of urinary norepinephrine/cortisol ratio in post traumatic stress disorder. *Journal of Nervous and Mental Disease, 176,* 498–502.

McDougle, C., Southwick, S. M., St. James, R., et al. (1991). An open trial of fluoxetine in the treatment of post traumatic stress disorder. *Journal of Clinical Psychopharmacology, 11,* 325–327.

McEwen, B. S. (1987). Glucocorticoid-biogenic amine interactions in relation to mood and behavior. *Biochemical Pharmacology, 36,* 1755–1763.

McEwen, B. S., DeKloet, E. R., & Rostene, W. (1986). Adrenal steroid receptors and actions in the nervous system. *Physiology Reviews, 66,* 1121–1188.

McFall, M., Murburg, M., Ko, G., et al. (1990). Autonomic responses to stress in Vietnam combat veterans with post traumatic stress disorder. *Biological Psychiatry, 27,* 1165–1175.

McGaugh, J. L. (1989). Involvement of hormonal and neuromodulatory systems in the regulation of memory storage. *Annual Review of Neuroscience, 12,* 255–287.

Meakins, J. C., & Wilson, R. M. (1918). The effect of certain sensory stimulation on the respiratory rate in case of so-called "irritable heart." *Heart, 7,* 17–22.

Melia, K. R., Nestler, E. J., Haycock, J., et al. (1991). Regulation of tyrosine hydroxylase (TH) in the locus coeruleus (LC) by corticotropin-releasing factor (CRF): Relation to stress and depression. *Neuroscience Abstracts, 16,* 444.

Milanes, F. J., Mack, C. N., Dennison, J., et al. (1984, June). Phenelzine treatment of post-Vietnam stress syndrome. *VA Practitioner,* pp. 40–47.

Morgan, W. W., Ruden, P. K., & Pfeil, K. A. (1975). Effect of immobilization stress on serotonin content and turnover in regions of the rat brain. *Life Science, 17,* 143–152.

Mueser, K. T., & Butler, R. W. (1987). Auditory hallucinations in combat-related chronic posttraumatic stress disorder. *American Journal of Psychiatry, 144,* 299–302.

Nemeth, M. C. (1960). Psychosis in a concentration camp survivor: A case presentation. In H. Krystal & W. G. Neiderland (Eds.), *Psychic traumatization aftereffects in individuals and communities* (Vol. 8). Boston: Little Brown.

Nisenbaum, L. K., Zigmond, M. J., Sved, A. F., et al. (1991). Prior exposure to chronic stress results in enhanced synthesis and release of hippocampal norepinephrine in response to a novel stressor. *Journal of Neuroscience, 11,* 1478–1484.

Nutt, D. J., Glue, P., Lawson, C., et al. (1990). Flumazenil provocation of panic attacks: Evidence for altered benzodiazepine receptor in panic disorder. *Archives of General Psychiatry, 47,* 917–925.

Orr, S. P. (1990). Psychophysiologic studies of posttraumatic stress disorder. In E. L. Giller (Ed.), *Biological assessment and treatment of posttraumatic stress disorder* (pp. 135–157). Washington, DC: American Psychiatric Press.

Perry, B. D., Giller, E. L., & Southwick, S. M. (1987). Altered platelet alpha-2 adrenergic binding sites in posttraumatic stress disorder. *American Journal of Psychiatry, 144,* 1511–1512.

Perry, B. D., Southwick, S. M., Yehuda, R., et al. (1990). Adrenergic dysregulation in PTSD. In E. L. Giller (Ed.), *Biological assessment and treatment of posttraumatic stress disorder* (pp. 87–114). Washington, DC: American Psychiatric Press.

Petty, F., & Sherman, D. (1983). Learned helplessness induction decreases in vivo cortical serotonin release. *Pharmacology, Biochemistry, and Behavior, 18,* 649–650.

Pitman, R., & Orr, S. (1990). Twenty-four hour urinary cortisol and catecholamine excretion in combat-related posttraumatic stress disorder. *Biological Psychiatry, 27,* 245–247.

Pitman, R. K., van der Kolk, B. A., Orr, S. P., et al. (1990). Naloxone-reversible analgesic response to combat-related stimuli in post traumatic stress disorder. *Archives of General Psychiatry, 47,* 541–544.

Rasmussen, K., Marilak, D. A., & Jacobs, B. L. (1986). Single unit activity of the locus coeruleus in the freely moving cat: I: During naturalistic behaviors and in response to simple and complex stimuli. *Brain Research, 371,* 324–334.

Redmond, D. E., Jr. (1987). Studies of the nucleus locus coeruleus in monkeys and hypotheses for neuropsychopharmacology. In H. Y. Meltzer (Ed.), *Psychopharmacology: The third generation of progress* (pp. 967–975). New York: Raven.

Reist, C., Kauffman, C. D., Haier, R. J., et al. (1989). A controlled trial of desipramine in 18 men with posttraumatic stress disorder. *American Journal of Psychiatry, 146,* 513–516.

Richardson, J. S., & Zaleski, W. A. (1983). Naloxone and self mutilation. *Biological Psychiatry, 18,* 99–101.

Robinson, T. E., Angus, A. L., & Becker, J. B. (1985). Sensitization to stress: The enduring effects of prior stress on amphetamine induced rotational behavior. *Life Science, 37,* 1039–1042.

Roth, R. H., Tam, S., Ida, Y., et al. (1988). Stress and the mesocorticolimbic dopamine systems. *Annals of the New York Academy of Science, 537,* 138–147.

Sapolsky, R. M., & Plotsky, P. M. (1990). Hypercortisolism and its possible neural bases. *Biological Psychiatry, 27,* 937–952.

Sapolsky, R. M., Uno, H., Rebert, C. S., et al. (1990). Hippocampal damage associated with prolonged glucocorticoid exposure in primates. *Journal of Neuroscience, 10,* 2897–2902.

Schwartz, R. D., Weiss, M. J., Labarca, R., et al. (1987). Acute stress enhances the activity of the GABA receptor-gated chloride ionophore ion channel in brain. *Brain Research, 411,* 151–155.

Seibyl, J. P., Krystal, J. H., Price, L. H., et al. (1991). Effects of ritanserin on the behavioral, neuroendocrine, and cardiovascular responses to m-chlorophenylipiperazine in healthy human subjects. *Psychiatry Research, 38,* 227–236.

Shatan, C. (1973). The grief of soldiers: Vietnam combat veterans self-help movement. *American Journal of Orthopsychiatry, 43,* 640–653.

Shen, W. W., & Park, S. (1983). The use of monoamine oxidase inhibitors in the treatment of traumatic war neurosis: A case report. *Military Medicine, 148,* 430–431.

Shestatzky, M., Greenberg, D., & Lerer, B. (1988). A controlled trial of phenelzine in post-traumatic stress disorder. *Psychiatry Research, 24,* 149–155.

Shors, T. J., Seib, T. B., Levine, S., et al. (1989). Inescapable versus escapable shock modulates long-term potentiation (LTP) in the rat hippocampus. *Science, 224,* 224–226.

Simson, P. E., & Weiss, J. M. (1988a). Altered activity of the locus coeruleus in an animal model of depression. *Neuropsychopharmacology, 1,* 287–295.

Simson, P. E., & Weiss, J. M. (1988b). Responsiveness of locus coeruleus neurons to excitatory stimulation is uniquely regulated by alpha-2 receptors. *Psychopharmacology Bulletin, 24,* 349–354.

Smith, M. A., Davidson, J., Ritchie, J. C., et al. (1989). The corticotropin releasing hormone test in patients with post traumatic stress disorder. *Biological Psychiatry, 26,* 349–355.

Soubrie, P. (1986). Reconciling the role of central serotonin neurons in human and animal behavior. *Behavioral and Brain Sciences, 9,* 319–364.

Southwick, S. M., Krystal, J. H., & Charney, D. S. (1991). Yohimbine in PTSD. In *New research program and abstracts of the American Psychiatric Association* (Abstract No. NR478). Washington, DC: American Psychiatric Association.

Southwick, S. M., Yehuda, R., Giller, E. L., et al. (1994). The use of tricyclics and monoamine oxidase inhibitors in the treatment of posttraumatic stress disorder: A quantitative review. In M. M. Murburg (Eds.), *Catecholamine function in posttraumatic stress disorder.* Washington, DC: American Psychiatric Press.

Squire, L. R. (1986). Mechanisms of memory. *Science, 232,* 1612–1619.

Stuckey, J., Marra, S., Minor, T., et al. (1989). Changes in mu opiate receptors following inescapable shock. *Brain Research, 476,* 167–169.

Teyler, T. J., & DiScenna, P. (1987). Long-term potentiation. *Annual Review of Neuroscience, 10,* 131–161.

Torda, T., Kvetnansky, R., & Petrikova, M. (1984). Effect of repeated immobilization stress on rat central and peripheral adrenoceptors. In E. Usdin, R. Dvetnansky, & J. Axelrod (Eds.), *Stress: The role of catecholamines and other neurotransmitters* (pp. 691–701). New York: Gordon & Breach.

Torda, T., Murgas, K., Cechova, E., et al. (1990). Adrenergic regulation of $_3$H-ketanserin binding sites during immobilization stress in the rat frontal cortex. *Brain Research, 527,* 198–203.

Tsuda, A., & Tanaka, M. (1985). Differential changes in noradrenaline turnover in specific regions of rat brain produced by controllable and uncontrollable shocks. *Behavior Neuroscience, 99,* 802–817.

Tsuda, A., Ida, Y., Satoh, H., et al. (1989). Stressor predictability and rat brain noadrenaline metabolism. *Pharmacology, Biochemistry, and Behavior, 32,* 569–572.

Uno, H., Tarara, R., Else, J., et al. (1989). Hippocampal damage associated with prolonged and fatal stress in primates. *Journal of Neuroscience, 9,* 1705–1711.

Valentino, R. J., Foote, S. L., & Aston-Jones, G. (1983). Corticotrophin-releasing factor activates noradrenergic neurons of the locus coeruleus. *Brain Research, 270,* 363–367.

van der Kolk, B. A., Greenberg, M. S., Orr, S. P., et al. (1989). Endogenous opioids, stress induced analgesia and post-traumatic stress disorder. *Psychopharmacology Bulletin, 25,* 417–421.

Walker, J. I. (1982). Chemotherapy of traumatic stress. *Military Medicine, 147,* 1029–1033.

Woods, S. W., Charney, D. S., Silver, J. M., et al. (1991). Behavioral, biochemical and cardiovascular responses to the benzodiazepine receptor antagonist flumazenil. *Psychiatry Research, 36,* 115–127.

Yehuda, R., Giller, E. L., Boisoneau, D., et al (1991b). Low dose DST in PTSD. In *New research abstracts of the American Psychiatric Association* (Abstract No. 144). Washington, DC: American Psychiatric Association.

Yehuda, R., Giller, E. L., Southwick, S. M., et al. (1991c). Hypothalamic pituitary adrenal axis dysfunction in PTSD. *Biological Psychiatry, 30,* 1031–1048.

Yehuda, R., Lowry, M. T., Southwick, S. M., et al. (1991a). Increased number of glucocorticoid receptors in post-traumatic stress disorder. *American Journal of Psychiatry, 144,* 499–504.

Yehuda, R., Southwick, S., Nussbaum, G., et al. (1990). Low urinary cortisol excretion in patients with post-traumatic stress disorder. *Journal of Nervous and Mental Disease, 178,* 366–369.

5

Victims of Violence

RONNIE JANOFF-BULMAN

Violence is an all too common feature of modern life. Media presentations are filled with images of people hurting one another, and although much attention is given to scenes depicting violence and even to perpetrators of violence, little is given to victims (Bard & Sangrey, 1979). Violence involves physical force with the intent to harm another, and from an observer's perspective, victims' injuries seem best measured in terms of physical harm. The plight of the victim, in other words, is generally understood in terms of physical violation. Yet injury to victims of violence involves not only physical violation but psychological violation as well. The aftermath of violence for victims must be understood by considering threats not only to their bodily integrity but to their psychological integrity. Victims are forced to confront directly the possible loss of physical functioning and even death. They are also forced to confront directly the possible breakdown of the cognitive structures that had been so instrumental in providing psychological stability.

The suffering of victims of violence varies from person to person, but it is generally far more intense than might be predicted from a simple examination of physical injury. Victims of rape, robbery, assault, sexual abuse, and physical abuse often have similar responses to their victimization (Janoff-Bulman & Frieze, 1983; Krupnick & Horowitz, 1980); they frequently feel helpless, out of control, depressed, ashamed, anxious, frightened, and disorganized. Behavioral reactions include sleep disturbances (e.g., insomnia, nightmares), uncontrollable crying, restlessness, deterioration of personal relationships, and

---

RONNIE JANOFF-BULMAN • Department of Psychology, University of Massachusetts, Amherst, Massachusetts 01003. Reprinted from S. Fisher and J. Reason (Eds.), *Handbook of Life Stress, Cognition and Health* (chapter 6, pp. 101–113).

Psychotraumatology, edited by George S. Everly, Jr. and Jeffrey M. Lating. Plenum Press, New York, 1995.

increased use of drugs (Frieze et al., 1984). For many victims, the trauma of violent victimization is resolved within 6 months to a year (Horowitz, 1976); for others, though, the stress of victimization persists. Research with rape victims, for example, has found that psychological symptoms often last beyond a year. Rape victims have been found to be more depressed a year after their victimization than a control sample of women (Ellis et al., 1981), and many feel they have not recovered as much as 4 to 6 years after the rape (Burgess & Holmstrom, 1976, 1979; also see Sales et al., 1984).

Persistent, severe, yet not uncommon responses of victims of violence are best described by post-traumatic stress disorder (PTSD), a diagnostic category of the *Diagnostic and Statistical Manual* (DSM-III) of the American Psychiatric Association (APA; 1980). In addition to a recognizable stressor, diagnostic criteria for PTSD include (a) reexperiencing the trauma via intrusive thoughts, dreams, or memories; (b) numbing of responsiveness, demonstrated by constricted affect, feelings of detachment from others, or diminished interest in important activities; and (c) the presence of at least two other symptoms, including sleep disturbance, exaggerated startle response, guilt, memory impairment, trouble concentrating, and phobias about activities triggering recollection of the event. In its discussion of PTSD, the APA (1980) does not make distinctions between different stressor events; rather, the stressor is simply presented as "a traumatic event that is generally outside the range of usual experience." Thus PTSD is intended to describe intense psychological responses of many types of victims—including not only victims of violence but also victims of natural disasters, accidents, and diseases. The only mention of any distinction to be drawn between these types of victimization is in a single sentence that reads, "The disorder is apparently more severe and longer lasting when the stressor is of human design" (APA, 1980, p. 236). Victims of violence (unlike those of natural disasters, accidents, or diseases) are victims of a stressor that is human induced and intended (i.e., designed) by a perpetrator. Such victims are particularly apt to experience severe psychological distress.

FEAR AND ANXIETY

One way to begin to understand the reactions of victims—and of victims of violence in particular—is to recognize that PTSD is classified as an anxiety disorder (APA, 1980). Anxiety and fear are clearly predominant emotional responses of victims of violence (Frederick, 1980; Krupnick & Horowitz, 1980). Among rape victims, for example, the most prominent, persistent reactions include general diffused anxiety and intense fears of rape-related situations (Calhoun et al., 1982; Nadelson et al., 1982). In their study of rape victims 3 to 6 months after the rape, Kilpatrick et al. (1979) found that the victims differed from nonvictims only on measures of fear and anxiety, and not on other distress measures.

Anxiety and fear are frequently presented as common reactions of victims, and the two emotional reactions often are not distinguished. This is understandable in light of the fact that fear and anxiety are generally indistinguishable from an observer's perspective. The manifestations of both include autonomic hyperactivity, apprehensive expectation, motor tension, and vigilance (APA, 1980). Nevertheless, they represent two distinct psychological responses by an individual.

Generally, the distinction drawn between fear and anxiety relates to the identifiability of the source of stimulation; in the case of fear, the source is readily identified, whereas in the case of anxiety it cannot be (see, e.g., Freud, 1926/1959; Rachman, 1978). In other words, victims can tell someone else what they fear, and it appears that victims of violence frequently report fears, particularly those of being alone, a recurrence of the victimization, and death (Frieze et al., 1984). In the case of fear, the threat of danger is consciously recognized and generally external (APA, 1980), and generally the fears of victims are strongly related to physical violation. In contrast, anxiety is more closely associated with psychological violation and does not involve a consciously recognized danger or an external threat. Yet a better understanding of anxiety can provide important clues to the psychological trauma often experienced by victims of violence.

The primary threat in the case of anxiety is internal, for the cardinal feature of anxiety is cognitive disintegration (Averill, 1976): "Many of the features commonly ascribed to anxiety can be traced directly or indirectly to the disintegration of cognitive systems. For example, a disruption of cognitive systems leaves the person feeling uncertain and helpless" (p. 120). Threats that produce anxiety are related to our symbolic systems of ideas, values, and concepts. Anxiety results when these symbols or cognitions no longer fit reality, when they no longer enable individuals to relate meaningfully to the world around them (Lazarus & Averill, 1972). Cognitive disintegration may arise in a number of ways; it could be a result of excessive stimulation that may tax the ability to process information, of intrapsychic conflict when two cognitions are incompatible, or of unusual information that is impossible to interpret (Averill, 1976; Lazarus & Averill, 1972). Violent victimization produces considerable anxiety in victims, suggesting that victims of violence experience cognitive disintegration. Understanding the reactions of victims of violence, then, involves better understanding the cognitive or symbolic systems that are affected by violent victimization.

ASSUMPTIVE WORLDS

Recent work in social psychology has stressed the importance of cognitive schemas for understanding people's perceptions, memories, and inferences (e.g., Abelson, 1981; Cantor, 1980; Fiske & Taylor, 1984; Markus, 1977). A schema is "a cognitive structure that represents organized knowledge about a given concept or type of stimulus" (Fiske & Taylor, 1984, p. 140). Our interactions in the world are primarily defined by top-down processing; that is, we start with schemas and understand phenomena through these cognitive structures. In processing information, we rely upon schemas without necessarily being aware of their content. Further, these schemas are generally resistant to major changes, for ordinarily we alter our perceptions and memories so as to render them schema consistent; we persevere in maintaining our schemas (see discussions in Fiske & Taylor, 1984; Nisbett & Ross, 1980).

Although work on schemas has generally dealt with our "theories" of particular categories of people or events, the psychological perspective represented by this work is consistent with the orientations of psychologists who have been interested in more global theories or assumptions people hold about themselves and their world. Parkes (1971, 1975), for example, maintains that people strongly hold a set of assumptions—their "assumptive world"—that represents their view of reality and is built and confirmed by years of experience. Bowlby's (1969) "world models," Marris's (1975) "structures of meaning" and Epstein's (1973, 1979, 1980) "theory of reality" all represent this same conceptual system that guides our perceptions and actions. As Epstein (1980) and Parkes (1971) maintain, we operate on the basis of these theories or assumptions, yet we are generally unaware of their content. Further, because we perceive the world through these assumptive lenses, it is very difficult to invalidate them. They generally persist and are resistant to change. Our assumptive world provides us with a stable conceptual system that affords us psychological equilibrium in a constantly changing actual world.

Although our basic assumptions about the world and ourselves are generally not questioned or challenged, occasionally particular events force us to objectify and confront them. In the realm of science, paradigms provide the basis for all work during "normal science" (Kuhn, 1962), just as our basic assumptions underlie normal (i.e., day-to-day) living. Yet there are occasions in science when crises arise. When anomalies call into question fundamental aspects of the paradigm and the old paradigm is "pushed too far," the result is a scientific revolution (Kuhn, 1962). Similarly, there are occasions in people's lives when their assumptive worlds are seriously challenged. Violent victimization represents one such experience. Victims of violence can no longer automatically rely upon their assumptive worlds to account for the data of their experience, and the stability of their conceptual system is threatened. The psychological trauma experienced by victims of violence can be understood in terms of the potential breakdown of their assumptive worlds. There is disorganization within their conceptual systems, and the individuals are thrown into a state of psychological crisis.

CORE ASSUMPTIONS

The threat to the victim's assumptive world occurs because victimization cannot readily be assimilated into his or her conceptual system. A cluster of assumptions (all of which relate to the general perception of relative invulnerability) are challenged by victimization, particularly by violent victimization. A very common reaction following victimization is an intense feeling of vulnerability. Most people, prior to any serious victimization, feel relatively invulnerable to negative events (Janoff-Bulman & Lang-Gunn, 1988; Perloff, 1983; Weinstein, 1980; Weinstein & Lachendro, 1982). Victims can no longer say, "It can't happen to me." Rather, they experience a lost sense of safety and security, whether they are victims of crime (e.g., Bard & Sangrey, 1979; Fischer, 1984; Krupnick, 1980; Notman & Nadelson, 1976), disease (e.g., Taylor, 1983; Weisman, 1979; Wortman & Dunkel-Schetter, 1979), or disasters (e.g., Lifton & Olson, 1976; Titchener et al., 1976; Wolfenstein, 1957). In his work with individuals exhibiting post-traumatic stress—including people who had been assaulted, had undergone a near-fatal experience, and had lost a loved one—Horowitz (1982) found that the most common theme expressed by these victims was discomfort over their own vulnerability.

This sense of vulnerability appears to be tied to the disruption of certain core assumptions about the self and the world. In particular, people generally seem to operate on the basis of three fundamental assumptions related to invulnerability: (a) the world is benevolent; (b) events in the world are meaningful; and (c) the self is positive and worthy. A benevolent world is not only one in which good things happen, but one in which people are good. A meaningful world is one in which events "make sense" because they predictably follow certain accepted "social laws" (Janoff-Bulman & Frieze, 1983; Silver & Wortman, 1980). In Western cultures, events are meaningful if they follow principles of justice (i.e., people get what they deserve; Lerner, 1980) or controllability (i.e., people's actions determine their outcomes; Seligman, 1975). A positive view of the self involves seeing oneself as decent and worthy, and thereby as deserving of good outcomes.

These three vulnerability-related assumptions may form a central core of our assumptive world. Work on the child's earliest experiences suggests that the groundwork for these assumptions is laid in the child's early interactions. Essentially, the development of the child during the first year involves learning to trust the world, learning that he or she is not vulnerable but rather is protected and secure (Erikson, 1950, 1968, 1980). The establishment of a sense of relative invulnerability seems grounded in early relationships with caregivers (Bowlby, 1969; Fairbairn, 1952; Sullivan, 1940, 1953). Typically the child comes to perceive the world as benevolent through predictable interactions with a responsible caregiver. Through positive interactions in which the child's needs (physical and emotional) are met, the child learns that his or her world is controllable, dependable, and just. Simultaneously the child begins to develop a sense of self-worth, in that he or she is the recipient of positive caregiving. The process is one of mutual regulation, in which the child perceives "friendly otherness" and "personal trustworthiness" through sensitive, dependable care. During the first year, as children learn that others are good, they also learn that they are good and that the world is orderly and predictable. Generally they come to believe that they are not helpless in a hostile environment (Horney, 1937, 1939), but capable and cared for in a benevolent world.

The assumptions of benevolence of the world, meaningfulness of events, and self-worth are grounded in the early preverbal experiences of the child and are therefore apt to be core assumptions in our conceptual system. Though certainly not the only assumptions an individual holds, these three vulnerability-related assumptions are no doubt very "high-order postulates" (Epstein, 1980) or, as Lakatos's (1974) terms, components of our "metaphysical hard-core." As such, their maintenance is essential to our psychological stability; threats to these core assumptions result in a great deal of psychological distress. Victimization threatens these assumptions, and the psychological responses of victims indicate their decreased sense of self-worth, coupled with a perception of the world that is malevolent and arbitrary.

Although these three basic assumptions are threatened by the experience of nonviolent victimization (e.g., disease, accidents, natural disasters), violent victimization seems to provide even greater threats and challenges to the assumptive worlds of victims (Janoff-Bulman, 1985). For victims of violence, the world is not only a place in which negative events occur (i.e., unfortunate outcomes become salient; Kahneman & Tversky, 1973), but people can no longer be trusted. Both the impersonal world and the personal world appear hostile. As Bard and Sangrey (1979) write, "Because crime is an interpersonal event, the victim's feeling of security in the world of other people is seriously upset" (p. 14). For those victimized by an individual they know well (e.g., a date, spouse, parent, friend), the breakdown in the assumption of a benign world is particularly acute. Considerable emotional trauma follows the experience of rape by a partner or friend (Burgess & Holmstrom, 1974; Medea & Thompson, 1974). Victims of rape and sexual abuse often have a great deal of difficulty establishing a sense of trust in subsequent close relationships (Miller et al., 1982; Nadelson & Notman, 1984). The individual who is victimized by a stranger often suffers a loss of trust in people as well, for the experience forces a direct confrontation with the realization that people can be malevolent; the world of people becomes suspect (Fischer, 1984).

Victims of violence, as well as victims of accidents, disease, and natural disasters, experience serious threats to their assumption of meaningfulness. They have been brought face to face with arbitrariness or randomness, and it is difficult to make sense of their victimization. Once again, however, the intent to harm by another human being suggests the possibility of unique difficulties for victims of violence. They must confront the existence of evil and the breakdown of a moral universe (see Lifton, 1967). Diseases, accidents, and natural disasters do not raise the question of evil; it is as if to be evil, something has to be intended, as is the case in violent victimizations (Janoff-Bulman, 1985).

There is considerable evidence that victims in general experience a marked decrease in their sense of self-worth (Horowitz et al., 1980; Krupnick, 1980). They perceive themselves as having been singled out for misfortune, and this leads to self-questioning, a perception of deviance, and self-stigma (Coates & Winston, 1983). Victims of violence are apt to experience the greatest threats to their self-worth, for being victimized by another who has intended harm is likely to exaggerate one's sense of powerlessness and helplessness, as well as one's sense of "losing" to another human being. One has been overpowered by another person and has thereby experienced a direct "violation of the self" (Bard & Sangrey, 1979). This sense of weakness and helplessness in contrast to the dominance of an evil other is apt to be experienced as humiliation, shame, and a loss of self-respect.

COPING AND "INAPPROPRIATE" REACTIONS

Coping with violent victimization involves coming to terms with the cognitive disorganization precipitated by the experience. Assumptions and personal theories that had provided psychological stability over the years are seriously challenged and often shattered. For victims of violence, intense anxiety—with all of its emotional, physiological, and behavioral manifestations—reflects the disruption in their cognitive systems, and the road to adjustment and decreased anxiety entails reorganizing and rebuilding their assumptive world.

The work of Horowitz (1976, 1980, 1982) is instructive in understanding the process of coping with victimization. According to Horowitz, people's "inner models" change as a result of serious life events, and he calls the tendency to integrate one's inner models and reality the *completion tendency*. Prior to this integration or completion, information from and reactions to the traumatic experience are stored in active memory and account for the intrusive thoughts experienced by victims. These intrusions cease when the information has been integrated and thereby is no longer stored in active memory.

From a cognitive perspective, the key to the victim's recovery process is the reestablishment of an integrated, organized set of basic assumptions or schemas. The traumatic event must be assimilated into the victim's assumptive world, or the assumptive world must accommodate to the new data (Piaget, 1971). In either case, anxiety will dissipate as the victim's cognitive system becomes integrated and viable as a means for understanding and responding to his or her world.

This focus on the victim's assumptive world renders the internal reality of the victim paramount in the process of understanding victims' reactions to traumatic events. Once the significance of this internal reality is recognized, certain reactions of victims that ordinarily appear inappropriate or maladaptive from an outsider's perspective begin to be comprehensible. Thus Janoff-Bulman and Timko (1987) maintain that the often-maligned process of denial is natural and often necessary and can, in fact, facilitate adaptation to traumatic experiences by modulating the attack on a victim's assumptive world. Denial allows the victim slowly and gradually to face the realities of the victimization and incorporate them into his or her internal world. Certainly it can be argued that it is easier to use denial in the case of victimization by disease than violent victimization, for the latter involves another person and a discrete event. Nevertheless, other apparently odd reactions of victims, particularly victims of violence, can better be understood by recognizing their role in the process of building and rebuilding a stable, integrated assumptive world for the victim.

The "Stockholm syndrome," sometimes found among hostages, is a case in point. The name derives from the case of a Stockholm bank robbery in which several of the hostages captured during the holdup defended their captors when released. It is now used to describe the alignment of positive affections by hostages toward their captors (Eitinger, 1982; Ochberg, 1986; Strentz, 1982; Symonds, 1982). Although typically explained via the psychoanalytic concept of identification with the aggressor, it seems possible that the victims' needs for a stable conceptual system may play a role in this phenomenon as well. By regarding their captors positively, hostages are able to maintain a belief in a benevolent environment in which their own safety and security are maximized. Their situation appears relatively benign, thereby minimizing the terror associated with their predicament.

Perhaps the best example of a victim response that may be better understood by noting the internal reality and cognitive needs of victims is that of self-blame. Self-blame is a common response by victims of violence (Bard & Sangrey, 1979; Frieze et al., 1984; Geis, 1981). Victims often seem unnecessarily willing to blame themselves for their victimization. The apparent inappropriateness of such a response is illustrated by Burgess and Holmstrom (1974) in their discussion of a woman who was assaulted outside her apartment one afternoon while searching through her purse for her keys. Although the woman fought back, even managing to take her assailant's knife, the man forced his way into her apartment, then beat and raped her. Surprisingly, the woman later engaged in self-blame and said she should have acted differently when she first saw the man; then neither she nor the rapist "would be in trouble." This tendency to accept blame is frequently found among victims of rape (Burgess & Holmstrom, 1974; Medea & Thompson, 1974; Weis & Weis, 1975). In a survey of rape crisis centers across the country, center workers reported that fully 74% of the women they saw blamed themselves at least in part for the rape (Janoff-Bulman, 1979). Battered women, too, often seem to engage in self-blame (Frieze, 1979; Hilberman &

Munson, 1978; Walker, 1979). Geis (1981), on the basis of his work with crime victims, writes, "It must be particularly appreciated that the crime victim rarely is able to see himself as an entirely guiltless person. . . . If nothing else, he must satisfactorily resolve questions relating to the lottery of human existence that resulted in injury being visited upon him rather than another" (p. 63). Geis goes on to note that too many alternative ways of behaving usually had been available to the crime victim (e.g., more care in choosing one's route, a better lock, staying aware from certain people), and "almost inevitably, then, some blame attaches to the self" (p. 61).

This focus on behavior as a basis for self-blaming is important in understanding the role of self-blame in the coping process of victims. There are (at least) two distinct types of self-blame, one of which has been labeled "behavioral self-blame," the other "characterological self-blame" (Janoff-Bulman, 1979). The former involves blaming one's behaviors for a negative outcome such as victimization, whereas the latter involves blaming one's character or enduring qualities. Thus a rape victim can blame herself by saying she should not have hitchhiked or should not have walked alone at night (behavioral self-blame), or she can say that she is too trusting, a bad person, or the type of person who attracts rapists (characterological self-blame). An important distinction between the two types of attributions concerns the perceived controllability (i.e., modifiability through one's own efforts) of the factor(s) blamed. This difference in perceived controllability has led Janoff-Bulman (1979; also see Wortman, 1976) to posit that behavioral self-blame may be an adaptive response to victimization, for it enables victims to minimize their perception of vulnerability by allowing them to believe that altering their behaviors in the future can minimize the likelihood of a recurrence. Behavioral self-blame may not only involve the avoidability of the particular negative outcome in question, but also promote a general belief in one's ability to avoid or control future negative outcomes in general (Janoff-Bulman, 1979; Janoff-Bulman & Lang-Gunn, 1988). Characterological self-blame, on the other hand, involves self-esteem deficits and is the type of self-blame generally associated with depression (Beck, 1967; Janoff-Bulman, 1979). Empirical support has been found for the adaptive value of behavioral self-blame (e.g., Affleck et al., 1985a, 1985b; Baum et al., 1983; Bulman & Wortman, 1977; Fischer, 1984; Peterson et al., 1981; Tennen et al., 1986; Tennen et al., 1984; Timko & Janoff-Bulman, 1985), although not consistently (e.g., Kiecolt-Glaser & Williams, 1987; Meyer & Taylor, 1986; Taylor et al., 1984; Witenberg et al., 1983).

Behavioral self-blame often seems to be psychologically adaptive; further, it is frequently manifested following victimization, perhaps especially by victims of violence who have been singled out for harm by another human being. Certainly any self-blame attribution provides a meaningful response to the question of selective incidence: "Why me?" A full understanding of why behavioral self-blame is so common and why it can be psychologically adaptive following victimization involves going beyond its control implications and considering, once again, the internal reality of victims and their need for a stable, integrated cognitive system. By engaging in behavioral self-blame, victims are able to minimize the threats and challenges to their assumptive worlds. They are essentially able to reestablish their conceptual systems such that cognitive disintegration can largely be avoided. Prior assumptions about the benevolence of the world, meaningfulness, and self-worth are not severely threatened when victims engage in behavioral self-blame. By maintaining that the event was attributable to their own behaviors (or behavioral omissions), victims need not change their view of how benign their environment is. Further, the victimization "makes sense" in that it was controllable via their own actions and can thus be avoided in the future; the event was not simply random and arbitrary. And behavioral self-blame generally does not result in decreased self-esteem in that it is an attribution to a specific behavior and does not involve generalizations to one's overall evaluation of the self, as does characterological self-blame. Engaging in behavioral self-blame, then, may be protective for the victim, who seeks to maintain cognitive stability in the face of an unexpected, negative, extreme event.

SUMMARY AND CONCLUSIONS

Reactions of victims of violence can be understood within a framework that emphasizes the significance of the victim's conceptual system following victimization. The intense anxiety experienced by victims of violence reflects their cognitive disintegration in the face of a traumatic external event. Basic unquestioned assumptions, built over years of experience, are suddenly challenged. In particular, assumptions about the benevolence of the world, the meaningfulness of events in the world, and self-worth are seriously threatened. Although these assumptions are no doubt threatened by the experience of any victimization, they are more severely challenged when an individual is the victim of harm by another person. The process of coping for victims involves reestablishing an integrated, stable system of basic assumptions that are viable in the face of their traumatic experience. Common victim reactions such as self-blame may appear inappropriate from the perspective of an observer; yet these responses become readily comprehensible when considered from the perspective of the victim's need to rebuild his or her assumptive world.

REFERENCES

Abelson, R. P. (1981). The psychological status of the script concept. *American Psychologist, 36,* 715–729.

Affleck, G., Allen, D. A., Tennen, H., McGrade, B. J., & Ratzan, S. (1985a). Causal and control cognitions in parent coping with a chronically ill child. *Journal of Social and Clinical Psychology, 3,* 369–379.

Affleck, G., McGrade, B. J., Allen, D. A., & McQueeney, M. (1985b). Mothers' beliefs about behavioral causes for their developmentally disabled infant's condition: What do they signify? *Journal of Pediatric Psychology, 10,* 193–303.

American Psychiatric Association. (1980). *Diagnostic and statistical manual of mental disorders* (3rd ed.). Washington, DC: Author.

Averill, J. (1976). Emotion and anxiety: Sociocultural, biological, and psychological determinants. In M. Zuckerman & C. D. Spielberger (Eds.), *Emotion and anxiety: New concepts, methods and applications.* New York: Erlbaum-Wiley.

Bard, M., & Sangrey, D. (1979). *The crime victim's book.* New York: Basic Books.

Baum, A., Flemming, R., & Singer, J. E. (1983). Coping with victimization by technological disaster. *Journal of Social Issues, 39,* 119–140.

Beck, A. T. (1967). *Depression: Clinical, experimental, and theoretical aspects.* New York: Harper & Row.

Bowlby, J. (1969). *Attachment and loss, vol. 1: Attachment.* London: Hogarth.

Bulman, R. J., & Wortman, C. B. (1977). Attributions of blame and coping in the "real world": Severe accident victims react to their lot. *Journal of Personality and Social Psychology, 35,* 351–363.

Burgess, A., & Holmstrom, L. (1974). Rape trauma syndrome. *American Journal of Psychiatry, 131,* 981–985.

Burgess, A., & Holmstrom, L. (1976). Coping behavior of the rape victim. *American Journal of Psychiatry, 13,* 413–417.

Burgess, A., & Holmstrom, L. (1979). Adaptive strategies and recovery from rape. *American Journal of Psychiatry, 136,* 1278–1282.

Calhoun, K. S., Atkeson, B. M., & Resick, P. A. (1982). A longitudinal examination of fear reactions in victims of rape. *Journal of Counseling Psychology, 29,* 665–661.

Cantor, N. (1980). Perceptions of situations: Situation prototypes and person–situation prototypes. In D. Magnusson (Ed.), *The situation: An interactional perspective.* Hillsdale, NJ: Erlbaum.

Coates, D., & Winston, T. (1983). Counteracting the deviance of depression: Peer support groups for victims. *Journal of Social Issues, 39,* 171–196.

Eitinger, L. (1982). The effects of captivity. In F. M. Ochberg & D. A. Soskis (Eds.), *Victims of terrorism.* Boulder, CO: Westview.

Ellis, E., Atkeson, B., & Calhoun, K. (1981). An assessment of long-term reaction to rape. *Journal of Abnormal Psychology, 90,* 263–266.

Epstein, S. (1973). The self-concept revisited, or a theory of a theory. *American Psychologist, 28,* 404–416.

Epstein, S. (1979). The ecological study of emotions in humans. In P. Pilner, K. R. Blanstein, & I. M. Spigel (Eds.), *Advances in the study of communication and affect, vol. 5: Perception of emotions in self and others.* New York: Plenum.

Epstein, S. (1980). The self-concept: A review and the proposal of an integrated theory of personality. In E. Staub (Ed.), *Personality: Basic issues and current research.* Englewood Cliffs, NJ: Prentice-Hall.

Erikson, E. (1950). *Childhood and society.* New York: Norton.

Erikson, E. (1968). *Identity: Youth and crisis.* New York: Norton.

Erikson, E. (1980). *Identity and the life cycle.* New York: Norton.

Fairbairn, W. R. D. (1952). *An object-relations theory of the personality.* New York: Basic Books.

Fischer, C. T. (1984). A phenomenological study of being criminally victimized: Contributions and constraints of qualitative research. *Journal of Social Issues, 40,* 161–178.

Fiske, S. T., & Taylor, S. E. (1984). *Social cognition.* Reading, MA: Addison-Wesley.

Frederick, C. (1980). Effects of natural vs. human-induced violence. *Evaluation and change.* [Special issue: Services for survivors], 71–75.

Freud, S. (1959). Inhibitions, symptoms, and anxiety. In J. Strachey (Ed. and Trans.), The standard edition of the complete psychological works of Sigmund Freud (Vol. 20). London: Hogarth. (Original work published 1926.)

Frieze, I. H. (1979). Perceptions of battered wives. In I. H. Frieze, D. Bar-Tal, & J. S.

Carroll (Eds.), *New approaches to social problems: Applications of attribution theory.* San Francisco, CA: Jossey-Bass.

Frieze, I. H., Hymer, S., & Greenberg, M. S. (1984). Describing the victims of crime and violence. In S. S. Kahn (Ed.), *Victims of crime and violence: Final report of the APA task force on the victims of crime and violence.* Washington, DC: American Psychological Association.

Geis, G. (1981). Victims of crimes of violence and the criminal justice system. In B. Galway & J. Hudson (Eds.), *Perspectives on crime victims.* St. Louis, MO: Mosby.

Hilberman, E., & Munson, K. (1978). Sixty battered women. *Victimology, 2,* 460–471.

Horney, K. (1937). *The neurotic personality of our time.* New York: Norton.

Horney, K. (1939). *New ways in psychoanalysis.* New York: Norton.

Horowitz, M. (1976). *Stress response syndromes.* New York: Aronson.

Horowitz, M. (1980). Psychological response to serious life events. In V. Hamilton & D. Warburton (Eds.), *Human stress and cognition.* New York: Wiley.

Horowitz, M. J. (1982). Stress response syndromes and their treatment. In L. Goldberger & S. Breznitz (Eds.), *Handbook of stress.* New York: Free Press.

Horowitz, M. J., Wilner, N., Marmar, C., & Krupnick, J. (1980). Pathological grief and the activation of latent self-images. *American Journal of Psychiatry, 137,* 1137–1162.

Janoff-Bulman, R. (1979). Characterological versus behavioral self-blame: Inquiries into depression and rape. *Journal of Personality and Social Psychology, 37*(10), 1798–1809.

Janoff-Bulman, R. (1985). Criminal vs. non-criminal victimization: Victims' reactions. *Victimology, 10,* 498–511.

Janoff-Bulman, R., & Frieze, I. H. (1983). A theoretical perspective for understanding reactions to victimization. *Journal of Social Issues, 39,* 1–17.

Janoff-Bulman, R., & Lang-Gunn, L. (1988). Coping with disease and accidents: The role of self-blame attributions. In L. Y. Abramson (Ed.), *Social cognition and clinical psychology* (pp. 116–147). New York: Guilford.

Janoff-Bulman, R., & Timko, C. (1987). Coping with traumatic life events: The role of denial in light of people's assumptive worlds. In C. R. Snyder & C. Ford (Eds.), *Coping with negative life events: Clinical and social psychological perspectives.* New York: Plenum.

Kahneman, D., & Tversky, A. (1973). On the psychology of prediction. *Psychological Review, 80,* 237–251.

Kiecolt-Glaser, J. K., & Williams, D. (1987). Self-blame, compliance, and distress among burn patients. *Journal of Personality and Social Psychology, 57,* 187–193.

Kilpatrick, D. G., Veronen, L. J., & Resick, P. A. (1979). The aftermath of rape: Recent empirical findings. *American Journal of Orthopsychiatry, 49,* 658–669.

Krupnick, J. (1980). Brief psychotherapy with victims of violent crime. *Victimology, 5,* 347–354.

Krupnick, J., & Horowitz, M. (1980). Victims of violence: Psychological responses, treatment implications. *Evaluation and change* [Special issue: Services for survivors], 42–46.

Kuhn, T. S. (1962). *The structure of scientific revolutions.* Chicago: University of Chicago Press.

Lakatos, I. (1974). Falsification and the methodology of scientific research programs. In I. Lakatos & A. Musgrave (Eds.), *Criticism and the growth of knowledge.* London: Cambridge University Press.

Lazarus, R. S., & Averill, J. R. (1972). Emotion and cognition: With special reference to anxiety. In C. D. Spielberger (Ed.), *Anxiety: Current trends in theory and research.* New York: Academic Press.

Lerner, M. J. (1980). *The belief in a just world.* New York: Plenum.

Lifton, R. J. (1967). *Death in life: Survivors of Hiroshima.* New York: Simon and Schuster.

Lifton, R. J., & Olson, E. (1976). Death imprint in Buffalo Creek syndrome: Symptoms and character change after a major disaster. In H. J. Parad, H. L. P. Resnik, & L. G. Parad (Eds.), *Emergency and disaster management.* Bowie, MD: Charles.

Markus, H. (1977). Self-schemata and processing information about the self. *Journal of Personality and Social Psychology, 35,* 63–78.

Marris, P. (1975). *Loss and change.* Garden City, NY: Anchor/Doubleday.

Medea, A., & Thompson, K. (1974). *Against rape.* New York: Farrar, Straus, & Giroux.

Meyer, C. B., & Taylor, S. E. (1986). Adjustment to rape. *Journal of Personality and Social Psychology, 50,* 1226–1234.

Miller, W. R., Williams, M., & Bernstein, M. H. (1982). The effects of rape on marital and sexual adjustment. *American Journal of Family Therapy, 10,* 51–58.

Nadelson, C. C., & Notman, M. T. (1984). Psychodynamics of sexual assault experiences. In I. R. Stuart & J. G. Greer (Eds.), *Victims of sexual aggression: Treatment of children, women, and men.* New York: Van Nostrand Reinhold.

Nadelson, C. C., Notman, M. T., Jackson, H., & Garnick, J. (1982). A follow-up study of rape victims. *American Journal of Psychiatry, 139,* 1266–1270.

Nisbett, R. E., & Ross, L. (1980). *Human inference: Strategies and shortcomings of social judgment.* Englewood Cliffs, NJ: Prentice-Hall.

Notman, M. T., & Nadelson, C. C. (1976). The rape victim: Psychodynamic considerations. *American Journal of Psychiatry, 133,* 408–413.

Ochberg, F. (1986). The victim of terrorism. In R. H. Moos (Ed.), *Coping with life crises.* New York: Plenum.

Parkes, C. M. (1971). Psycho-social transitions: A field of study. *Social Science and Medicine, 5,* 101–115.

Parkes, C. M. (1975). What becomes of redundant world models? A contribution to the study of adaptation to change. *British Journal of Medical Psychology, 48,* 131–137.

Perloff, L. S. (1983). Perceptions of vulnerability to victimization. *Journal of Social Issues, 39*(2), 41–62.

Peterson, C., Schwartz, S. M., & Seligman, M. E. P. (1981). Self-blame and depressive symptoms. *Journal of Personality and Social Psychology, 41,* 253–259.

Piaget, J. (1971). *The construction of reality in the child.* New York: Basic Books.

Rachman, S. J. (1978). *Fear and courage.* San Francisco: Freeman.

Sales, E., Baum, M., & Shore, B. (1984). Victim readjustment following assault. *Journal of Social Issues, 40,* 117–136.

Seligman, M. E. P. (1975). *Helplessness: On depression, development, and death.* San Francisco: Freeman.

Silver, R. L., & Wortman, C. B. (1980). Coping with undesirable life events. In J. Garber & M. E. P. Seligman (Eds.), *Human helplessness: Theory and application.* New York: Academic Press.

Strentz, T. (1982). The Stockholm syndrome: Law enforcement policy and hostage behavior. In F. M. Ochberg & D. A. Soskis (Eds.), *Victims of terrorism.* Boulder, CO: Westview.

Sullivan, H. S. (1940). *Conceptions of modern psychiatry.* New York: Norton.

Sullivan, H. S. (1953). *The interpersonal theory of psychiatry.* New York: Norton.

Symonds, M. (1982). Victim responses to terror: Understanding and treatment. In F. M. Ochberg & D. A. Soskis (Eds.), *Victims of terrorism.* Boulder, CO: Westview.

Taylor, S. E. (1983). Adjustment to threatening events: A theory of cognitive adaptation. *American Psychologist, 38,* 1161–1173.

Taylor, S. E., Wood, J. V., & Lichtman, R. R. (1983). It could be worse: Selective evaluation as a response to victimization. *Journal of Social Issues, 39*(2), 19–40.

Tennen, H., Affleck, G., & Gerschman, K. (1986). Self-blame among parents of infants with perinatal complications: The role of self-protective motives. *Journal of Personality and Social Psychology, 50,* 690–696.

Tennen, H., Affleck, G., Allen, D. A., McGrade, B. J., & Ratzan, S. (1984). Causal attributions and coping with insulin-dependent diabetes. *Basic and Applied Social Psychology, 5,* 131–142.

Timko, C., & Janoff-Bulman, R. (1985). Attributions, vulnerability, and psychological adjustment: The case of breast cancer. *Health Psychology, 4,* 521–544.

Titchener, J. L., Kapp, F. T., & Winget, C. (1976). The Buffalo Creek syndrome: Symptoms and character change after a major disaster. In H. J. Parad, H. L. P. Resnik & L. G. Parad (Eds.), *Emergency and disaster management.* Bowie, MD: Charles.

Walker, L. E. (1979). *The battered woman.* New York: Harper & Row.

Weinstein, N. D. (1980). Unrealistic optimism about future life events. *Journal of Personality and Social Psychology, 39,* 806–820.

Weinstein, N. D., & Lachendro, E. (1982). Egocentrism as a source of unrealistic optimism. *Personality and Social Psychology Bulletin, 8,* 195–200.

Weis, K., & Weis, S. (1975). Victimology and the justification of rape. In I. Drapkin & E. Viano (Eds.), *Victimology: A new focus* (Vol. 3). Lexington, MA: Lexington Books.

Weisman, A. D. (1979). *Coping with cancer.* New York: McGraw-Hill.

Witenberg, S. H., Blanchard, E. B., Suls, J., Tennen, H., McCoy, G., & McGoldrick, M. D. (1983). Perceptions of control and causality as predictors of compliance and coping in hemodialysis. *Basic and Applied Social Psychology, 40,* 650–663.

Wolfenstein, M. (1957). *Disaster: A psychological essay.* Glencoe, IL: Free Press.

Wortman, C. B. (1976). Causal attributions and personal control. In J. H. Harvey, W. J. Ickes, & R. F. Kidd (Eds.), *New directions in attributions research* (Vol. 1). Hillsdale, NJ: Erlbaum.

Wortman, C. B., & Dunkel-Schetter, C. (1979). Interpersonal relationships and cancer: A theoretical analysis. *Journal of Social Issues, 3*(5), 120–155.

6

Complex PTSD

A Syndrome in Survivors of Prolonged and Repeated Trauma

JUDITH LEWIS HERMAN

The current diagnostic formulation of PTSD derives primarily from observations of survivors of relatively circumscribed traumatic events: combat, disaster, and rape. It has been suggested that this formulation fails to capture the protean sequelae of prolonged, repeated trauma. In contrast to the circumscribed traumatic event, prolonged, repeated trauma can occur only where the victim is in a state of captivity, unable to flee, and under the control of the perpetrator. Examples of such conditions include prisons, concentration camps, and slave labor camps. Such conditions also exist in some religious cults, in brothels and other institutions of organized sexual exploitation, and in some families.

Captivity, which brings the victim into prolonged contact with the perpetrator, creates a special type of relationship—one of coercive control. This is equally true whether the victim is rendered captive primarily by physical force (as in the case of prisoners and hostages), or by a combination of physical, economic, social, and psychological means (as in the case of religious cult members, battered women, and abused children). The psychological impact of subordination to coercive control may have many common features, whether that subordination occurs within the public sphere of politics or within the supposedly private (but equally political) sphere of sexual and domestic relations.

JUDITH LEWIS HERMAN • 61 Roseland Street, Somerville, Massachusetts 02143. Reprinted from *Journal of Traumatic Stress,* Vol. 5, No. 3, 1992.

Psychotraumatology, edited by George S. Everly, Jr. and Jeffrey M. Lating. Plenum Press, New York, 1995.

This chapter reviews the evidence for the existence of a complex form of post-traumatic disorder in survivors of prolonged, repeated trauma. A preliminary formulation of this complex post-traumatic syndrome is currently under consideration for inclusion in DSM-IV under the name of *disorders of extreme stress* (DESNOS). In the course of a larger work in progress, I have recently scanned literature of the past 50 years on survivors of prolonged domestic, sexual, or political victimization (Herman, 1992). This literature includes first-person accounts of survivors themselves, descriptive clinical literature, and, where available, more rigorously designed clinical studies. In the literature review, particular attention was directed toward observations that did not fit readily into the existing criteria for PTSD. Though the sources include works by authors of many nationalities, only works originally written in English or available in English translation were reviewed.

The concept of a spectrum of post-traumatic disorders has been suggested independently by many major contributors to the field. Kolb (1989), in a letter to the editor of the *American Journal of Psychiatry,* writes of the "heterogeneity" of PTSD. He observes that "PTSD is to psychiatry as syphilis was to medicine. At one time or another PTSD may appear to mimic every personality disorder," and notes further that "it is those threatened over long periods of time who suffer the long-standing severe personality disorganization." Niederland, on the basis of his work with survivors of the Nazi Holocaust, observes that "the concept of traumatic neurosis does not appear sufficient to cover the multitude and severity of clinical manifestations" of the survivor syndrome (in Krystal, 1968, p. 314). Tanay, working with the same population, notes that "the psychopathology may be hidden in characterological changes that are manifest only in disturbed object relationships and attitudes towards work, the world, man and God" (Krystal, 1968, p. 221). Similarly, Kroll and his colleagues (1989), on the basis of their work with Southeast Asian refugees, suggest the need for an "expanded concept of PTSD that takes into account the observations [of the effects of] severe, prolonged, and/or massive psychological and physical traumata." Horowitz (1986) suggests the concept of a "post-traumatic character disorder," and Brown and Fromm (1986) speak of "complicated PTSD."

Clinicians working with survivors of childhood abuse also invoke the need for an expanded diagnostic concept. Gelinas (1983) describes the "disguised presentation" of the survivor of childhood sexual abuse as a patient with chronic depression complicated by dissociative symptoms, substance abuse, impulsivity, self-mutilation, and suicidality. She formulates the underlying psychopathology as a complicated traumatic neurosis. Goodwin (1988) conceptualizes the sequelae of prolonged childhood abuse as a severe post-traumatic syndrome that includes fugue and other dissociative states, ego fragmentation, affective and anxiety disorders, reenactment and revictimization, somatization and suicidality.

Clinical observations identify three broad areas of disturbance that transcend simple PTSD. The first is symptomatic: the symptom picture in survivors of prolonged trauma often appears to be more complex, diffuse, and tenacious than in simple PTSD. The second is characterological: Survivors of prolonged abuse develop characteristic personality changes, including deformations of relatedness and identity. The third area involves the survivor's vulnerability to repeated harm, both self-inflicted and at the hands of others.

SYMPTOMATIC SEQUELAE OF PROLONGED VICTIMIZATION

Multiplicity of Symptoms

The pathological environment of prolonged abuse fosters the development of a prodigious array of psychiatric symptoms. A history of abuse, particularly in childhood, appears to be one of the major factors predisposing a person to become a psychiatric patient. Though only a minority of survivors of chronic childhood abuse become psychiatric patients, a large proportion (40–70%) of adult psychiatric patients are survivors of abuse (Briere & Runtz, 1987; Briere & Zaidi, 1989; Bryer et al., 1987; Carmen et al., 1984; Jacobson & Richardson, 1987).

Survivors who become patients present with a great number and variety of complaints. Their general levels of distress are higher than those of patients who do not have abuse histories. Detailed inventories of their symptoms reveal significant pathology in multiple domains: somatic, cognitive, affective, behavioral, and relational. Bryer and his colleagues (1987), studying psychiatric inpatients, report that women with histories of physical or sexual abuse have significantly higher scores than other patients on standardized measures of somatization, depression, general and phobic anxiety, interpersonal sensitivity, paranoia, and "psychoticism" (dissociative symptoms were not measured specifically). Briere (1988), studying outpatients at a crisis intervention service, reports that survivors of childhood abuse display significantly more insomnia, sexual dysfunction, dissociation, anger, suicidality, self-mutilation, drug addiction, and alcoholism than other patients. Perhaps the most impressive finding of studies employing a symptom-checklist approach is the sheer length of the list of symptoms found to be significantly related to a history of childhood abuse (Browne & Finkelhor, 1986). From this wide array of symptoms, I have selected three categories that do not readily fall within the classic diagnostic criteria for PTSD: the somatic, dissociative, and affective sequelae of prolonged trauma.

Somatization

Repetitive trauma appears to amplify and generalize the physiologic symptoms of PTSD. Chronically traumatized people are hypervigilant, anxious, and agitated, without any recognizable baseline state of calm or comfort (Hilberman, 1980). Over time, they begin to complain not only of insomnia, startle reactions, and agitation but also of numerous other somatic symptoms. Tension headaches, gastrointestinal disturbances, and abdominal, back, or pelvic pain are extremely common. Survivors also frequently complain of tremors, choking sensations, or nausea. In clinical studies of survivors of the Nazi Holocaust, psychosomatic reactions were found to be practically universal (De Loos, 1990; Hoppe, 1968; Krystal & Niederland, 1968). Similar observations are now reported in refugees from the concentration camps of Southeast Asia (Kinzie et al., 1990; Kroll et al., 1989). Some survivors may conceptualize the damage of their prolonged captivity primarily in somatic terms. Nonspecific somatic symptoms appear to be extremely durable and may in fact increase over time (van der Ploerd, 1989).

The clinical literature also suggests an association between somatization disorders and childhood trauma. Briquet's initial descriptions of the disorder that now bears his name are filled with anecdotal references to domestic violence and child abuse. In a study of 87 children under age 12 with hysteria, Briquet noted that one third had been "habitually mistreated or held constantly in fear or had been directed harshly by their parents." In another 10%, he attributed the children's symptoms to traumatic experiences other than parental abuse (Mai & Merskey, 1980). A controlled study of 60 women with somatization disorder (Morrison, 1989) found that 55% had been sexually molested in childhood, usually by relatives. The study focused only on early sexual experiences; patients were not asked about physical abuse or about the more general climate of violence in their families. Systematic investigation of the childhood histories of patients with somatization disorder has yet to be undertaken.

Dissociation

People in captivity become adept practitioners of the arts of altered consciousness. Through the practice of dissociation, voluntary thought suppression, minimization, and sometimes outright denial, they learn to alter an unbearable reality. Prisoners frequently instruct one another in the induction of trance states. These methods are consciously applied to withstand hunger, cold, and pain (Partnoy, 1986; Sharansky, 1988). During prolonged confinement and isolation, some prisoners are able to develop trance capabilities ordinarily seen only in extremely hypnotizable people, including the ability to form positive and negative hallucinations and to dissociate parts of the personality. (See first-person accounts by Elaine Mohamed in Russell, 1989, and by Mauricio Rosencof in Weschler, 1989.) Disturbances in time sense, memory, and concentration are almost universally reported (Allodi, 1985; Kinzie et al., 1984; Tennant et al., 1986). Alterations in time sense begin with the obliteration of the future but eventually progress to the obliteration of the past (Levi, 1958). The rupture in continuity between present and past frequently persists even after the prisoner is released. The prisoner may give the appearance of returning to ordinary time while psychologically remaining bound in the timelessness of the prison (Jaffe, 1968).

In survivors of prolonged childhood abuse, these dissociative capacities are developed to the extreme. Shengold (1989) describes the "mind-fragmenting operations" elaborated by abused children in order to preserve "the delusion of good parents"; he notes the "establishment of isolated divisions of the mind in which contradictory images of the self and of the parents are never permitted to coalesce." The virtuosic feats of dissociation seen, for example, in multiple personality disorder are almost always associated with a childhood history of massive and prolonged abuse (Putnam, 1989; Putnam et al., 1986; Ross et al., 1990). A similar association between severity of childhood abuse and extent of dissociative symptomatology has been documented in subjects with borderline personality disorder (Herman et al., 1989), and in a nonclinical college student population (Sanders et al., 1989).

There are people with very strong and secure belief systems who can endure the ordeals of prolonged abuse and emerge with their faith intact, but these are the extraordinary few. The majority experience the bitterness of being forsaken by man and God (Wiesel, 1960). These staggering psychological losses most commonly result in a tenacious state of depression. Protracted depression is reported as the most common finding in virtually all clinical studies of chronically traumatized people (Goldstein et al., 1987; Herman, 1981; Hilberman, 1980; Kinzie et al., 1984; Krystal, 1968; Walker, 1979). Every aspect of the experience of prolonged trauma combines to aggravate depressive symptoms. The chronic hyperarousal and intrusive symptoms of PTSD fuse with the vegetative symptoms of depression, producing what Niederland calls the "survivor triad" of insomnia, nightmares, and psychosomatic complaints (in Krystal, 1968, p. 313). The dissociative symptoms of PTSD merge with the concentration difficulties of depression. The paralysis of initiative of chronic trauma combines with the apathy and helplessness of depression. The disruptions in attachments of chronic trauma reinforce the isolation and withdrawal of depression. The debased self-image of chronic trauma fuels the guilty ruminations of depression. And the loss of faith suffered in chronic trauma merges with the hopelessness of depression.

The humiliated rage of the imprisoned person also adds to the depressive burden (Hilberman, 1980). During captivity the prisoner cannot express anger at the perpetrator; to do so would jeopardize survival. Even after release, the survivor may continue to fear retribution for any expression of anger against the captor. Moreover, the survivor carries a burden of unexpressed anger against all those who remained indifferent and failed to help. Efforts to control this rage may further exacerbate the survivor's social withdrawal and paralysis of initiative. Occasional outbursts of rage against others may further alienate the survivor and prevent the restoration of relationships. And internalization of rage may result in a malignant self-hatred and chronic suicidality. Epidemiological studies of returned POWs consistently document increased mortality as the result of homicide, suicide, and suspicious accidents (Segal et al., 1976). Studies of battered women similarly report a tenacious suicidality; in one clinical series of 100 battered women, 42% had attempted suicide (Gayford, 1975). Although major depression is frequently diagnosed in survivors of prolonged abuse, the connection with the trauma is frequently lost. Patients are incompletely treated when the traumatic origins of the intractable depression are not recognized (Kinzie et al., 1990).

CHARACTEROLOGICAL SEQUELAE OF PROLONGED VICTIMIZATION

Pathological Changes in Relationship

In situations of captivity, the perpetrator becomes the most powerful person in the life of the victim, and the psychology of the victim is shaped over time by the actions and beliefs of the perpetrator. The methods that enable one human being to control another are remarkably consistent. These methods were first systematically detailed in reports of so-called brainwashing in American prisoners of war (Biderman, 1957; Farber et al., 1957). Subsequently, Amnesty International (1973) published a systematic review of methods of coercion, drawing upon the testimony of political prisoners from widely differing cultures. The accounts of coercive methods given by battered women (Dobash & Dobash, 1979; NiCarthy, 1982; Walker, 1979), abused children (Rhodes, 1990), and coerced prostitutes (Lovelace & McGrady, 1980) bear an uncanny resemblance to those hostages, political prisoners, and survivors of concentration camps. Whereas perpetrators of organized political or sexual exploitation may instruct each other in coercive methods, perpetrators of domestic abuse appear to reinvent them.

The methods of establishing control over another person are based upon the systematic, repetitive infliction of psychological trauma. These methods are designed to instill terror and helplessness, to destroy the victim's sense of self in relation to others, and to foster a pathological attachment to the perpetrator. Although violence is a universal method of instilling terror, the threat of death or serious harm—either to the victim or to others close to her—is much more frequent than the actual resort to violence. Fear is also increased by unpredictable outbursts of violence and by inconsistent enforcement of numerous trivial demands and petty rules.

In addition to inducing terror, the perpetrator seeks to destroy the victim's sense of autonomy. This is achieved by control of the victim's body and bodily functions. Deprivation of food, sleep, shelter, exercise, personal hygiene, or privacy are common practices. Once the perpetrator has established this degree of control, he becomes a potential source of solace as well as humiliation. The capricious granting of small indulgences may undermine the psychological resistance of the victim far more effectively than unremitting deprivation and fear.

As long as the victim maintains strong relationships with others, the perpetrator's power is limited; invariably, therefore, he seeks to isolate his victim. The perpetrator will attempt not only to prohibit communication and material support but to destroy the victim's emotional ties to others. The final step in the "breaking" of the victim is not completed until she has been forced to betray her most basic attachments by witnessing or participating in crimes against others.

As the victim is isolated, she becomes increasingly dependent upon the perpetrator not only for survival and basic bodily needs, but also for information and even for emotional sustenance. Prolonged confinement in fear of death and in isolation reliably produces a bond of identification between captor and victim. This is the "traumatic bonding" that occurs in hostages, who come to view their captors as their saviors and to fear and hate their rescuers. Symonds (1982) describes this process as an enforced regression to "psychological infantilism" that "compels victims to cling to the very person who is endangering their life." The same traumatic bonding may occur between a battered women and her abuser (Dutton & Painter, 1981; Graham et al., 1988) or between an abused child and abusive parent (Herman, 1981; van der Kolk, 1987). Similar experiences are also reported by people who have been inducted into totalitarian religious cults (Halperin, 1983; Lifton, 1987).

With increased dependency on the perpetrator comes a constriction in initiative and planning. Prisoners who have not been entirely "broken" do not give up the capacity for active engagement with their environment. On the contrary, they often approach the small daily tasks of survival with extraordinary ingenuity and determination. But the field of initiative is increasingly narrowed within confines dictated by the perpetrator. The prisoner no longer thinks of how to escape but rather of how to stay alive, or how to make captivity more bearable. This narrowing in the range of initiative becomes habitual with prolonged captivity, and it must be unlearned after the prisoner is liberated. (See, e.g., the testimony of Hearst, 1982, and Rosencof in Weschler, 1989.)

Because of this constriction in the capacities for active engagement with the world, chronically traumatized people are often described as passive or helpless. Some theorists have in fact applied the concept of "learned helplessness" to the situation of battered women and other chronically traumatized people (van der Kolk, 1987; Walker, 1979). Prolonged captivity undermines or destroys the ordinary sense of a relatively safe sphere of initiative in which there is some tolerance for trial and error. To the chronically traumatized person, any independent action is insubordination, which carries the risk of dire punishment.

The sense that the perpetrator is still present, even after liberation, signifies a major alteration in the survivor's relational world. The enforced relationship, which of necessity monopolizes the victim's attention during captivity, becomes part of her inner life and continues to engross her attention after release. In political prisoners, this continued relationship may take the form of a brooding preoccupation with the criminal careers of specific perpetrators or with more abstract concerns about the unchecked forces of evil in the world. Released prisoners continue to track their captors, and to fear them (Krystal, 1968). In sexual, domestic, and religious cult prisoners, this continued relationship may take a more ambivalent form: The survivor may continue to fear her former captor and to expect that he will eventually hunt her down; she may also feel empty, confused, and worthless without him (Walker, 1979).

Even after escape, it is not possible simply to reconstitute relationships of the sort that existed prior to captivity. All relationships are now viewed through the lens of extremity. Just as there is no range of moderate engagement or risk for initiative, there is no range of moderate engagement or risk for relationship. The survivor approaches all relationships as though questions of life and death are at stake, oscillating between intense attachment and terrified withdrawal.

In survivors of childhood abuse, these disturbances in relationship are further amplified. Oscillations in attachment—with formation of intense, unstable relationships—are frequently observed. These disturbances are described most fully in patients with borderline personality disorder (BPD), the majority of whom have extensive histories of childhood abuse. A recent empirical study, confirming a vast literature of clinical observations, outlines in detail the specific pattern of relational difficulties. Such patients find it very hard to tolerate being alone but are also exceedingly wary of others. Terrified of abandonment on the one hand, and domination on the other, they oscillate between extremes of abject submissiveness and furious rebellion (Melges & Swartz, 1989). They tend to form "special" dependent relations with idealized caretakers in which ordinary boundaries are not observed (Zanarini et al., 1990). Very similar patterns are described in patients with multiple personality disorder, including the tendency to develop intense, highly "special" relationships ridden with boundary violations, conflict, and potential for exploitation (Kluft, 1990).

Pathological Changes in Identity

Subjection to a relationship of coercive control produces profound alterations in the victim's identity. All the structures of the self—the image of the body, the internalized images of others, and the values and ideals that lend a sense of coherence and purpose—are invaded and systematically broken down. In some totalitarian system (political, religious, or sexual/domestic), this process reaches the extent of taking away the victim's name (Hearst & Moscow, 1982; Lovelace & McGrady, 1980). Whereas the victim of a single acute trauma may say she is "not herself" since the event, the victim of chronic trauma may lose the sense that she has a self. Survivors may describe themselves as reduced to a nonhuman life form (Lovelace & McGrady, 1980; Timerman, 1981). Niederland (1968), in his clinical observations of concentration camp survivors, noted that alterations of personal identity were a constant feature of the survivor syndrome. Whereas the majority of his patients complained, "I am now a different person," the most severely harmed stated simply, "I am not a person."

Survivors of childhood abuse develop even more complex deformations of identity. A malignant sense of the self as contaminated, guilty, and evil is widely observed. Fragmentation in the sense of self is also common, reaching its most dramatic extreme in multiple personality disorder (MPD). Ferenczi (1932) describes the "atomization" of the abused child's personality. Rieker and Carmen (1986) describe the central pathology in victimized children as a "disordered and fragmented identity deriving from accommodations to the judgments of others." Disturbances in identity formation are also characteristic of patients with borderline and multiple personality disorders, the majority of whom have childhood histories of severe trauma. In MPD, the fragmentation of the self into dissociated alters is, of course, the central feature of the disorder (Bliss, 1986; Putnam, 1989). Patients with BPD, though they lack the dissociative capacity to form fragmented alters, have similar difficulties in the formation of an integrated identity. An unstable sense of self is recognized as one of the major diagnostic criteria for BPD, and the "splitting" of inner representations of self and others is considered by some theorists to be the central underlying pathology of the disorder (Kernberg, 1967).

REPETITION OF HARM FOLLOWING PROLONGED VICTIMIZATION

Repetitive phenomena have been widely noted to be sequelae of severe trauma. The topic has been reviewed in depth by van der Kolk (1989). In simple PTSD, these repetitive phenomena may take the form of intrusive memories, somato-sensory reliving experiences, or behavioral reenactments of the trauma (Brett & Ostroff, 1985; Terr, 1983). After prolonged and repeated trauma, by contrast, survivors may be at risk for repeated harm, either self-inflicted or at the hands of others. These repetitive phenomena do not bear a direct relation to the original trauma; they are not simple reenactments or reliving experiences. Rather, they take a disguised symptomatic or characterological form.

About 7% to 10% of psychiatric patients are thought to injure themselves deliberately (Favazza & Conterio, 1988). Self-mutilation is a repetitive behavior that appears to be quite distinct from attempted suicide. This compulsive form of self-injury appears to be strongly associated with a history of prolonged repeated trauma. Self-mutilation, which is rarely seen after a single acute trauma, is a common sequel of protracted childhood abuse (Briere, 1988; van der Kolk et al., 1991). Self-injury and other paroxysmal forms of attack on the body have been shown to develop most commonly in those victims whose abuse began early in childhood.

The phenomenon of repeated victimization also appears to be specifically associated with histories of prolonged childhood abuse. Widescale epidemiological studies provide strong evidence that survivors of childhood abuse are at increased risk for repeated harm in adult life. For example, the risk of rape, sexual harassment, and battering, though very high for all women, is approximately doubled for survivors of childhood sexual abuse (Russell, 1986). One clinical observer goes so far as to label this phenomenon the "sitting duck syndrome" (Kluft, 1990).

In the most extreme cases, survivors of childhood abuse may find themselves involved in abuse of others, either in the role of passive bystander or, more rarely, as a perpetrator. Burgess and her collaborators (1984), for example, report that children who had been exploited in a sex ring for more than 1 year were likely to adopt the belief system of the perpetrator and to become exploitative toward others. A history of prolonged childhood abuse does appear to be a risk factor for becoming an abuser, especially in men (Herman, 1988; Hotaling & Sugarman, 1986). In women, a history of witnessing domestic violence (Hotaling & Sugarman, 1986), or sexual victimization (Goodwin et al., 1982) in childhood appears to increase the risk of subsequent marriage to an abusive mate. It should be noted, however, that contrary to the popular notion of a "generational cycle of abuse," the great majority of survivors do not abuse others (Kaufman & Zigler, 1987). For the sake of their children, survivors frequently mobilize caring and protective capacities that they have never been able to extend to themselves (Coons, 1985).

CONCLUSIONS

The review of the literature offers unsystematized but extensive empirical support for the concept of a complex post-traumatic syndrome in survivors of prolonged, repeated victimization. This previously undefined syndrome may coexist with simple PTSD, but extends beyond it. The syndrome is characterized by a pleomorphic symptom picture, enduring personality changes, and high risk for repeated harm, either self-inflicted or at the hands of others.

Failure to recognize this syndrome as a predictable consequence of prolonged, repeated trauma contributes to the misunderstanding of survivors, a misunderstanding shared by the general society and the mental health professions alike. Social judgment of chronically traumatized people has tended to be harsh (Biderman & Zimmer, 1961; Wardell et al., 1983). The propensity to fault the character of victims can be seen even in the case of politically organized mass murder. Thus, for example, the aftermath of the Nazi Holocaust witnessed a protracted intellectual debate regarding the "passivity" of the Jews and even their "complicity" in their fate (Dawidowicz, 1975). Observers who have never experienced prolonged terror, and who have no understanding of coercive methods of control, often presume that they would show greater psychological resistance than the victim in similar circumstances. The survivor's difficulties are all too easily attributed to underlying character problems, even when the trauma is known. When the trauma is kept secret, as is frequently the case in sexual and domestic violence, the survivor's symptoms and behavior may appear quite baffling not only to lay people but also to mental health professionals.

The clinical picture of a person who has been reduced to elemental concerns of survival is still frequently mistaken for a portrait of the survivor's underlying character. Concepts of personality developed in ordinary circumstances are frequently applied to survivors without an understanding of the deformations of personality that occur under conditions of coercive control. Thus patients who suffer from the complex sequelae of chronic trauma commonly risk being misdiagnosed as having personality disorders. They may be described as "dependent," "masochistic," or "self-defeating." Earlier concepts of masochism or repetition compulsion might be more usefully supplanted by the concept of a complex traumatic syndrome.

Misapplication of the concept of personality disorder may be the most stigmatizing diagnostic mistake, but it is by no means the only one. In general, the diagnostic concepts of the existing psychiatric canon—including simple PTSD—are not designed for survivors of prolonged, repeated trauma and do not fit them well. The evidence reviewed in this chapter offers strong support for expanding the concept of PTSD to include a spectrum of disorders (Brett, 1993) ranging from the brief, self-limited stress reaction to a single acute trauma, through simple PTSD, to the complex disorder of extreme stress (DESNOS) that follows upon prolonged exposure to repeated trauma.

REFERENCES

Allodi, F., et al. (1985). Physical and psychiatric effects of torture: Two medical studies. In E. Stover & E. Nightingale (Eds.), *The breaking of bodies and minds: Torture, psychiatric abuse, and the health profession.* New York: Freeman. (pp. 58–78).

Amnesty International. (1973). *Report on torture.* New York: Farrar, Straus and Giroux.
Biderman, A. D. (1957). Communist attempts to elicit false confessions from Air Force prisoners of war. *Bull. New York Acad. Med., 33,* 616–625.
Biderman, A. D., & Zimmer, H. (1961). *The manipulation of human behavior.* New York: Wiley.
Bliss, E. L. (1986). *Multiple personality, allied disorders, and hypnosis.* New York: Oxford University Press.
Brett, E. A. (1993). Classifications of posttraumatic stress disorder in DSM-IV: Anxiety disorder, dissociative disorder, or stress disorder? In J. Davidson & E. Foa (Eds.), *Posttraumatic stress disorder: DSM-IV and beyond* (pp. 191–204). Washington, DC: American Psychiatric Press.
Brett, E. A., & Ostroff, R. (1985). Imagery in post-traumatic stress disorder: An overview. *American Journal of Psychiatry, 142,* 417–424.
Briere, J. (1988). Long-term clinical correlates of childhood sexual victimization. *Annals of the New York Academy of Sciences, 528,* 327–334.
Briere, J., & Runtz, M. (1987). Post sexual abuse trauma: Data and implications for clinical practice. *J. Interpers. Viol., 2,* 367–379.
Briere, J., & Zaidi, L. (1989). Sexual abuse histories and sequelae in female psychiatric emergency room patients. *American Journal of Psychiatry, 146,* 1602–1606.
Brown, D. P., & Fromm, E. (1986). *Hypnotherapy and hypnoanalysis.* Hillsdale, NJ: Erlbaum.
Browne, A., & Finkelhor, D. (1986). Impact of child sexual abuse: A review of the literature. *Psychological Bulletin, 99,* 55–77.
Bryer, J. B., Nelson, B. A., Miller, J. B., & Krol, P. A. (1987). Childhood sexual and physical abuse as factors in adult psychiatric illness. *American Journal of Psychiatry, 144,* 1426–1430.
Burgess, A. W., Hartman, C. R., McCausland, M. P., et al. (1984). Response patterns in children and adolescents exploited through sex rings and pornography. *American Journal of Psychiatry, 141,* 656–662.
Carmen, E. H., Rieker, P. P., & Mills, T. (1984). Victims of violence and psychiatric illness. *American Journal of Psychiatry, 141,* 378–383.
Coons, P. M. (1985). Children of parents with multiple personality disorder. In R. P. Kluft (ed.), *Childhood antecedents of multiple personality disorder* (pp. 151–166). Washington, DC: American Psychiatric Press.
Dawidowicz, L. (1975). *The war against the Jews.* London: Weidenfeld and Nicolson.
De Loos, W. (1990). Psychosomatic manifestations of chronic PTSD. In M. E. Wolf & A. D. Mosnaim (Eds.), *Posttraumatic stress disorder: Etiology, phenomenology, and treatment* (pp. 94–105). Washington, DC: American Psychiatric Press.
Dobash, R. E., & Dobash, R. (1979). *Violence against wives: A case against the patriarchy.* New York: Free Press.
Dutton, D., & Painter, S. L. (1981). Traumatic bonding: The development of emotional attachments in battered women and other relationships of intermittent abuse. *Victimology, 6,* 139–155.
Farber, I. E., Harlow, H. F., & West, L. J. (1957). Brainwashing, conditioning, and DDD (debility, dependency, and dread). *Sociometry, 23,* 120–147.
Favazza, A. R., & Conterio, K. (1988). The plight of chronic self-mutilators. *Community Mental Health Journal, 24,* 22–30.
Ferenczi, S. (1932/1955). Confusion of tongues between adults and the child: The language of tenderness and of passion. In *Final contributions to the problems and methods of psychoanalysis.* New York: Basic Books.
Gayford, J. J. (1975). Wife-battering: A preliminary survey of 100 cases. *British Medical Journal, 1,* 194–197.
Gelinas, D. (1983). The persistent negative effects of incest. *Psychiatry, 46,* 312–332.
Goldstein, G., van Kammen, V., Shelley, C., et al. (1987). Survivors of imprisonment in the Pacific theater during World War II. *American Journal of Psychiatry, 144,* 1210–1213.
Goodwin, J., McMarty, T., & DiVasto, P. (1982). Physical and sexual abuse of the children of adult incest victims. In J. Goodwin (Ed.), *Sexual abuse: Incest victims and their families.* Boston: John Wright. (pp. 139–154).

Goodwin, J. (1988). Evaluation and treatment of incest victims and their families: A problem oriented approach. In J. G. Howells (Ed.), *Modern perspectives in psycho-social pathology,* New York: Brunner/Mazel.

Graham, D. L., Rawlings, E., & Rimini, N. (1988). Survivors of terror: Battered women, hostages, and the Stockholm syndrome. In K. Yllo & M. Bograd (eds.), *Feminist perspectives on wife abuse* (pp. 217–233). Beverly Hills, CA: Sage.

Halperin, D. A. (1983). Group processes in cult affiliation and recruitment. In *Psychodynamic perspectives on religion, sect, and cult.* Boston: John Wright.

Hearst, P. C., & Moscow, A. (1982). *Every secret thing.* New York: Doubleday.

Herman, J. L. (1981). *Father-daughter incest.* Cambridge, MA: Harvard University Press.

Herman, J. L. (1988). Considering sex offenders: A model of addiction. *Signs: Journal of Women in Culture and Society, 13,* 695–724.

Herman, J. L. (1992). *Trauma and recovery.* New York: Basic Books.

Herman, J. L., Perry, J. C., & van der Kolk, B. A. (1989). Childhood trauma in borderline personality disorder. *American Journal of Psychiatry, 146,* 490–495.

Hilberman, E. (1980). The "wife-beater's wife" reconsidered. *American Journal of Psychiatry, 137,* 1336–1347.

Hoppe, K. D. (1968). Resomatization of affects in survivors of persecution. *International Journal of Psychoanalysis, 49,* 324–326.

Horowitz, M. (1986). *Stress response syndromes.* Northvale, NJ: Aronson.

Hotaling, G., & Sugarman, D. (1986). An analysis of risk markers in husband to wife violence: The current state of knowledge. *Viol. Vict., 1,* 101–124.

Jacobson, A., & Richardson, B. (1987). Assault experiences of 100 psychiatric inpatients: Evidence of the need for routine inquiry. *American Journal of Psychiatry, 144,* 908–913.

Jaffe, R. (1968). Dissociative phenomena in former concentration camp inmates. *Int. J. Psychoanal., 49,* 310–312.

Kaufman, J., & Zigler, E. (1987). Do abused children become abusive parents? *American Journal of Orthopsychology, 57,* 186–192.

Kernberg, O. (1967). Borderline personality organization. *Journal of the American Psychoanalytic Association, 15,* 641–685.

Kinzie, J. D., Boehnlein, J. K., Leung, P. K., et al. (1990). The prevalence of posttraumatic stress disorder and its clinical significance among Southeast Asian refugees. *American Journal of Psychiatry, 147,* 913–917.

Kinzie, J. D., Fredrickson, R. H., Ben, R. et al. (1984). PTSD among survivors of Cambodian concentration camps. *American Journal of Psychiatry, 141,* 645–650.

Kluft, R. P. (1990). Incest and subsequent revictimization: The case of therapist-patient sexual exploitation, with a description of the sitting duck syndrome. In *Incest-related syndromes of adult psychopathology* (pp. 263–289). Washington, DC: American Psychiatric Press.

Kolb, L. C. (1989). Letter to the editor. *American Journal of Psychiatry, 146,* 811–812.

Kroll, J., Habenicht, M., Mackenzie, T. et al. (1989). Depression and posttraumatic stress disorder in Southeast Asian refugees. *American Journal of Psychiatry, 146,* 1592–1597.

Krystal, H. (Ed.) (1968). *Massive psychic trauma.* New York: International Universities Press.

Krystal, H., & Niederland, W. (1968). Clinical observations on the survivor syndrome. In H. Krystal (Ed.), *Massive Psychic Trauma* (pp. 327–348). New York: International Universities Press.

Levi, P. (1961). *Survival in Auschwitz: The Nazi Assault on Humanity* (S. Woolf, Trans. New York: Collier. (Original work published 1958).

Lifton, R. J. (1987). Cults: Religious totalism and civil liberties. In *The future of immortality and other essays for a nuclear age.* New York: Basic Books.

Lovelace, L., & McGrady, M. (1980). *Ordeal.* Secaucus, NJ: Citadel.

Mai, F. M., & Merskey, H. (1980). Briquet's treatise on hysteria: Synopsis and commentary. *Archives of General Psychiatry, 37,* 1401–1405.

Melges, F. T., & Swartz, M. S. (1989). Oscillations of attachment in borderline personality disorder. *American Journal of Psychiatry, 146,* 1115–1120.

Morrison, J. (1989). Childhood sexual histories of women with somatization disorder. *American Journal of Psychiatry, 146,* 239–241.

NiCarthy, G. (1982). *Getting free: A handbook for women in abusive relationships.* Seattle: Seal

Niederland, W. G. (1968). Clinical observations on the "survivor syndrome." *International Journal of Psychoanalysis, 49,* 313–315.
Partnoy, A. (1986). *The little school: Tales of disappearance and survival in Argentina.* San Francisco: Cleis.
Putnam, F. W. (1989). *Diagnosis and treatment of multiple personality disorder.* New York: Guilford.
Putnam, F. W., Guroff, J. J., Silberman, E. K. *et al.* (1986). The clinical phenomenology of multiple personality disorder: Review of 100 recent cases. *Journal of Clinical Psychiatry, 47,* 285–293.
Rhodes, R. (1990). *A hole in the world.* New York: Simon and Schuster.
Rieker, P. P., & Carmen, E. (1986). The victim-to-patient process: The disconfirmation and transformation of abuse. *American Journal of Orthopsychiatry, 56,* 360–370.
Ross, C. A., Miller, S. D., Reagor, P. et al. (1990). Structured interview data on 102 cases of multiple personality disorder from four centers. *American Journal of Psychiatry, 147,* 596–601.
Russell, D. (1986). *The secret trauma.* New York: Basic Books.
Russell, D. (1989). *Lives of courage: Women for a new South Africa.* New York: Basic Books.
Sanders, B., McRoberts, G., & Tollefson, C. (1989). Childhood stress and dissociation in a college population. *Dissociation, 2,* 17–23.
Segal, J., Hunter, E. J., & Segal, Z. (1976). Universal consequences of captivity: Stress reactions among divergent populations of prisoners of war and their families. *International Journal of Social Science, 28,* 593–609.
Sharansky, N. (1988). *Fear no evil* (S. Hoffman, Trans.). New York: Random House.
Shengold, L. (1989). *Soul Murder: The Effects of Childhood Abuse and Deprivation.* New Haven, CT: Yale University Press.
Strentz, T. (1982). The Stockholm syndrome: Law enforcement policy and hostage behavior. In F. M. Ochberg & D. A. Soskis (Eds.), *Victims of terrorism* (pp. 149–163). Boulder, CO: Westview.
Symonds, M. (1982). Victim responses to terror: Understanding and treatment. In F. M. Ochberg & D. A. Soskis (Eds.), *Victims of terrorism* (pp. 95–103). Boulder, CO: Westview.
Tennant, C. C., Gouston, K. J., & Dent, O. F. (1986). The psychological effects of being a prisoner of war: Forty years after release. *American Journal of Psychiatry, 143,* 618–622.
Terr, L. C. (1983). Chowchilla revisited: The effects of psychic trauma four years after a school-bus kidnapping. *American Journal of Psychiatry, 140,* 1543–1550.
Timerman, J. (1981). *Prisoner without a name, cell without a number* (T. Talbot, Trans.). New York: Vintage.
van der Kolk, B. A. (1987). *Psychological trauma.* Washington, DC: American Psychiatric Press.
van der Kolk, B. A. (1989). Compulsion to repeat the trauma: Reenactment, revictimization, and masochism. *Psychiatr. Clin. North Am, 12,* 389–411.
van der Kolk, B. A., Perry, J. C., & Herman, J. L. (1991). Childhood origins of self-destructive behavior. *American Journal of Psychiatry, 148,* 1665–1671.
van der Ploerd, H. M. (1989). Being held hostage in the Netherlands: A study of long-term aftereffects. *Journal of Traumatic Stress, 2,* 153–170.
Walker, L. (1979). *The battered woman.* New York: Harper and Row.
Wardell, L., Gillespie, D., & Leffler, A. (1983). Science and violence against wives. In Finkelhor, D., Gelles, R., Hotaling, G., et al. (eds.), *The dark side of families: Current family violence research* (pp. 69–84). Beverly Hills, CA: Sage.
Weschler, L. (1989, April 3). The great exception: I. Liberty, *New Yorker.*
Wiesel, E. (1960). *Night* (S. Rodway, Trans.), New York: Hill and Wang.
Zanarini, M., Gunderson, J., Frankenburg, F., et al. (1990). Discriminating borderline personality disorder from other Axis II disorders. *American Journal of Psychiatry, 147,* 161–167.

II

Assessment of Post-Traumatic Stress

In Part I we described post-traumatic stress and PTSD from historical, conceptual, biological, and psychological perspectives. By now the reader should have a sense of the nature of the phenomenon under discussion. Chapter 3, in an integrative effort, presented post-traumatic stress from a unifying two-factor perspective. Neurological hypersensitivity and overarousal have been identified as the constituents of the first factor; psychological hypersensitivity in the form of an inability to assimilate the traumatic event represents the second factor. In effect, the traumatic event represents a contradiction or violation to the individual's worldview regarding safety, security, and/or sense of self. Now that we have posited the phenomenological nature of post-traumatic stress, the next logical step in an examination of any given taxonomic construction is assessment.

The purpose of Part II is to examine and yield insight into the specific assessment of PTSD, but to also provide assessment insight into post-traumatic stress as a broader phenomenon. Chapter 7 reviews the use of standardized psychological tests to assess the psychological domain as it relates to PTSD. This chapter also raises issues relevant to differential diagnosis. Chapter 8 introduces and reviews the concept of psychophysiological assessment, both as it reflects the neurological hypersensitivity factor of post-traumatic stress and as it increases diagnostic efficiency. Finally, Chapter 9 introduces the notion that post-traumatic stress may result in neuropsychological impairments. The rationale and process of neuropsychological assessment as it relates to post-traumatic stress are addressed.

7

Psychological Assessment of PTSD

JEFFREY M. LATING, AMOS ZEICHNER, and TERENCE M. KEANE

Behavioral and psychological reactions following a traumatic event are an inherent part of the human condition (Jones & Barlow, 1990), and the effects of traumatic stressors have been clinically observed since the Civil War (Ettedgui & Bridges, 1985). Not until 1980, however, did posttraumatic stress disorder (PTSD) become nosologically defined within the *Diagnostic and Statistical Manual of Mental Disorders,* Third Edition (DSM-III; American Psychiatric Association [APA], 1980) as a disorder. As a result of this recognition, research efforts have grown considerably, generating a substantial amount of information on assessment and treatment.

PTSD research received further credibility when DSM-III-R and now DSM-IV (APA, 1987, 1994) provided additional clarity of diagnostic criteria. Despite progress in the validation of the diagnosis of PTSD (Keane, Wolfe, & Taylor, 1987; Zimering, Caddell, Fairbank, & Keane, 1993), consensus is currently lacking regarding optimal assessment strategies. Part of the complication in accurately assessing PTSD is the high frequency of Axis I and Axis II comorbidity in PTSD patients (Keane & Wolfe, 1990; Solomon,

---

JEFFREY M. LATING • Division of Psychology and Behavioral Medicine, Union Memorial Hospital, Baltimore, Maryland 21218. **AMOS ZEICHNER** • Department of Psychology, University of Georgia, Athens, Georgia 30602. **TERENCE M. KEANE** • Outpatient Clinics, Department of Veterans Affairs Medical Center, Boston, Massachusetts 02130.

Psychotraumatology, edited by George S. Everly, Jr. and Jeffrey M. Lating. Plenum Press, New York, 1995.

Bleich, Koslowsky, Kron, & Lerer, 1991). Therefore, the purpose of this chapter is to review the prevailing techniques used in psychological assessment of PTSD, as well as to evaluate critically the criteria utilized in making differential diagnoses and concurrent Axis I and Axis II diagnoses.

FUNDAMENTAL CONCEPTS IN MEASUREMENT THEORY

Before addressing the instruments used in the psychological assessment of PTSD, we will provide a brief overview of the fundamental measurement concepts of reliability and validity. This cursory review will permit the reader to evaluate the quality of PTSD assessment instruments more critically.

Reliability

In general, *reliability* refers to the consistency or stability of a measurement process. With regard to psychological indices, reliability refers to the "extent of unsystematic variation in the quantitative description of some characteristics of an individual when the same individual is measured a number of times" (Ghiselli, Campbell, & Zedeck, 1981, p. 191). In this definition, *unsystematic variation* refers to fluctuations in measurement from one occasion to the next that occur in an inconsistent manner and lead to errors in measurement. Sources of unsystematic variation are limitless in number and variety; they range from such factors as the individual's emotional and physical state while taking an inventory to such environmental factors as time of day or room temperature.

Reliability is the most fundamental aspect of psychological measurement; there is no need to consider validity or utility of a measurement process if reliability cannot first be established. Therefore a particular measurement process may be reliable without being valid, but no such process can be valid without being reliable (Everly & Sobelman, 1987).

There are several different forms of reliability, and the ones most applicable for a better understanding of the review of PTSD instrumentation will be briefly addressed. *Test-retest reliability* is the consistency of a given measure over time. When a given instrument is administered two or more times to the same group of individuals while all factors theoretically are kept constant, the intercorrelations among the scores on the administrations are reported as the *reliability coefficient* (Ghiselli et al., 1981). Accordingly, the higher the reliability, the less vulnerable the scores are to indiscriminate changes occurring in the examinee or in the testing environment.

Internal consistency is another form of reliability; it typically refers to the homogeneity (or similarity) of the components or individual items of an instrument. If an assessment instrument is considered relatively homogeneous, the data it provides usually permit unambiguous interpretation. A general statistical expression of internal consistency used when a test has no right or wrong answers is known as *coefficient alpha;* this provides a reliability estimate that simultaneously considers all the possible ways of splitting the test items in an interitem correlational matrix.

Another statistical procedure frequently reported in the PTSD literature is a *kappa coefficient.* Kappa is a useful index for measuring interobserver reliability for categorical data. Kappa indicates the rate of agreements corrected for chance agreements. For example, when kappa is positive, the proportion of observed agreement is more than the proportion of chance agreement.

Alternate-form reliability refers to the use of distinctive, yet comparable forms of the same test. The same individual can complete both forms of the test at varying times, and the correlation between the scores obtained on the two forms represents the reliability coefficient for that test. Having alternate forms of the same test is valuable when repeated testing is planned and carryover effects are anticipated if the same instrument is used.

Validity

The most common definition of validity is the extent to which a test or an assessment procedure measures what it purports to measure. Stated differently, the validity of a test is the degree of accuracy and appropriateness of its data in answering diagnostic questions. Validity is established with reference to other independently observable facts about the criterion or construct of interest; simply put, validity must be earned. Common forms of validity include construct validity, content validity, and criterion-related (concurrent and predictive) validity.

Construct validity is the extent to which a technology can assess or measure a theoretical or hypothetical trait (e.g., intelligence, stress, anxiety). High correlations with other accepted measures of the same construct are a method to assess the convergent validity of a new measure of the construct under investigation. In addition to high correlations, the assessment tool should possess characteristics superior to other existing tests in areas such as ease of administration, brevity, or applicability to a specific population. In this regard, the new test is not merely a superfluous duplication of other accepted measures (Anastasi, 1982). Moreover, the new test should have low correlations with tests that measure a different construct; this is evidence of the test's divergent or discriminant validity.

Content validity refers to the fit between the measurement operations and the characteristics they are intended to represent. This type of validity is typically established by the judgment of subject matter experts, who determine the extent to which each test item relates to the construct of interest, as well as to which the entire set of items accurately represents the domain of possible items measuring the construct (Ghiselli et al., 1981).

Concurrent criterion-related validity refers to the capacity of the measure to discriminate accurately between presence and absence of the investigated construct (Everly & Sobelman, 1987). Specifically, scores obtained during one condition are used to estimate scores expected in another condition, with both conditions measuring co-occurring properties in the individual.

The concepts of sensitivity and specificity are worth noting at this time. These concepts are included in analyses of the effectiveness of tests in identifying cases and noncases of a given disorder. *Sensitivity* is the capacity of the measurement process to identify correctly individuals who actually possess the construct under investigation; this type of classification is known as a *true positive*. *Specificity* is the capacity of the measurement process to identify correctly individuals who do not possess the construct under investigation; this type of classification is known as a *true negative*. Both sensitivity and specificity are receiving increasing use in the development of psychological tests developed to identify specific diagnostic categories (e.g., depression, PTSD, panic).

Predictive criterion-related validity refers to the extent to which the criterion of interest will be manifested in the future. For example, it relates to how well grades in high school predict performance in college, or how well an employee selection test predicts later job performance.

PSYCHODIAGNOSTIC ASSESSMENT OF PTSD

This section briefly reviews some of the instruments used most often in PTSD assessment, and it provides available psychometric data. The reader is encouraged to use this overview as a means to become familiar with existing pertinent research data on PTSD assessment. Specifically, structured interviews, traditional batteries, and psychometric assessment tools uniquely developed for PTSD will be reviewed.

Structured Clinical Interviews

Despite the rapid advances made in the use of psychometric instruments in PTSD assessment, primary diagnostic emphasis is still placed on the results of clinical interviews (Lyons, 1991). The most common structured clinical interviews include the Diagnostic Interview Schedule (DIS; Robins & Helzer, 1985), the Structured Clinical Interview for DSM-III (SCID; Spitzer & Williams, 1986), the Structured Interview for PTSD (SI-PTSD; Davidson, Smith, & Kudler, 1989), and the PTSD Interview (PTSD-I; Watson, Juba, Manifold, Kucala, & Anderson, 1991). More recently, the Clinician-Administered PTSD Scale (CAPS; Blake et al., 1990) has been developed to address limitations in available structured interviews.

SCID and DIS. The SCID and DIS are highly structured interviews used to obtain information on the presence of Axis I disorders. The SCID, which is modeled after the clinical interview, allows the clinician to use symptom-specific questions and clinical judgment to determine whether the interviewee meets diagnostic criteria for an Axis I diagnosis. The SCID has a PTSD module that has considerable sensitivity (.81), powerful specificity (.98), and a robust kappa (.82) when compared to other diagnostic criteria, including the SCID (Kulka et al., 1988, cited in Watson, 1990). Although the inclusion of the PTSD module may have inflated these statistical indices, other investigators have reported similar results using the SCID to validate other diagnostic instruments (Davidson, Smith, & Kudler, 1989; McFall, Smith, Mackay, & Tarver, 1990).

The DIS is a structured interview designed to be administered by paraprofessionals who are required not to deviate from the fully explained questions and probes. Like the SCID, the DIS also has stress-disorder modules that in two validation studies (Schlenger & Kulka, 1987; Watson et al., 1991), using clinical charts, SCIDs, and other diagnostic data, have reported sensitivities of .87 and .92, specificities of .73 and .91, and overall categorical agreement of .64 and .84, respectively. The DIS reportedly performed poorly, however, in the National Vietnam Veterans Readjustment Study (NVVRS; Kulka et al., 1988), the most comprehensive epidemiological study of PTSD to date. Although its specificity was superior (r = .98), its sensitivity was poor (r = .22), leading Kulka et al. (1988) to caution researchers about the use of DIS-type instruments in PTSD assessment. Thus, whereas the SCID appears to be the superior structured interview in PTSD assessment, this tool should not be used as the sole criterion for establishing or conferring the PTSD diagnosis (Litz, Penk, Gerardi, & Keane, 1992).

Structured Interview for PTSD (SI-PTSD). The SI-PTSD (Davidson et al., 1989) is an operationally defined 13-item scale of DSM-III items that the interviewer rates from 0 (absent) to 4 (extremely severe). The total score ranges from 0 to 52, with an option to rate each symptom individually. This approach has a distinct advantage over scales that simply rate a symptom dichotomously.

A factor analysis of SI-PTSD items revealed three components. Factor 1 items related to arousal and intrusiveness (e.g., recurrent recollections and dreams, and increased startle reaction). Factor 2 consisted of items describing detached behavior, avoidance, and survival guilt. Factor 3 included items related to decreased sleep, impaired concentration and memory, and constricted affect.

Psychometric data reported by Davidson and colleagues (1989) on the SI-PTSD included internal consistency ratings of r = .94 and test-retest reliability of r = .71. Additionally, two measures of interrater reliability between psychiatrist and nurse raters were reported. On an assessment of continuous measures for each item, Pearson correlation coefficients ranged from r = .73 to r = 1.00 (median r = .95). On an estimate of category agreement (i.e., symptom presence or absence), kappa ranged from .42 to 1.00, with cutoff = 2/3 (median = .72). Psychiatrist and nurse raters also evidenced high agreement on SI-PTSD total scores (intraclass r = .97 to .99) and 100% agreement on the presence or absence of PTSD.

Concurrent validity was evaluated by comparing the results of 41 Vietnam War veterans who completed the SI-PTSD in addition to the SCID. Kappa was .79, overall diagnostic sensitivity was .96, and specificity was .80. Because the scoring of the SI-PTSD allows for the quantification of severity, various cutoff scores were examined to determine whether the patient met PTSD diagnosis on the SCID. Whereas a cutoff score of more than 16 resulted in diagnostic sensitivity of .93 and specificity of 1.0, a cutoff score of more than 18 resulted in diagnostic sensitivity of .96 and specificity of .93. Such strong psychometric properties of the SI-PTSD, if replicated in other controlled settings, would enhance its inclusion in subsequent research.

PTSD Interview (PTSD-I). The PTSD-I, developed by Watson and colleagues (1991), consists of 20 items that closely reflect DSM-III-R criteria. The first question inquires whether the interviewee has experienced an event that DSM-III-R would classify as a "trauma." The next 19 items, which are scored on a Likert rating scale ranging from 1 ("no" or "never") to 7 ("extremely" or "always"), address symptoms of Sections B (trauma reexperiencing), C (avoidance), D (arousal), and E (duration). A summary section is then completed by the interviewer, and a frequency/severity score is calculated.

Watson and associates (1991) reported results of a reliability assessment on the PTSD-I from a sample of 31 Vietnam War veterans. High ratings of internal consistency (alpha = .92) and high total score test-retest reliability (r = .95) were observed. In addition, concurrent validities of the PTSD-I ratings were compared with corresponding items from the DIS-III PTSD section on a sample of 61 Vietnam veterans. The point-biserial correlation between PTSD-I total scores and a diagnosis of PTSD from the DIS was .94; sensitivity was .89, specificity was .94, and its overall hit rate was 91.8%. The mean PTSD-I total score for the stress group was 58.2 (*SD* = 14.5).

Clinician-Administered PTSD Scale (CAPS-1). The CAPS-1 (Blake et al., 1990) was developed to provide continuous measurement of PTSD symptomatology and to determine the extent of social and vocational impairment attributable to the symptom clusters that make up the PTSD condition. It is a 30-item scale that uses explicit behavioral criteria as the basis for clinical ratings, and it includes items that assess each of the 17 core symptoms of DSM-III-R-defined PTSD. Furthermore, eight items that have been identified as associated features of adult PTSD have been included. The CAPS-1 also includes frequency and intensity ratings on a 5-point continuum (0 to 4, from lowest to highest frequency or intensity) and is designed to ascertain the current and lifetime prevalence of PTSD symptoms.

Now being used by researchers and clinicians alike, the initial ratings of the psychometric properties of the CAPS are strongly encouraging (Blake et al., 1990), and a more comprehensive evaluation of reliability and validity has recently been completed (Weathers et al., 1992). In a sample of 123 Vietnam veterans, test-retest reliabilities for three unique pairs of raters for 60 of the Vietnam subjects (i.e., each pair interviewed 20 subjects) yielded r's ranging from .77 to .96 for the three symptom-criterion subgroups (reexperiencing, numbing and avoidance, and hyperarousal) and .90 to .98 for the total CAPS severity scores. Internal consistency ratings (Cronbach's alpha) ranged from .85 to .87 for the subgroups and was .94 for the total score. Concurrent validity ratings with accepted indices of PTSD, such as the Mississippi Scale for Combat-Related PTSD (M-PTSD; r = .91) and the SCID PTSD module (r = .89), indicate that the CAPS has excellent agreement. Finally, a CAPS severity score of 65 was found to have 95% specificity, 84% sensitivity, and 89% hit rate, and a kappa of .78 when compared with the SCID PTSD diagnosis. The flexibility of this instrument to conform to the needs and objectives of the individual clinician and researcher, in addition to its impressive diagnostic utility, are its primary strengths.

Objective Batteries

Within the past 10 years the field of PTSD has witnessed an immense growth in sophistication of quantifiable assessment data. Although several scales have been developed specifically to assess PTSD, traditional batteries such as the MMPI, MCMI, and the Impact of Event Scale (IES) continue to be employed when clinicians are evaluating this disorder.

MMPI. Studies employing the MMPI to assess Vietnam War veterans with PTSD have consistently shown elevations in certain validity and clinical scales (Fairbank, Keane, & Malloy, 1983; Foy, Sipprelle, Rueger, & Carroll, 1984; Penk et al., 1981). Two of the three validity scales, the *F* scale and the *K* scale, and two of the ten clinical scales, the Depression scale (2) and the Schizophrenic scale (8), often demonstrate a pattern that is characteristic of PTSD patients.

The *F* scale was developed to detect atypical ways of responding to test items (Meehl & Hathaway, 1946). Elevated scores on the *F* scale may be interpreted as an attempt by the examinee to exaggerate symptoms as a plea for help, as faking illness or malingering, as a manifestation of unusual forms of thinking, or as an indication of general dissatisfaction (Graham, 1987). The *K* scale was developed as a subtle index to detect attempts of the examinee to present favorably. Low scores on the *K* scale are indicative of an exaggeration of problems, as a feeling of self-dissatisfaction, as a suspiciousness of others, or as a reflection of ineffectiveness in dealing with problems of daily life (Graham, 1987). High scores on scale 2 reflect symptomatic depression and are considered to be associated with the negative symptoms of PTSD (avoidance, dysphoria, withdrawal), whereas elevations on scale 8 reflect the possibility of psychotic symptoms (e.g., hallucinations or delusions) or the indication of the positive symptoms of the disorder (reexperiencing, dissociation; Graham, 1987; Litz, Penk, Gerardi, & Keane, 1992).

Keane, Malloy, and Fairbank (1984), in a study designed to develop empirically based criteria for use of the MMPI in the assessment of PTSD, noted a consistent MMPI 8-2 elevation pattern in a sample of 100 Vietnam War veterans with PTSD compared to 100 psychiatric patients serving as controls. In addition, the *F* scale was consistently and significantly elevated, whereas the *K* scale was significantly lower. Based on the sample data available, Keane et al. (1984) calculated the following MMPI cutoff *T* scores to diagnose PTSD:

$F \geq 66$
Depression (2) ≥ 78
Schizophrenia (8) ≥ 79

Subjects with scores above these points were classified as having PTSD with an accuracy rate of 74%.

MMPI Subscale to Assess PTSD. In order to determine endorsement patterns, Keane and associates (1984) conducted an item analysis of the MMPI, comparing the PTSD and control groups using chi-square analyses. The results produced 49 items that related directly to DSM-III criteria for PTSD and improved diagnostic hit rates to 82%. The cutoff score used to separate the PTSD and control groups in this sample of combat veterans was 30. When using the PTSD scale of the MMPI (or *PK* scale) with survivors of other traumatic life experiences, these authors recommended the development of population specific norms and cutoff scores.

Other studies comparing Vietnam veterans to psychiatric populations have found that cutoffs as low as 13 have differentiated the two groups (Orr et al., 1990; Schlenger & Kulka, 1987; Watson, Kucala, Manifold, 1986). In a recent effort to validate and cross-validate the MMPI scale on an accident/disaster sample, Koretzky and Peck (1990) correctly classified 87% of validation subjects and 88% of cross-validation subjects using a cutoff score of 19 in a total sample of 69 subjects. Watson (1990), in a review of PTSD measurement studies, suggested that a cutoff of about 25 may yield the best balance of sensitivity and specificity.

In an effort to identify individuals who were instructed to fake PTSD symptoms, Fairbank, McCaffrey, and Keane (1985) reported that subjects with a *T* score above 88 on the *F* scale were likely to possess a factitious disorder (the issue of differential diagnoses will be discussed below). As a result, the *F* scale decision rule became $66 \leq F \leq 88$ and correctly identified 93% of the sample when combined with the previously reported cutoffs of (2) ≥ 78 and (8) ≥ 79. In an attempt to replicate these findings, McCaffrey and Bellamy-Campbell (1989), using a functional analysis on the *F* and PTSD subscale, correctly classified 91.4% of their 35 subjects as having either real or factitious PTSD.

With the recent restandardization of the MMPI (MMPI-2; Butcher, Dahlstrom, Graham, Tellegen, & Kaemmer, 1989), Litz and colleagues (1991) addressed the question of whether the MMPI-2 is comparable to the original MMPI in assessment applicability of PTSD. The *PK* scale (Keane et al., 1984) was only slightly modified in the revised MMPI-2; however, a new experimental scale, the Schlenger and Kulka PTSD scale (or *PS* scale), has been added to the MMPI-2 (Schlenger & Kulka, 1989). The *PS* scale contains 60 items; these include the *PK* items in addition to MMPI items that were shown to best differentiate non-treatment-seeking Vietnam veterans with PTSD from non-treatment-seeking Vietnam veterans without PTSD (Kulka et al., 1988).

Litz and associates (1991) administered the MMPI and MMPI-2 on two separate occasions (about 1 month apart) to the same sample of 29 Vietnam combat veterans meeting DSM-III-R criteria for PTSD. Though the majority of clinical *T* scores for the MMPI-2 were lower than the MMPI scores, significant test-retest correlations were reported between *T* scores across the validity and clinical scales, with *r* ranging from .46 on the *K* validity scale to .90 on the Schizophrenia scale.

Multiple discriminant function analyses demonstrated that for both the MMPI and MMPI-2, the clinical scales of Depression and Schizophrenia were found to discriminate the PTSD subjects best from other groups. Though the test-retest correlation between the MMPI and the MMPI-2 was $r = .80$ for *PK* raw scores, the mean MMPI *PK* raw score ($M = 43.2$, $SD = 9.0$) was significantly higher than the mean MMPI-2 raw score ($M = 36.2$, $SD = 7.9$). The PTSD group's mean *T* scores were 97 ($SD = 13.2$) for the MMPI-2 *PK* scale and 97.3 ($SD = 13.2$) for the MMPI-2 *PS* scale. Combining the clinical scales with the *PK* scale correctly classified 86.2% and 82.8% of the PTSD veterans using the MMPI and MMPI-2, respectively. Although it will be important to cross-validate these findings, these results provide preliminary evidence that the MMPI-2 and the MMPI are roughly equivalent in measuring PTSD.

Millon Clinical Multiaxial Inventory (MCMI). The MCMI (Millon, 1983) was developed to assess maladaptive personality styles and various clinical syndromes. The 11 personality scales are compatible with each of the DSM-III Axis II personality categories and are considered to measure pervasive traits (Hyer, Woods, Boudewyns, Bruno, & O'Leary, 1988). In addition, nine symptom scales are included that are congruent with DSM-III Axis I categories.

Using the MCMI, McDermott (1986) evaluated 22 Vietnam War combat veterans, 11 of whom had been diagnosed with PTSD. The results indicated that PTSD patients may present with elevations on the Schizoid and Avoidant scales and with a concomitant decrease on the Histrionic scale. In another study using the MCMI, 60 PTSD Vietnam War veteran inpatients were found to have a profile characterized by prominent elevations on the Passive-Aggressive and Avoidant scales (Hyer et al., 1988). In addition, the Schizoid and Borderline scales were considered influencing styles, as were the symptom scale disorders of Anxiety and Dysthymia. The latest edition of the MCMI (MCMI-III) now contains a PTSD scale (Millon, Millon, and Davis, 1994).

Beck Depression Inventory (BDI) and State-Trait Anxiety Inventory (STAI). Fairbank, Keane, and Malloy (1983), noting that many of the symptoms of PTSD were theoretically related to both clinical depression and anxiety, administered both the BDI (Beck, Ward, Mendelson, Mock, & Erbaugh, 1961) and STAI (Spielberger, Gorsuch, & Lushene, 1970) as part of a comprehensive battery to assess PTSD in a group of 36 male Vietnam War veterans (12 combat veterans patients in a PTSD treatment program; 12 combat veterans without postcombat adjustment problems or other psychological disorders; 12 noncombat veterans with other psychiatric disorders). They found that PTSD subjects reported significantly more depression on the BDI (M = 25, SD = 9.3) than did both normals (M = 3, SD = 4.0) and psychiatric controls (M = 14, SD = 9.6). Regarding scores on the STAI, PTSD subjects endorsed significantly more state anxiety items (M = 56, SD = 14.2) and trait anxiety items (M = 54, SD = 11.7) than did normal controls on the state (M = 35, SD = 11.4) and trait measures (M = 34, SD = 7.8). PTSD subjects also scored higher than did the psychiatric group on state (M = 46, SD = 13.8) and trait anxiety (M = 50, SD = 10.6); however, this difference did not reach statistical significance.

Impact of Event Scale (IES). The IES (Horowitz, Wilner, & Alvarez, 1979), although developed more than a dozen years ago and not designed to assess DSM-III criteria, is still a widely applicable diagnostic instrument for providing PTSD data (Schwarzwald, Solomon, Weisenberg, & Mikulincer, 1987). The IES is a 15-item scale used to assess current subjective distress caused by any life event, and its items are theoretically related to the view of stress responses initially posited by Horowitz (1976). The 15 items provide data on the symptoms of intrusive thinking (7 items) and avoidance (8 items) in addition to a total stress score. The scale was originally normed on a sample of 66 subjects admitted to an outpatient clinic for treatment of stress (Horowitz et al., 1979). The mean Intrusive subscale score was 21.4 (SD = 9.6, range 0–35), and the mean Avoidance subscale score was 18.2 (SD = 10.8, range 0–38). Internal consistency, calculated using Cronbach's alpha, was .78 for Intrusive items and .82 for Avoidance items. Test-retest reliability on a different sample of 25 students was r = .87 for Total Stress scores, r = .89 for the Intrusive subscale, and r = .79 for the Avoidance subscale.

Mississippi Scale for Combat-Related PTSD (M-PTSD). Keane, Caddell, and Taylor (1988) developed the M-PTSD, a 35-item scale based on DSM-III criteria for PTSD. A 5-point Likert scale (from 1 to 5) is used by the examinee to rate each item, for a total score ranging from 35 to 175. The index also has six factors (one for intrusive memories, a second for interpersonal adjustment, a third for affect lability and memory disturbances, a fourth and fifth for ruminative features, and a sixth for sleep difficulties). A validation study on a sample of 92 combat veterans revealed that a cutoff score of 107 correctly identified 90% of subjects as either PTSD or non-PTSD. Keane and associates (1988) reported a test-retest correlation of r = .97 in combat veterans, and an internal consistency alpha coefficient of .94. Two separate validity studies (Keane et al., 1988; Schlenger & Kulka, 1987) comparing Vietnam-combat PTSD patients with mixed non-PTSD veteran patients and well-adjusted veterans reported sensitivities of .93 and .94 and specificities of .89 and .80, respectively.

Penn Inventory for Posttraumatic Stress Disorder. As the interest in PTSD assessment continues to develop, it is important that empirically based instruments that possess utility for both veteran and civilian populations evolve (Kulka et al., 1991). The Penn Inventory for PTSD (Hammarberg, 1992), which measures the severity of a traumatic event, appears to be such an instrument. This 26-item scaled-sentences inventory, with three options per statement as in the BDI, is based on DSM-III and DSM-III-R criteria and provides a continuous total score that ranges from 0 to 78.

The psychometric properties of this scale appear promising. On a sample of 83 subjects that consisted of Vietnam War combat veterans diagnosed with PTSD, veterans without a diagnosis of PTSD, and nonveterans without PTSD, overall internal consistency measured by alpha was .94, and overall test-retest reliability was .96 (Hammarberg, 1992).

Using a cutoff score of 35 on two additional samples—one consisting of 98 Vietnam War veterans (with and without a diagnosis of PTSD) and nonveterans, and the other consisting of 57 Vietnam War veterans and 19 survivors of the Piper Alpha oil rig disaster—differential and concurrent validity of the Penn Inventory for PTSD were examined (Hammarberg, 1992). Results of the first sample revealed a sensitivity rate of 98%, a specificity rate of 94%, and an overall hit rate of 97% when the Penn Inventory was compared to a diagnosis of PTSD based on a structured interview.

For the 57 Vietnam War veterans in the second sample, results revealed sensitivity to be .97, specificity to be .61, and an overall hit rate to be .86 for the Penn Inventory compared to sensitivity of .95, specificity of .72, and an overall hit rate of .88 for the M-PTSD (Keane et al., 1988). Hammarberg (1992) noted that "its lower specificity suggests some caution when it is used in settings where prevalence is low, but this possible limitation needs to be studied empirically" (p. 75). With respect to the 19 Piper Alpha survivors, 16 of whom were diagnosed by a team of evaluators using DSM-III-R criteria to have PTSD, the Penn Inventory had a sensitivity rate of 94%, a specificity rate of 100%, and an overall hit rate of 95%. These results are encouraging and suggest that the Penn Inventory may be responsive to severity of PTSD symptoms, in addition to being useful for diagnosing "civilian" as well as combat-related PTSD.

Projective Techniques and the Psychological Assessment of the Two-Factor Model

Part I of this book has argued for the existence of a two-factor phenomenology of post-traumatic stress, with the factors being (a) neurological hypersensitivity and overarousal and (b) contradiction of one's worldview pertaining to safety and/or sense of self. Although the psychological assessment techniques reviewed have shown diagnostic efficiency, the process of placing an individual in a diagnostic category without understanding the foundational phenomenology of that category may have questionable value. The assessment techniques reviewed above are largely criterion based, with the extant DSM as the standard for validation. Yet what do these technologies tell us about the specific nature of the post-traumatic stress reaction that adds phenomenological form and substance that may be of value in treatment planning?

To assist in such an endeavor, the diagnostician may consider adding projective assessment techniques to the assessment battery. Technologies such as the Thematic Apperception Test (Murray, 1943), the Rorschach Ink Blot Test (Rorschach, 1921), and the Incomplete Sentences Test (Rotter, 1950) serve to place the symptom criteria within a contextual framework that will prove of value to the clinician who is faced with not only diagnosis but also treatment planning and implementation. More specifically, projective techniques (as well as narrative diary techniques) allow the symptoms to "come to life," thus providing the clinician with insight into the meaning of the traumatic event in the patient's eyes.

It appears that the process of healing a psychological injury is usually predicated on determining the nature of that injury. Referring back to the two-factor model of post-traumatic stress proposed in Chapter 3, a projectively or narratively derived analysis of the contradiction to the patient's worldview (factor 2) engendered by the trauma may prove essential phenomenological data in the overall treatment process. Using the Rorschach with PTSD patients, van der Kolk and Ducey (1989) confirmed the failure of the patients to assimilate the traumatic event into some meaningful schema or worldview. If stressors (like beauty) reside in the eye of the beholder, the clinician needs to obtain a glimpse of the world through the patient's eyes. Projective and narrative diary techniques provide just a prospective.

In sum, PTSD, not unlike other diagnostic categories, lacks a "gold standard" (Gerardi, Keane, & Penk, 1989) or definitive test for the true status of the individual. Until such a methodologically precise, comprehensive, and sophisticated instrument is developed and agreed on, it is inadvisable to purport that one assessment tool is superior to another. What we suggest, however, is that in the psychological assessment of PTSD a multidimensional approach should be used that includes a structured interview, objective psychometric data (Lyons, Gerardi, Wolfe, & Keane, 1988), and even projectively derived data. The inclusion of psychophysiological assessment (to be discussed in Chapter 8) may add another dimension of credibility to the other measures of this psychological disorder.

DIFFERENTIAL DIAGNOSIS

The symptoms that constitute PTSD are protean, ranging from those that are clearly anxiety related to those that appear psychotic in nature (Lucking, 1986). In order to assess PTSD accurately, it is imperative to recognize that other DSM-IV diagnoses are frequently associated with trauma and must be differentiated from PTSD or diagnosed concomitantly with it. For instance, in a community sample of 1,200 Vietnam veterans, approximately 16% of whom had a diagnosis of PTSD, Kulka and associates (1988) reported that 98.8% of those with current PTSD met criteria for at least one additional Axis I diagnosis.

Despite this frequently observed complexity, it is important to acknowledge that not all individuals exposed to traumatic events develop symptoms associated with PTSD. The issue of how the stress response may be influenced by such person variables as unique vulnerabilities, individual resilience, and personal "hardiness" is currently a prominent concern in the PTSD literature, albeit beyond the scope of this chapter (see Bartone, Ursano, Wright, & Ingraham, 1989; Kobasa, 1979; McFarlane, 1990; Sutker, Uddo-Crane, & Allain, 1991). The purpose of this section is to address some of the most common psychiatric diagnoses that are often given in conjunction with, and differentiated from, PTSD.

Depression

Patients with a diagnosis of PTSD frequently report experiencing depressed mood. Analogous to the DSM-III-R (Rundell, Ursano, Holloway, & Silberman, 1989), three diagnostic criteria in DSM-IV—loss of interest in activities, concentration impairment, and sleep disturbances—are shared by both major depression and PTSD.

Several studies have reported that many PTSD patients have a concurrent diagnosis of depression or a past history of the disorder (Behar, 1984; Escobar, Randolph, Puente, et al., 1983; Sierles, Chen, McFarland, & Taylor, 1983). In a recent investigation of 536 male veteran inpatients who received a diagnosis of PTSD, Faustman and White (1989) reported that nearly 20% had a concurrent affective-related diagnosis (major depressive episode, dysthymic disorder, bipolar-depressed). Sierles and associates (1986) reported that in their sample of 25 outpatients who fit criteria for PTSD, 84% had a history of some type of depression. In a larger sample of 404 Southeast Asian refugees seen at a community clinic, Kroll and colleagues (1989) reported that nearly 75% of these patients met DSM-III criteria for a major depressive episode, and 14% had a diagnosis of PTSD. Moreover, Hryvniak and Rosse (1989) reported that nearly 37% of 63 inpatients diagnosed as having PTSD also had a concurrent diagnosis of major depression.

Although the literature is replete with acknowledgments of the concurrence of affective disorders and PTSD, this view has not always been accepted. It was previously considered uncommon for a major depressive episode to be diagnosed in the presence of the defining features of PTSD, even if several criteria for the affective disorder had been met (Helzer, Robins, & Davis, 1976; Nardial, 1983). The dysphoric mood of PTSD was thought to be associated with the stress responses of guilt and grief. Additionally, the mood shifts ranging among anger, anxiety, and depression seen in PTSD have been contrasted with the pervasive anhedonia seen in depression (Arnold, 1985).

Lucking (1986), however, reported three case studies in which the patient with the primary diagnosis of PTSD also had an unrecognized concurrent diagnosis of bipolar disorder. These patients were treated with lithium carbonate (the most readily accepted pharmacological treatment for bipolar disorder), which substantially decreased the intensity of the symptoms and improved the patients' daily functioning. Such changes may have been a function of lithium's well-accepted effects on anger and labile mood. It is noteworthy that when two of these patients were treated with antidepressants, they evidenced minimal modifications of symptoms. Other case studies have been reported, though, where some PTSD patients evinced amelioration of depressive symptomatology with the proper use of antidepressant medication (Birkhimer, DeVane, & Muniz, 1985; Shen & Park, 1983; van der Kolk, 1983; Walker, 1982). These cases highlight the importance of discriminating the presence and absence of other comorbid diagnoses that tend to occur with PTSD. Corrective therapies may need to address both PTSD and the other major disorders present in order to enhance overall psychological and interpersonal functioning.

Schizophrenia

Prior to the publication of detailed diagnostic criteria for PTSD and schizophrenia in DSM-III, many Vietnam War veterans who experienced behavioral and emotional problems subsequent to a trauma received a diagnosis of schizophrenia, usually paranoid type (Arnold, 1985). Because the clinical presentation of visual and auditory flashbacks of prior traumatic events and intrusive thoughts mimic the hallucinations observed in schizophrenia, these errors were understandable. In addition, the suspicious and intermittent hostility often displayed by patients with PTSD may have been considered paranoid in nature.

With the increased emphasis on empirically derived theoretical conceptualizations and validation of the PTSD construct, however, there is less ambiguity in differentiating PTSD from schizophrenia. Arnold (1985) noted that the distinguishing factor between the traumatic flashbacks of PTSD patients and the hallucinations experienced in schizophrenia is the content. He suggested that for PTSD patients the content of the flashback reproduces prior traumatic experiences, whereas the hallucinations of schizophrenics are likely to be sundry in content. Thus detailed inquiry regarding the content of hallucinations should be undertaken prior to making a differential diagnosis.

Another distinguishing feature between schizophrenia and PTSD is in affect. PTSD individuals, not unlike schizophrenics, frequently evince a restricted or flat affect characterized by diminished responsiveness and feelings of avoidance and detachment. Unlike schizophrenics (who generally fail to recognize their inappropriate affect), however, PTSD patients frequently anguish at their incapacity to experience the same degree of emotion they were capable of premorbidly (Arnold, 1985). A thorough psychosocial history may therefore be particularly relevant for the formulation of an accurate differential diagnosis.

It is possible, though, that schizophrenia can occur concurrently with PTSD. Hryvniak and Rosse (1989) found in their sample that approximately 16% of 63 veterans diagnosed with PTSD had a concomitant diagnosis of schizophrenia. Faustman and White (1989) have also reported the possible concurrence of PTSD and schizophrenia. Given the rates of trauma exposure in our society, it is not surprising that individuals who have schizophrenia when exposed to high-magnitude stressors would be likely to develop PTSD in addition to their primary disorder.

In addition to considering the differentiation and concomitance of PTSD and schizophrenia, McGorry and colleagues (1991) have suggested that PTSD may be an unrecognized syndrome that develops during the recovery phase of a recent-onset psychotic illness. In their study, the authors cogently argued that the experience of acute psychosis satisfies criterion A of DSM-III. They then provided prospective data on 36 inpatients recovering from recent-onset psychosis during the first year following discharge. The data revealed that the prevalence of PTSD, assessed by objective measures linked to DSM-III criteria, was found to be 46% at four months and 35% at 11 months, at which time a significant number of the diagnosed veterans were no longer manifesting psychotic symptoms. These results, suggesting that the comorbidity of schizophrenia and PTSD may at times occur sequentially, are intriguing and warrant further investigation.

Anxiety Disorders

PTSD is categorized within the anxiety disorders in DSM-IV. Therefore it is not surprising that there is symptom overlap between PTSD and generalized anxiety disorder (GAD), panic disorder, and the phobias (Breslau & Davis, 1987). The overlap includes symptoms of hyperalertness, sleep disturbance, impaired memory or concentration, and avoidance. DSM-IV has also introduced acute stress disorder which is in essence a temporal precursor to PTSD. For a comprehensive discussion of the symptom similarities and differences, as well as proposed etiology of PTSD and the other anxiety disorders, the reader is referred to the work of Jones and Barlow (1990).

DSM-IV has made advancements in clarifying the nature and extent of traumatic events which are used to differentiate PTSD from other anxiety disorders since this issue was recurrently contested during the tenure of DSM-III-R. Breslau and Davis (1987) argued that no empirical evidence existed to support the DSM-III distinction between extraordinary and more common stressors; consequently, they questioned whether a qualitatively separate category for PTSD was justified. In rebuttal, Horowitz and associates (1987) acknowledged the necessity to consider individual vulnerabilities when interpreting whether stressors are extreme or ordinary. They reported, however, that this issue did not detract from nor alter the usefulness of the PTSD diagnosis to explain the psychological processes of adaptation to the stressors.

In part because of the overlap of fundamental components of PTSD and other anxiety disorders, there is a proclivity for concurrent diagnoses. In a sample of 48 Vietnam War veterans with chronic PTSD, Roszell, McFall, and Malas (1991) reported that 25% had an additional Axis I diagnosis of generalized anxiety. Also, 25% had an additional diagnosis of social phobia, whereas 10.4% had a diagnosis of simple phobia. In a retrospective study based on self-report accounts of 62 former World War II POWs, Engdahl and colleagues (1991) reported that 50% met DSM-III PTSD criteria within 1 year of release and 29% continued to meet the criteria 40 years later at the time this study was conducted. A lifetime diagnosis of GAD was found in 38% of those who reportedly recovered from PTSD and in 94% of those who still had the primary diagnosis. Other studies have reported similar data regarding concurrent anxiety disorders and PTSD diagnoses (Davidson, Swartz, Storck, et al., 1985; Horowitz, Wilner, Kaltreider, et al., 1980; Kroll, Habenicht, Mackenzie, et al., 1989).

Antisocial Personality Disorder

The multiple characteristics of PTSD also share features associated with the antisocial personality disorder (ASPD). These include substance abuse, marital dysfunction, long periods of unemployment, and legal problems (Jordan, Howe, Gelsomino, & Lockert, 1986). The similarities between the two disorders may further hamper proper differential diagnosing by the presence of comparable emotional symptoms (e.g., impulsivity, hostile attitudes, financial irresponsibility, and sexual dysfunctions). Walker (1981) has noted that it may be difficult at times to differentiate between actual PTSD and an individual with an antisocial personality disorder who is feigning the symptoms of PTSD. It may also be that ASPD individuals may lead lives that place them at increased risk of exposure to traumatic life experiences. This would in part account for the frequent observation of PTSD and ASPD comorbidity (Keane & Wolfe, 1990; Kulka et al., 1991).

Procedures have been suggested, however, to differentiate PTSD from antisocial personality (Arnold, 1985; Bailey, 1985). For example, a thorough developmental and social history designed to assess irresponsible behavior during childhood and adolescence is considered to be essential. In order to be diagnosed as having an antisocial personality disorder, the person must have a history of some symptoms of conduct disorder before age 15 (see DSM-IV for a comprehensive description of conduct disorder diagnosis).

Examining these differences in Vietnam War veterans, Bailey (1985) noted that individuals with a diagnosis of antisocial personality often had a poor premilitary history, including truancy and institutionalization. For these individuals, the military often served as a way to evade domestic or legal problems. Upon examination of the military records of those with a diagnosis of sociopathy, Bailey noted that the combat histories of these veterans tended to be more vague, and their complaints more general, than those of veterans with confirmed PTSD. In contrast, he reported that PTSD veterans often have a good premilitary history, including satisfactory school performance and patriotic reasons given for joining the service. Moreover, PTSD veterans often had their symptom onset in conjunction with the intrusive recollections of a specific combat-related event and had adjustment difficulties mostly following their military experience.

In addition to premilitary history, current behavioral symptomatology can be used to differentiate antisocial personality from PTSD. Antisocial individuals frequently evince a lack of remorse or guilt, a lack of emotional response commensurate with the reported PTSD symptoms, little or no improvement with treatment, and the ability to describe severe war trauma without noticeable difficulty (Bailey, 1985; Jordan et al., 1986). In contrast, PTSD patients most often experience survivor guilt, emotional numbing, and a reluctancy to disclose the details and severity of their combat experiences.

The noted differences between PTSD and antisocial personality do not, however, preclude the possibility that these two diagnoses can occur concomitantly. Sierles and associates (1986), for example, put the occurrence of antisocial personality in a sample of 25 inpatients and 25 outpatients (each with a diagnosis of PTSD) at 48% and 64%, respectively. Furthermore, in a comparison between 30 incarcerated and 31 community Vietnam War veterans, the prevalence of PTSD was found to be similar (39% and 37%, respectively; Shaw, Churchill, Noyes, & Loeffelholz, 1987). It was noted, though, that a significantly greater portion of the incarcerated sample met criteria for an antisocial personality disorder.

Factitious Disorders and Malingering

Factitious disorders and malingering are both characterized by psychological or physical symptoms that are feigned or intentionally produced (APA, 1994). Factitious disorders differ from malingering primarily in the motivation for the production of the symptoms. In factitious disorders, the primary purpose for the individual in developing the symptoms appears to be a need to assume the role of the patient. Conversely, malingering is characterized by the intentional production of symptoms for an external incentive or goal, such as monetary compensation, evasion of legal difficulties, or to obtain prescription medication.

The differential diagnosis for these two disorders is not nearly as relevant as determining whether an individual actually possesses PTSD or whether the symptoms are fabricated. The importance of accurately differentiating PTSD from malingering and factitious disorder is often a financial issue. The amount of money involved can be substantial (Peterson, Prout, & Schwarz, 1991): Victim cases, civil litigation cases, and compensation awards are often decided upon the presence or absence of PTSD and the severity of its effects on an individual's social, marital, and vocational functioning. Discriminating the presence of PTSD, its course, and the extent of impairment is a multidimensional process that requires considerable information from various sources to arrive at a competent and reasonable clinical judgment.

The ability to make an accurate differential diagnosis, however, is often affected by several contextual determinants. For example, some individuals may educate themselves regarding the diagnostic criteria needed to receive a compensable diagnosis of PTSD. This material is readily available from books, journals, newspapers, and "survival manuals" issued to individuals that provide detailed criteria on how to apply for compensation (Eldridge, 1991).

There are other contextual issues that ought to be considered part of the process of evaluating veterans and civilians for compensation. As previously mentioned, it is necessary to consider individual vulnerabilities and idiosyncratic responses to trauma. For example, a trauma survivor may experience recurrent intrusive recollections and persistent avoidance of stimuli associated with the trauma; however, the individual may not meet additional criteria needed for a diagnosis of PTSD. Furthermore, since PTSD symptoms vary over time (McFarlane, 1986), it reasonably follows that empirical evidence is currently lacking regarding the specific frequency, severity, or time course of normal and abnormal reactions to traumatic events. Therefore, more research on the longitudinal course of PTSD is needed to assist in understanding the normal course of recovery from exposure to traumatic life events.

Fortunately, there are some measures that can be employed to assist in making an accurate differential diagnosis (Eldridge, 1991). One is to obtain and verify the social, academic, occupational, medical, and legal history of the patient. Individuals who are malingering or who possess a factitious disorder are often referred by an attorney and are likely to have a past that suggests manipulation of the health care system. Additionally, these patients often have several brief admissions to numerous facilities, show noncompliance with previous treatment, and have inconsistent recollections of their illness (Burstein, 1986; Sparr & Atkinson, 1986).

Another technique to arrive at an accurate clinical decision is to employ multimodal assessment techniques, particularly those that provide indicators of exaggeration, like the *F* scale from the MMPI (reviewed previously) and psychophysiological assessment (see review in following chapter). Furthermore, the clinician should carefully observe the behavioral and affective responses during his or her interviews of the patients (Keane et al., 1987) and use clinical judgment to assist in making the appropriate differential diagnosis.

Adjustment Disorders

According to DSM-IV, "The essential feature of an adjustment disorder is the development of clinically significant emotional or behavioral symptoms in response to an identifiable psychosocial stressor or stressors" (APA, 1994, p. 623). To satisfy the definition of an adjustment disorder, the stressor may be of *any severity* and may involve an array of possible symptoms. In contrast, PTSD stressors by definition must be extreme (life-threatening) in nature, involve actual or threatened serious injury, or be a "threat to the physical integrity of self or others" (APA, 1994, p. 427). In addition, PTSD is characterized by a specific and unique constellation of symptoms, such as "reexperiencing the trauma." This may take the form of dissociative flashbacks, intrusive recollections, or nightmares. Therefore, an individual evidencing only limited difficulty in daily social or occupational functioning, while following an extreme stressor, would appropriately receive a diagnosis of an adjustment disorder. Moreover, an individual exhibiting a symptom pattern consistent with PTSD in response to a stressor that is not extreme would also receive a diagnosis of an adjustment disorder. Therefore, according to DSM-IV criteria, the dimensions on which PTSD and adjustment disorders differ are stressor and symptom variability.

Regarding symptom duration, an adjustment disorder has an onset within three months of the stressor, and the reaction does not persist for longer than six months after the stressor (or its consequences) has terminated. Symptoms of PTSD can, however, arise months or years after the traumatic experience; this fact presents some potentially interesting diagnostic issues in determining a differential or concurrent diagnosis with an adjustment disorder. For example, a woman may seek treatment because she has had difficulty sleeping and has been depressed since losing her job two weeks ago. In addition, she experienced the breakup of a four-year relationship over the past weekend. What appears to be diagnostically indicative of an adjustment disorder may become equivocal when she discloses that the sleep difficulties include nightmares about a violent rape that occurred seven years ago. She may further report symptoms of increased heart rate and feelings of impending panic, in addition to having difficulty concentrating and experiencing outbursts of anger. If the symptoms ascribed to PTSD have been occurring before the current identified stressors, then a diagnosis of both conditions may be appropriate. If diagnostic assessment reveals that her current symptoms are the result of unsuccessful avoidance efforts to avert or diminish her from reexperiencing the rape for the past several years, then the principal diagnosis is likely to be PTSD (Arnold, 1985).

DSM-III-R criteria for adjustment disorders made no reference to PTSD in developing a differential diagnosis. DSM-IV acknowledges, however, that the two disorders overlap, which gives credence to Arnold's statement a decade ago that "adjustment disorder and PTSD may be thought of as a continuum with interactive elements" (1985, p. 120). For example, a study of 536 male veteran inpatients with PTSD reported a concurrent adjustment disorder in 54% (Faustman & White, 1989).

Alcoholism

Although alcohol abuse or alcohol dependence presents few difficulties in making a differential diagnosis with PTSD, the extent of comorbidity between the two diagnoses is considerable. In several studies, 23% to 76% of PTSD patients were found to have a concurrent diagnosis of alcohol abuse (Engdahl, Speed, Eberly, & Schwartz, 1991; Faustman & White, 1989; Hyrvniak & Rosse, 1989; Sierles et al., 1986). Although these results cannot be ignored, it is often difficult to determine whether substance abuse is primary or secondary to PTSD (Blank, 1986). For example, alcohol may often be used as a form of self-medication for individuals with PTSD. As van der Kolk (1983) suggested, alcohol has the potential effect of suppressing nightmares, decreasing autonomic activity, and promoting nontraumatic fantasies. Substance abuse more generally may be the factor responsible for bringing many patients with trauma histories into treatment. Ongoing research studies are beginning to document the high rate of trauma exposure and PTSD among those seeking help for substance abuse.

SUMMARY

PTSD assessment has progressed remarkably in the dozen years since DSM-III appeared. The assortment of structural interviews available, some of which are reviewed above, and the steadily growing number of psychological instruments attest to the growing interest in this important field of clinical work and research. Epidemiological data suggest that the incidence of PTSD in the general population may be as high as 1% (Helzer, Robins, & McEvoy, 1987). This information makes it increasingly vital that newly developed assessment instruments, such as the Penn Inventory for PTSD (Hammarberg, 1992) and the CAPS (Blake, et al., 1990), have utility for both civilian and combat populations.

Future research in this area needs to address the utility of instruments across different forms of traumatic events, occurring at different developmental phases, and in different populations. Cross-cultural studies, for example, would provide valuable new information on how different societies process and recover from high-magnitude traumatic events. Such studies may shed light on the active ingredients that are part of successful patient- and provider-initiated interventions.

Currently, the assessment of PTSD remains an art as well as a science. Clinicians and researchers alike are encouraged to employ multiple measures of PTSD derived from various sources when evaluating presumed cases of the disorder. Confidence and accuracy of judgment in distinguishing the complexity of PTSD from the myriad of other psychiatric conditions will be enhanced through the use of such an approach.

REFERENCES

American Psychiatric Association. (1980). *Diagnostic and statistical manual of mental disorders* (3rd ed.). Washington, DC: Author.

American Psychiatric Association. (1987). *Diagnostic and statistical manual of mental disorders* (3rd ed. rev.). Washington, DC: Author.

American Psychiatric Association. (1994). *Diagnostic and statistical manual of mental disorders* (4th ed.). Washington, DC: Author.

Anastasi, A. (1982). *Psychological testing* (5th ed.). New York: Macmillan.

Arnold, A. L. (1985). Diagnosis of post-traumatic stress disorder. In S. M. Sonnenberg, A. S. Blank, & J. A. Talbott (Eds.), *The trauma of war: Stress and recovery in Viet Nam veterans* (pp. 101–123). Washington, DC: American Psychiatric Press.

Bailey, J. E. (1985). Differential diagnosis of post-traumatic stress and antisocial personality disorders. *Hospital and Community Psychiatry, 36,* 881–883.

Bartone, P. T., Ursano, R. J., Wright, K. M., & Ingraham, L. H. (1989). The impact of a military air disaster on the health of assistance workers: A prospective study. *Journal of Nervous and Mental Disease, 177,* 317–328.

Beck, A. T., Ward, C. H., Mendelson, M., Mock, J., & Erbaugh, J. (1961). An inventory for measuring depression. *Archives of General Psychiatry, 4,* 561–571.

Behar, D. (1984). Confirmation of concurrent illnesses in post-traumatic stress disorder [letter]. *American Journal of Psychiatry, 141,* 1311.

Birkhimer, L. J., DeVane, L. C., & Muniz, C. E. (1985). Post-traumatic stress disorder: Characteristics and pharmacological response in the veteran population. *Comprehensive Psychiatry, 26,* 304–310.

Blake, D. D., Weathers, F. W., Nagy, L. M., Kaloupek, D. G., Klauminzer, G., Charney, D., & Keane, T. M. (1990). A clinician rating scale for assessing current and lifetime PTSD: The CAPS-1. *Behavior Therapist, 18,* 187–188.

Blank, A. S. (1986). Irrational reactions to post-traumatic stress disorder and Vietnam veterans. In S. M. Sonnenberg, A. S. Blank, & J. A. Talbott (Eds.), *The trauma of war:*

Stress and recovery in Vietnam veterans (pp. 69–98). Washington DC: American Psychiatric Press.

Breslau, N., & Davis, G. C. (1987). Post-traumatic stress disorder: The stressor criterion. *Journal of Nervous and Mental Disease, 175,* 255–263.

Burstein, A. (1986). Treatment of noncompliance in patients with post-traumatic stress disorder. *Psychosomatics, 27,* 37–40.

Butcher, J. N., Dahlstrom, W. G., Graham, J. R., Tellegen, A., & Kaemmer, B. (1989). *Manual for the restandardized Minnesota Multiphasic Personality Inventory: MMPI-2. An administrative and interpretive guide.* Minneapolis: University of Minnesota Press.

Davidson, J., Smith, R., & Kudler, H. (1989). Validity and reliability of the DSM-III criteria for post-traumatic stress disorder: Experience with a structured interview. *Journal of Nervous and Mental Disease, 177,* 336–341.

Davidson, J., Swartz, M., Storck, M., Krishnan, R. R., & Hammett, E. (1985). A diagnostic and family study of post-traumatic stress disorder. *American Journal of Psychiatry, 142,* 90–93.

Eldridge, G. D. (1991). Contextual issues in the assessment of post-traumatic stress disorder. *Journal of Traumatic Stress, 1,* 7–23.

Engdahl, B. E., Speed, N., Eberly, R. E., & Schwartz, J. (1991). Comorbidity of psychiatric disorders and personality profiles of American World War II prisoners of war. *Journal of Nervous and Mental Disease, 179,* 181–187.

Escobar, J. I., Randolph, E., Puente, G., Spiwak, F., Asamen, J. K., Hill, M., & Hough, R. L. (1983). Post-traumatic stress disorder in Hispanic Vietnam veterans: Clinical phenomenology and sociocultural characteristics. *Journal of Nervous and Mental Disease, 171,* 585–596.

Ettedgui, E., & Bridges, M. (1985). Post-traumatic stress disorder. *Psychiatric Clinics of North America, 8,* 89–103.

Everly, G. S., & Sobelman, S. H. (1987). *The assessment of the human stress response: Neurological, biochemical, and psychological foundations.* New York: AMS.

Fairbank, J. A., Keane, T. M., & Malloy, P. F. (1983). Some preliminary data on the psychological characteristics of Vietnam veterans with posttraumatic stress disorders. *Journal of Consulting and Clinical Psychology, 51,* 912–919.

Fairbank, J. A., McCaffrey, R. J., & Keane, T. M. (1985). Psychometric detection of fabricated symptoms of post-traumatic stress disorder. *American Journal of Psychiatry, 14,* 501–503.

Faustman, W. O., & White, P. A. (1989). Diagnostic and psychopharmacological treatment characteristics of 536 inpatients with post-traumatic stress disorder. *Journal of Nervous and Mental Disease, 177,* 154–159.

Foy, D. W., Sipprelle, R. C., Rueger, D. P., & Carroll, E. M. (1984). Etiology of post-traumatic stress disorder in Vietnam veterans: Analysis of premilitary, military, and combat exposure influences. *Journal of Consulting and Clinical Psychology, 52,* 79–87.

Gerardi, R., Keane, T. M., & Penk, W. E. (1989). Utility: Sensitivity and specificity in developing diagnostic tests of combat-related post-traumatic stress disorder (PTSD). *Journal of Clinical Psychology, 44,* 691–703.

Ghiselli, E. E., Campbell, J. P., & Zedeck, S. (1981). *Measurement theory for the behavioral sciences.* San Francisco: Freeman.

Graham, J. R. (1987). *The MMPI: A practical guide* (2nd ed). New York: Oxford.

Hammarberg, M. (1992). Penn Inventory for Post-traumatic Stress Disorder: Psychometric properties. *Psychological Assessment, 4,* 67–76.

Helzer, J. E., Robins, L. N., & Davis, D. H. (1976). Depressive disorders in Vietnam returnees. *Journal of Nervous and Mental Disease, 163,* 177–185.

Helzer, J. E., Robins, L. N., & McEvoy, L. (1987). Post-traumatic stress disorder in the general population: Findings of the Epidemiological Catchment Area survey. *New England Journal of Medicine, 317,* 1630–1634.

Horowitz, M. J. (1976). *Stress response syndromes.* New York: Aronson.

Horowitz, M. J., Weiss, D. S., & Marmar, C. (1987). Diagnosis of post-traumatic stress disorder. *Journal of Nervous and Mental Disease, 175,* 267–268.

Horowitz, M. J., Wilner, N., & Alvarez, W. (1979). Impact of Event Scale: A measure of subjective stress. *Psychosomatic Medicine, 41,* 209–218.

Horowitz, M. J., Wilner, N., Kaltreider, N., & Alvarez, W. (1980). Signs and symptoms of post-traumatic stress disorder. *Archives of General Psychiatry, 37,* 85–90.

Hryvniak, M. R., & Rosse, R. B. (1989). Concurrent psychiatric illness in inpatients with post-traumatic stress disorder. *Military Medicine, 154,* 399–401.

Hyer, L., Woods, M. G., Boudewyns, P. A., Bruno, R., & O'Leary, W. C. (1988). Concurrent validation of the Millon Clinical Multiaxial Inventory among Vietnam veterans with post-traumatic stress disorder. *Psychological Reports, 63,* 271–278.

Jones, J. C., & Barlow, D. H. (1990). The etiology of post-traumatic stress disorder. *Annual Psychology Review, 10,* 299–328.

Jordan, H. W., Howe, G. L., Gelsomino, J., & Lockert, E. W. (1986). Post-traumatic stress disorder: A psychiatric defense. *Journal of the National Medical Association, 78,* 119–126.

Keane, T. M., Caddell, J. M., & Taylor, K. L. (1988). Mississippi Scale for combat-related post-traumatic stress disorder: Three studies in reliability and validity. *Journal of Consulting and Clinical Psychology, 56,* 85–90.

Keane, T. M., Malloy, P., & Fairbank, J. (1984). The empirical development of an MMPI subscale for the assessment of combat-related post-traumatic stress disorders. *Journal of Consulting and Clinical Psychology, 52,* 888–891.

Keane, T. M., & Wolfe, J. A. (1990). Comorbidity in post-traumatic stress disorder: An analysis of community and clinical studies. *Journal of Applied Social Psychology, 20,* 1776–1788.

Keane, T. M., Wolfe, J. A., & Taylor, K. L. (1987). Post-traumatic stress disorder: Evidence for diagnostic validity and methods of psychological assessment. *Journal of Clinical Psychology, 43,* 32–43.

Keane, T. M., Zimering, R. T., & Caddell, J. M. (1985). A behavioral formulation of post-traumatic stress disorder in Vietnam veterans. *Behavior Therapist, 8,* 9–12.

Kobassa, S. C. (1979). Stressful life events, personality, and health: An inquiry into hardiness. *Journal of Personality and Social Psychology, 37,* 1–11.

Koretzky, M. B., & Peck, A. H. (1990). Validation and cross-validation of the PTSD subscale of the MMPI with civilian trauma victims. *Journal of Clinical Psychology, 46,* 296–300.

Kroll, J., Habenicht, M., MacKenzie, T., Yang, M., Chan, S., Vang, T., Nguyen, T., Ly, M., Phommasouvanh, B., Hguyen, H., Vang, Y., Souvannasoth, L., & Cabugao, R. (1989). Depression and post-traumatic stress disorder in Southeast Asian refugees. *American Journal of Psychiatry, 146,* 1592–1597.

Kulka, R. A., Schlenger, W. E., Fairbank, J. A., Hough, R. L., Jordan, B. K., Marmar, C. R., & Weiss, D. S. (1988). *National Vietnam Veterans Readjustment Study (NVVRS): Description, current status, and initial PTSD prevalence estimates.* Research Triangle Park, NC: Research Triangle Park Institute.

Kulka, R. A., Schlenger, W. E., Fairbank, J. A., Jordan, B. K., Hough, R. L., Marmar, C. R., & Weiss, D. S. (1991). Assessment of post-traumatic stress disorder in the community: Prospects and pitfalls from recent studies of Vietnam veterans. *Psychological Assessment, 3,* 547–560.

Litz, B. T., Penk, W. E., Gerardi, R. J., & Keane, T. M. (1992). The assessment of post-traumatic disorder. In P. Saigh (Ed.), *Post-traumatic stress disorder: A behavioral approach to assessment and treatment* (pp. 50–84). New York: Pergamon.

Litz, B. T., Penk, W. E., Walsh, S., Hyer, L., Blake, D. D., Marx, B., Keane, T. M., & Bitman, D. (1991). Similarities and differences between MMPI and MMPI-2 applications to the assessment of post-traumatic stress disorder. *Journal of Personality Assessment, 57,* 238–253.

Lucking, R. G. (1986). Bipolar disorder in post-traumatic stress disorder–A difficult diagnosis: Case reports. *Military Medicine, 151,* 282–284.

Lyons, J. A. (1991). Issues to consider in assessing the effects of trauma: Introduction. *Journal of Traumatic Stress, 4,* 3–6.

Lyons, J. A., Gerardi, R. J., Wolfe, J., & Keane, T. M. (1988). Multidimensional assessment of combat-related PTSD: Phenomenological, psychometric, and psychophysiological considerations. *Journal of Traumatic Stress, 1,* 373–394.

McCaffrey, R. J., & Bellamy-Campbell, R. (1989). Psychometric detection of fabricated symptoms of combat-related post-traumatic stress disorder: A systematic replication. *Journal of Clinical Psychology, 45,* 76–79.

McDermott, W. (1986). *The influence of Vietnam combat on subsequent psychopathology.* Paper presented at the Conference on the Millon Clinical Inventories, Miami.

McFall, M. E., Smith, D. E., Mackay, P. W., & Tarver, D. J. (1990). Reliability and validity of the Mississippi Scale for combat-related PTSD. *Psychological Assessment, 2,* 114–121.

McFarlane, A. C. (1986). Post-traumatic morbidity of a disaster: A study of cases presenting problems for psychiatric treatment. *Journal of Nervous and Mental Diseases, 174,* 4–13.

McFarlane, A. C. (1990). Vulnerability to post-traumatic stress disorder. In M. E. Wolf & A. D. Mosnam (Eds.), *Post-traumatic stress disorder: Etiology, phenomenology, and treatment* (pp. 2–20). Washington, DC: American Psychiatric Press.

McGorry, P. D., Chanen, A., McCarthy, E., Van Riel, R., McKenzie, D., & Singh, B. S. (1991). Post-traumatic stress disorder following recent-onset psychosis: An unrecognized postpsychotic syndrome. *Journal of Nervous and Mental Disease, 179,* 253–258.

Meehl, P. E., & Hathaway, S. R. (1946). The K factor as a suppressor variable in the MMPI. *Journal of Applied Psychology, 30,* 525–564.

Millon, T. (1983). *Millon Clinical Multiaxial Inventory manual* (2nd ed.). Minneapolis, MN: National Computer Systems.

Millon, T., Millon, C. M., & Davis, R. (1994). *Millon Clinical Multiaxial Inventory Manual* (3rd ed.). Minneapolis, MN: National Computer Systems.

Murray, H. A. (1943). *Thematic Apperception Test manual.* Cambridge, MA: Harvard University Press.

Nardial, J. E. (1983, June 23). Diagnosis: Depressive disorder. *Stars and Stripes,*

Orr, S. P., Claiborn, J. M., Altman, B., Forgue, D. F., de Long, J. B., Pitman, R. K., & Herz, L. R. (1990). Psychometric profile of post-traumatic stress disorder, anxious, and healthy Vietnam veterans: Correlations with psychophysiologic responses. *Journal of Consulting and Clinical Psychology, 58,* 329–335.

Penk, W. E., Robinowitz, R., Roberts, W. R., Patterson, E. T., Dolan, M. P., & Atkins, H. G. (1981). Adjustment differences among male substance abusers varying in degree of combat experience in Vietnam. *Journal of Consulting and Clinical Psychology, 49,* 426–437.

Peterson, K. C., Prout, M. F., & Schwarz, R. A. (1991). *Post-traumatic stress disorder: A clinician's guide.* New York: Plenum.

Robins, L. N., & Helzer, J. E. (1985). *Diagnostic Interview Schedule (DIS) version III-A.* St. Louis, MO: Department of Psychiatry, Washington University.

Rorschach, H. (1981). *Psychodiagnostics: A diagnostic test based on perception* (P. Lemkau & B. Kronenberg, Eds. & Trans.; 9th ed.). New York: Grune & Stratton. (Original work published 1921)

Roszell, D. K., McFall, M. E., & Malas, K. L. (1991). Frequency of symptoms and concurrent psychiatric disorder in Vietnam veterans with chronic PTSD. *Hospital and Community Psychiatry, 42,* 293–296.

Rotter, J. B. (1950). *Incomplete Sentences Blank.* New York: Psychological Corporation.

Rundell, J. R., Ursano, R. J., Holloway, H. C., & Silberman, E. K. (1989). Psychiatric responses to trauma. *Hospital and Community Psychiatry, 40,* 68–74.

Schlenger, W. E., & Kulka, R. A. (1987, August). *Performance of the Fairbank-Keane MMPI scale and other self-report measures in identifying post-traumatic stress disorder.* Paper presented at the 95th annual convention of the American Psychological Association, New York.

Schlenger, W. E., & Kulka, R. A. (1989). *PTSD scale development for the MMPI-2.* Research Triangle Park, NC: Research Triangle Institute.

Schwarzwald, J., Solomon, Z., Weisenberg, M., & Mikulincer, M. (1987). Validation of the impact of event scale for psychological sequelae of combat. *Journal of Consulting and Clinical Psychology, 55,* 251–256.

Shaw, D. M., Churchill, C. M., Noyes, R., & Loeffelholz, P. L. (1987). Criminal behavior and post-traumatic stress disorder in Vietnam veterans. *Comprehensive Psychiatry, 28,* 403–411.
Shen, W. W., & Park, S. (1983). The use of monoamine oxidase inhibitors in the treatment of traumatic war neurosis: Case report. *Military Medicine, 148,* 430–431.
Sierles, F. S., Chen, J. J., McFarland, R. E., & Taylor, M. A. (1983). Post-traumatic stress disorder and concurrent psychiatric illness: A preliminary report. *American Journal of Psychiatry, 140,* 1177–1179.
Sierles, F. S., Chen, J. J., Messing, M. L., Besyner, J. K., & Taylor, M. A. (1986). Concurrent psychiatric illness in non-Hispanic outpatients diagnosed as having post-traumatic stress disorder. *Journal of Nervous and Mental Disease, 174,* 171–173.
Solomon, Z., Bleich, A., Koslowsky, M., Kron, S., & Lerer, B. (1991). Post-traumatic stress disorder: Issues of co-morbidity. *Journal of Psychiatric Research, 25,* 89–94.
Sparr, L. F., & Atkinson, R. M. (1986). Post-traumatic stress disorder as an insanity defense: Medicolegal quicksand. *American Journal of Psychiatry, 143,* 608–613.
Spielberger, C. D., Gorsuch, R. L., & Lushene, R. E. (1970). *Manual for the State-Trait Anxiety Inventory (self-evaluation questionnaire).* Palo Alto, CA: Consultant Psychologists Press.
Spitzer, R. L., & Williams, J. B. W. (1986). *Structured Clinical Interview for DSM-III-R—non-patient version* [modified for Vietnam Veterans Readjustment study 4/1/87]. New York: Biometrics Research Department, New York State Psychiatric Institute.
Sutker, P. B., Uddo-Crane, M., & Allain, A. N. (1991). Clinical and research assessment of PTSD: A conceptual overview. *Psychological Assessment, 3,* 520–530.
van der Kolk, B. A. (1983). Psychopharmacological issues in post-traumatic stress disorder. *Hospital and Community Psychiatry, 34,* 683–684, 691.
van der Kolk, B. A., & Ducey, C. P. (1989). The psychological processing of traumatic experience: Rorschach patterns in PTSD. *Journal of Traumatic Stress, 2,* 259–274.
Walker, I. (1981). Vietnam combat veterans with legal difficulties: A psychiatric problem? *American Journal of Psychiatry, 138,* 1384–1385.
Walker, I. (1982). Chemotherapy of traumatic war stress. *Military Medicine, 147,* 1029–1033.
Watson, C. G. (1990). Psychometric post-traumatic stress disorder measurement techniques: A review. *Psychological Assessment, 2,* 460–469.
Watson, C. G., Juba, M. P., Manifold, V., Kucala, T., & Anderson, P. E. D. (1991). The PTSD Interview: Rationale, description, reliability, and concurrent validity of a DSM-III-based technique. *Journal of Clinical Psychology, 47,* 179–188.
Watson, C. G., Kucala, T., & Manifold, V. (1986). A cross-validation of the Keane and Penk MMPI scales as measures of post-traumatic stress disorder. *Journal of Clinical Psychology, 42,* 727–732.
Weathers, F. W., Blake, D. D., Krinsley, K. E., Haddad, W., Huska, J. A., & Keane, T. M. (1992). *The Clinician-Administered PTSD Scale: Reliability and construct validity.* Paper presented at the Association for the Advancement of Behavior Therapy, Boston.
Zimering, R. T., Caddell, J. M., Fairbank, J. A., & Keane, T. M. (1993). Post-traumatic stress disorder in Vietnam veterans: An experimental validation of the DSM-III diagnostic criteria. *Journal of Traumatic Stress, 6,* 327–342.

8

Psychophysiological Assessment of PTSD

JEFFREY M. LATING and GEORGE S. EVERLY, JR.

The authors of the previous chapter reviewed technologies that may be used to assess post-traumatic stress disorder as evidenced in the psychological domain. They argued for a multidimensional battery in the assessment of PTSD; clearly, there is value in combining DSM-criteria-based interviews and objective tests to create a diagnostic opinion. These authors also suggested that the use of projective assessment techniques adds a unique richness and context to the discovery of diagnostic criteria. Finally, the authors of Chapter 7 suggested that psychophysiological assessment technologies may be considered when completing the assessment battery. Our purpose in this chapter is to introduce and examine the use of psychophysiological technologies in the assessment of PTSD.

Psychophysiological assessment of post-traumatic stress, as discussed in this chapter, serves two functions:

1. It allows direct assessment of the physiological tone and reactivity of the neurologically mediated arousal factor of post-traumatic stress, as discussed in chapter 3.
2. It may be used as part of a larger multidimensional assessment battery in order to discriminate PTSD more accurately from other dis-

JEFFREY M. LATING • Division of Psychology and Behavioral Medicine, Union Memorial Hospital, Baltimore, Maryland 21218. **GEORGE S. EVERLY, JR.** • International Critical Incident Stress Foundation, Ellicott City, Maryland 21042; Union Memorial Hospital, Baltimore, Maryland 21218; and Department of Psychology, Loyola College, Baltimore, Maryland 21210.

Psychotraumatology, edited by George S. Everly, Jr. and Jeffrey M. Lating. Plenum Press, New York, 1995.

orders (Keane, Fairbank, Caddell, Zimering, & Bender, 1985; Wolfe, Keane, Lyons, & Gerardi, 1987), given the issues of differential diagnosis raised in Chapter 7.

To assist the reader in the review of psychophysiological data as presented in this chapter, we will first provide a brief overview of the concepts that undergird psychophysiological assessment.

BASIC CONCEPTS OF PSYCHOPHYSIOLOGY

The underlying premise in the field of psychophysiology is to identify and measure specific configurations of electrical or chemical events occurring in the nervous system that correspond to particular behaviors. Psychophysiological assessment has historically been involved in the noninvasive quantification of electrophysiological events as they relate to distinctive psychological variables (Kallman & Feuerstein, 1986). The basic assessment protocol generally involves exposing the individual to controlled evocative stimuli while recording bioelectrical or physical responses (e.g., viscera, cardiovascular, electrodermal) via psychometric instruments (e.g., polygraphs, blood pressure monitors, thermistors) that typically provide objective measures of the covert events. Generally speaking, there are two primary, rapid psychophysiological response axes that are commonly measured: the neural axes, and the neuroendocrine axis.

Neural Axes

The human nervous system is divided into the central nervous system (CNS) and the peripheral nervous system (PNS). The CNS consists of the brain and spinal cord, each of which is further divided along anatomical lines. The PNS is also divided into two main parts: the somatic system and the autonomic system. The somatic component of the PNS transmits sensory and motor signals to and from the CNS and is broadly concerned with the body's adjustment with the external environment.

The autonomic nervous system (ANS) is involved in the regulation of the body's internal function and the preservation of homeostasis. The interaction between the ANS and the CNS has been of particular interest in the study of psychophysiology because of its prominent role in the experience and expression of the stress response. The ANS is divided into the sympathetic and parasympathetic branches, which work in conjunction to regulate the functioning of such target organs as the heart, the intestines, and the lungs. Symptoms of ANS alteration, particularly dysregulation of the sympathetic nervous system (SNS), are considered the characteristic outcome of stressful encounters. When a person is aroused, direct SNS innervation leads primarily to the release of the neurotransmitter norepinephrine, which is responsible for increased heart rate, increased respiration, increased blood pressure, increased blood glucose concentrations, increased muscle tension, and decreased digestive and eliminative processes (Guyton, 1987). The effects of neural activation via the parasympathetic system lead primarily to slowing and "restorative" functions, such as decreased heart rate and increased digestion.

Neuroendocrine Axis

Although excitation and discharge of the neurological arm of the human stress response is sudden and often dramatic, as in the case of orienting and defense reflexes, it fails to explain chronic, continued arousal. The two adrenal medullae (the central core of the adrenal glands) serve as the anatomical bases for the neuroendocrine stress response axis. The neuroendocrine axis was the subject of considerable research conducted by Cannon (1914), who termed this axis the "fight or flight response." This mechanism, as one might assume, serves to functionally continue arousal of a sympathetic, ergotropic nature.

Upon stimulation of the adrenal medullary cells, two hormones—collectively called meduallary catecholamines—are released. These hormones are epinephrine (adrenaline) and norepinephrine (noradrenaline). Activation of these neuroendorcrine hormones includes (a) increased arterial blood pressure, (b) diminished renal blood flow, (c) increased cardiac output, (d) increased contraction of the skeletal muscular system, (e) increased triglyceride levels, (f) increased cholesterol levels, and (g) diminished blood flow to the skin and gastrointestinal system (see Everly, 1989).

ORIGINS OF THE PSYCHOPHYSIOLOGY–PTSD INTERFACE

The interest in assessing the psychophysiological responses of individuals exposed to trauma is not a new endeavor. More than 50 years ago, Kardiner (1941), who identified the psychological sequelae of war as a physioneurosis because of the biological markers he observed, identified five clinical features of what we now refer to as PTSD. He considered these features—which included irritability, a startle pattern, a fixation on the trauma, an atypical dream life, and a propensity to experience an explosive aggressive reaction—to be an automatically recurring physiological pattern of behavior. Gillespie (1942) also considered distinct psychophysiological responses to be an integral part of the disorder. In his clinical observations of traumatized World War II veterans, he described circumstances of increased generalized muscle tension and palpitations.

These clinical observations helped to formulate a model based on classical conditioning that is designed to explain the etiology of the psychophysiological symptoms of PTSD. According to this model, unconditioned behavioral, physiological, and emotional reactions to traumatic events become classically conditioned to otherwise neutral stimuli, resulting in these conditioned stimuli eliciting the initial ANS response (Kolb, 1984; van der Kolk & Greenberg, 1987).

Keane, Zimering, and Caddell (1985) broadened this formulation when they proposed that Mower's (1960) two-factor theory could be used as the basis for explaining the etiology and maintenance of PTSD symptoms. This model contends that both classical conditioning and instrumental learning occur in the acquisition of avoidance and fear. The temporal contiguity, second-order conditioning, and stimulus generalization associated with classical conditioning are followed by the development of instrumentally learned escape responses that decrease the discomfort generated by the conditioned stimuli (negative reinforcement). Keane, Zimering, and Caddell (1985) suggested that this theory may account for the contradiction regarding why repeated exposures (or reexperiences) by PTSD individuals to conditioned stimuli fail to alleviate their anxiety. The authors contended that the relatively short duration of the exposures, coupled with the strong propensity of the PTSD individual to escape the unpleasant situation, precludes a modification of the fear structure.

PSYCHOPHYSIOLOGICAL INVESTIGATIONS OF PTSD: COMBAT POPULATIONS

Wenger (1948) is often credited with the first controlled investigation of physiological responses associated with PTSD. He performed extensive physiological testing to explore the hypothesis that 225 World War II combat flyers who were recovering from what the Air Force had labeled "operational fatigue" differed in ANS arousal and muscular tension from 98 "psychoneurotics" and 488 aviation students and cadets who had not yet flown in combat. The combat flyers who were suffering from operational fatigue manifested one or more of the following symptoms: insomnia, night terror, anorexia, tremors, tenseness, nervousness, anxiety, extreme startle reactions, asocial tendencies, fatigue, and general emotional instability. Wenger's results, taken at baseline conditions, revealed that the recovering combat pilots evidenced significantly greater sympathetic nervous activity than the students on measures such as salivary output (3.8 vs. 4.2 cc/3 min), salivary pH (7.1 vs. 7.2), palmar skin conductance level (19.8 vs. 16.8 micromhos), systolic blood pressure (115.6 vs. 111.1 mm Hg), diastolic blood pressure (74.9 vs. 70.0 mm Hg), heart rate or shorter heart period (147.5 vs. 160.4) millimin/10 periods), respiration period (4.1 vs. 5.1 secs/respiration cycle), and tidal air mean (18.9 vs. 21.8 mm).

Wenger (1948) also compared the 225 operational-fatigue pilots with a group of 166 asymptomatic individuals who had recently returned from combat. The group with operational fatigue, evidenced significantly higher palmar skin conductance (19.8 vs. 15.8 micromhos), diastolic (but not systolic) blood pressure (74.9 vs. 69.0 mm Hg), sinus arrhythmia (0.07 vs. 1.0 rating unit), heart period (147.5 vs. 154.8 millimin/10 periods), and lower finger temperature (34.1 vs. 35.2 °C). Moreover, in a comparison of the fatigued pilots with 98 individuals with a diagnosis of anxiety or psychoneurosis, the results demonstrated that the pilots had significantly higher palmar skin conductance (19.8 vs. 17.2 micromhos) and skin conductance change between stress and rest (31.2 vs. 25.7 log units). The two groups did not differ in blood pressure or heart rate measures.

In another reported psychophysiological study of PTSD, Dobbs and Wilson (1960) compared heart rate, EEG, and respiration responses of three diverse groups to combat-related audiovisual stimuli. The first group consisted of 8 WWII combat veterans who were considered "decompensated" because they had residual symptoms of combat neurosis; the second group consisted of 13 "compensated" combat veterans from World War I, World War II, and the Korean War who had no evidence of emotional difficulty; and the last group consisted of 10 university students who had not been in combat and were considerably younger than the other groups.

After a 5- to 7-minute baseline period, the subjects were told that a tape recording of combat noises would be played, and that it would be discontinued at any time if they chose. The subjects were then exposed to approximately 8 minutes of audiotaped sounds of an artillery barrage, small arms fire, and aerial bombardment. During the second half of the recording, synchronized single light flashes from a photic stimulator were presented to intensify the stimuli; however, they were found to have minimal additional effect.

Baseline pulse rates for the decompensated and compensated veterans were 79.4/min and 77.3/min, respectively. Although not differing significantly from each other, these scores were significantly higher than the mean pulse rate of 66.5/min for the 10 students. Baseline measures of respiration for the decompensated group, compensated group, and student group were 20.5/min, 15.3/min, and 12.3/min, respectively. The percentage of alpha activity on the EEG during baseline was highest for the compensated group (55.6%) followed by the decompensated group (38.9%) and was lowest for the student group (25.8%).

The mean pulse rate and respiration responses to the combat recording were significantly greater in the compensated group than in the student group. The mean pulse rate change for the compensated group was 6.1/min compared to 2.5/min for the student controls. For the respiration responses, the change for the compensated veterans was a 2.8/min increase compared to an increase of only 0.8/min for the controls. Percentage of alpha activity for EEG decreased in both the compensated veterans and the student controls. For the former the mean decrease was to 38.4% (or a decrease of 31% from baseline), and for the latter the mean decrease was to 16.3% (or a decrease from baseline of 37%).

Because of the decompensated subjects' behavioral agitation during the presentation of the combat stimuli, physiological measures could not be reliably attained. Dobbs and Wilson (1960) reported that 5 of the decompensated veterans were unable to listen to the full length of the recording, turning it off after periods ranging from a few seconds to 4 minutes. Furthermore, while the recording was being played, they were observed to be restless, and some appeared to be trying to remove themselves from the experimental condition. By the end of the experimental phase, all the men in this group were observed to be overtly anxious, some were noticeably shaky, and others were tearful.

Blanchard, Kolb, Pallmeyer, and Gerardi (1982) replicated the work of Dobbs and Wilson (1960) with several methodological changes. For example, the diagnostic criteria for patients with PTSD were made more explicit by using DSM-III, the nonveteran control group was matched for age with the veteran combat group, and a "neutral" stressor (strident music) was added to the combat sounds. The study compared psychophysiological reactivity of 11 male Vietnam veterans with 11 age- and sex-matched nonveterans with no psychiatric diagnoses. Skin resistance level, blood pressure, heart rate, skin temperature, and forehead EMG were recorded during five trials, each consisting of mental arithmetic followed by a 6-minute return to baseline, 30 seconds of music, 30 seconds of silence, and 30 seconds of combat sounds. Over the course of the five trials, the volume of the music and combat noises gradually increased from 42 to 82 dB. Lastly, the subjects were exposed to another combat tape that lasted for 8 minutes and gradually increased in intensity from 41 to 78 dB.

The results revealed that the control and PTSD groups both evidenced increased heart rate and systolic pressure during mental arithmetic. Only the PTSD veterans, however, had significantly greater increased systolic blood pressure, heart rate, and forehead EMG during the combat sounds. For example, the mean heart rate increased from 77.5 bpm during baseline to 86.6 bpm during exposure to the combat sounds for the PTSD veteran group, compared to a mean decrease from baseline to combat sounds of 70.2 to 68.6 bpm for the controls. Systolic blood pressure increased from 134 mm Hg during baseline to 141.8 mm Hg during exposure to combat sounds for the PTSD veteran group, whereas it decreased from 125.5 mm Hg to 124.7 mm Hg for the control group. Although the descriptive statistics were not presented, an extrapolation from the presented figure suggests that EMG increased from a baseline of around 875 microvolt sec/min after mental arithmetic to around 1150 microvolt sec/min during the last exposure to the combat noises for the PTSD group, whereas the control group decreased from a baseline of around 875 microvolt sec/min after mental arithmetic to around 760 microvolt sec/min during the last exposure to the combat noises. A discriminant function analysis revealed that nearly 96% of subjects could be correctly classified by heart rate measures alone. Although these results are compelling, the lack of a non-PTSD combat veteran group makes it difficult to determine whether the outcome was attributable to PTSD or whether the differences were caused by combat exposure (Lyons, Gerardi, Wolfe, & Keane, 1988).

Malloy, Fairbank, and Keane (1983) directly addressed this question when they administered an audiovisual protocol and collected heart rate and skin resistance data on 10 Vietnam veterans with PTSD, 10 combat veterans without a psychiatric diagnosis, and 10 noncombat psychiatric patients who were screened to rule out combat exposure, psychosis, and organicity. While listening to relevant sounds (e.g., car noises, crowd noises), subjects were first shown a series of neutral photographs of a couple embarking on a trip to a shopping mall. They were then shown pictures of combat scenes of a platoon loading onto helicopters and flying over rice paddies; these scenes were accompanied by engine noises and sounds of machine gun fire. Each videotape segment lasted 60 seconds, with an accompanying sound level increase in 10 dB increments to a maximum of 80 dB.

Psychophysiological results of the PTSD, normal, and psychiatric groups revealed no significant differences in heart rate or skin resistance data during either of the baseline periods preceding the videos. Unlike the other groups, however, the PTSD group increased their mean heart rate from 93 bpm during the neutral tape to 104 bpm during the combat tape. Additionally, 8 of the 10 PTSD subjects, but none of the veterans without PTSD, chose to terminate the combat scene. The 2 subjects who did not end the session were observed averting their eyes from the monitor and weeping continuously during the final combat scenes. The average number of scenes completed by the PTSD group was six, and the authors noted observable agitation usually beginning by scene four. A discriminant function analyses revealed that the four physiological responses could accurately classify 80% of subjects as PTSD or non-PTSD.

Other studies have attempted to refine further the methodology used in the psychophysiological assessment of PTSD. Pallmeyer, Blanchard, and Kolb (1986) incorporated five groups of subjects, including 12 Vietnam veterans with PTSD based on DSM-III criteria, 10 Vietnam veterans with combat experience but no DSM-III diagnoses, 5 Vietnam veterans with other DSM-III disorders (3 alcoholism, 1 bipolar disorder, 1 generalized anxiety disorder), 5 Vietnam-era veterans (individuals free of psychiatric disorders who served in the military but never saw active duty in Asia), and 8 nonveteran patients with a specific phobia. The psychophysiological responses of heart rate, systolic and diastolic blood pressure, skin conductance level, and forehead EMG for each group were compared during rest, a 30-second period following a 2-second startle condition (80 dB white noise), mental arithmetic, and combat sounds (helicopters, AK-47 firing, mortars, and screaming wounded).

The results revealed that PTSD veterans had higher basal heart rates and systolic blood pressure levels across experimental conditions, and that they showed an accelerated heart rate response to the combat noises. Despite significant group-by-condition interactions for heart rate, systolic blood pressure, diastolic blood pressure, and skin conductance, Pallmeyer and associates (1986) presented only the heart rate effects in detail. Extrapolating from the presented figure, baseline heart rates were as follows: the 12 PTSD veterans, 81 bpm; the 10 Vietnam combat veterans without PTSD, 69.5 bpm; the 5 Vietnam veterans with a psychiatric diagnosis, 73 bpm; the 5 Vietnam veterans who never saw duty in Southeast Asia, 62.5 bpm; and the 8 nonveteran patients with an anxiety disorder, 73 bpm.

All the groups showed a significant increase in heart rate during mental arithmetic, but only the PTSD group evidenced a significant increase in heart rate in response to the combat stimuli (calculated by change scores in heart rate between listening to music and listening to the combat sounds). For example, when the combat noise was presented for the first time, the PTSD group showed a significantly greater increase in heart rate (of about 6 bpm) compared to the Vietnam-era veterans, who showed the second highest increase (of around 2 bpm).

Discriminant function analyses using six parameters derived from different scores of heart rate revealed correct classification of 75% of the PTSD veterans and 100% of the combat veterans without PTSD, for an overall hit rate of 86.4%. Using the single parameter of a difference score between maximum heart rate response to combat sounds and heart rate response to mental arithmetic, and setting the cutoff score at −3.5 bpm (combat sounds − mental arithmetic), resulted in correct classification of 83% of PTSD veterans, and 89% of other subjects.

In a large study investigating the psychophysiological reactivity of combat-related PTSD, Blanchard, Kolb, Gerardi, Ryan, and Pallmeyer (1986) assessed 91 Vietnam veterans, 57 of whom met DSM-III criteria for PTSD. The other 34 subjects were combat veterans free from psychiatric disturbance. The cardiac responses of the Vietnam veterans were examined in the same way as in the study reported above. Once again, heart rate proved to be an important discriminating variable between the PTSD and non-PTSD veterans.

The graphic data presented by Blanchard et al. indicate that the baseline measures for heart rate for the PTSD veterans and the non-PTSD veterans were about 77 bpm and 65 bpm, respectively. The average heart rate response to mental arithmetic, calculated as a change score from baseline, did not differ between the two groups. The difference in average heart rate during the combat sounds, calculated by subtracting the heart rate value during music at the comparable sound level, was, however, highly significant for each decibel level of combat sounds (40 dB, 50 dB, 60 dB, 70 dB, and the highest individual level tolerated), with the PTSD veterans showing the greater change. For example, the largest change for both groups was to the combat sounds at the highest level tolerated. Whereas the PTSD veterans showed a heart rate response of +10.6, the non-PTSD veterans showed a heart rate response of +3.5. An examination of the distribution of scores of the single largest response to any of the combat sounds from 40 to 80 dB revealed that a heart rate change cutoff score of +7 bpm could accurately discern 88.2% of non-PTSD combat veterans and 70.2% of those with PTSD.

Pitman, Orr, Forgue, de Jong, and Clairborn (1987), in an innovative and well-designed study, utilized psychophysiological techniques to assess emotional arousal while scripts describing individual combat experiences were being read to 33 Vietnam combat veterans (18 of whom met DSM-III-R criteria for PTSD). The scripts included individualized portrayals of actual combat experiences in the subject's past, a premilitary stressful experience, a positive experience, and a neutral situation. In addition to the personal scripts, standardized scripts were also developed that portrayed hypothetical experiences, including a combat experience, a positive experience, a neutral situation, and a noncombat stress experience (public speaking).

Following a baseline period, the scripts were read to the subjects for 30 seconds; the subjects were then told to continue imagining the events being portrayed. Heart rate (HR), skin conductance (SC), and frontalis electromyogram (EMG) were recorded during each 30-second phase (baseline, read, imagery, and recovery) for the 11 script presentations. A comparison of the baseline physiological levels between the PTSD veterans and the non-PTSD veterans, respectively, revealed the following: a significant heart rate difference of 75.3 bpm versus 66.3 bpm, a nonsignificant skin conductance (SC) difference of 1.45 versus 1.34 micromhos, and a nonsignificant frontalis EMG difference of 2.71 versus 3.70 microvolts.

An examination of the physiological responses to individualized combat scripts revealed highly significant SC and EMG responses for the PTSD veterans compared to the non-PTSD veterans. Extrapolations from the graphic data presented showed there was an approximate skin conductance change of 0.6 micromhos for the PTSD veterans compared to less than 0.1 micromhos for the non-PTSD veterans, and a frontalis EMG change of about 1.8 microvolts for the PTSD veterans compared to less than 0.25 microvolts for the non-PTSD veterans. Although HR responses were not significant, there was a trend for the PTSD veterans to show a greater change. Discriminant function analyses indicated that SC alone successfully classified 73%, EMG 67%, and heart rate 64% of the veterans. A stepwise discriminant analysis employing all three physiological responses correctly classified 100% of the PTSD subjects and 61% of the non-PTSD subjects, for an overall hit rate of 79%.

Whereas the above studies employed visual and auditory stimuli, Kline and Rausch (1985) described two case reports in which olfaction was a prominent component in triggering PTSD symptomatology in combat veterans. Odors such as certain plants, burning food, diesel fuel, and blood elicited distinct and painful memories in these subjects; this led the authors to conclude that clinicians should routinely inquire about meaningful odors when assessing PTSD.

As evidence steadily accumulated to support the hypothesis of heightened cardiac response to relevant stimuli among veterans with PTSD, and because PTSD is a disorder in which veterans may seek financial compensation from the Veterans Administration, the question arose regarding the ability of psychophysiological assessment procedures to detect faking in Vietnam veterans with and without PTSD (Blanchard et al., 1986). Gerardi, Blanchard, and Kolb (1989) directly addressed this question in a study of 36 combat Vietnam veterans, 18 diagnosed with PTSD and 18 without PTSD.

All subjects were exposed to six trials consisting of adaptation, baseline, mental arithmetic (a "neutral" stressor), return to baseline, music, silence, and then combat sounds (taken from the soundtrack of the movie *Apocalypse Now*) while heart rate, blood pressure, peripheral surface temperature, frontalis EMG, and skin resistance level (SRL) were monitored. After the sixth trial, the experimenter reentered the subject room and asked the subjects if they would be willing to listen to the entire tape again. Eight of the PTSD subjects were given "fake good" instructions, which consisted of a description of the physiological responses (e.g., faster heart rate, higher blood pressure, and increased muscle tension) typically seen in PTSD patients. These subjects were then asked to control their bodily responses to present themselves as *not* having PTSD. Conversely, for the veterans without PTSD, half ($N = 9$) were given "fake bad" instructions, which consisted of the same description of the physiological responses given to the PTSD patients; however, they were asked to present themselves as having PTSD. The other subjects were simply asked to listen to the tape again.

Gerardi and colleagues (1989) reported a significant difference in baseline heart rate and DBP for the PTSD veterans and non-PTSD veterans, with the former having a mean heart rate of 76 bpm and a mean DBP of 69 mm Hg and the latter having a mean heart rate of 63 bpm and a mean DBP of 62 mm Hg. Although the raw data were not presented, significant difference scores during the combat sounds (calculated by subtracting the raw physiological response score obtained during the music condition from that obtained during the combat condition) were reported for heart rate, SCL, and frontal EMG, but not for SBP, DBP, or peripheral temperature. Discriminant function analyses revealed that heart rate correctly classified 72.2% of PTSD and 88.9% of non-PTSD veterans, for a total classification of 80.6%.

Regarding the capability to alter physiological responses to the combat sounds, PTSD subjects were unable to do so. Their responses were not statistically different from those who simply listened to the tape twice. The results indicated, however, that the veterans without PTSD were quite capable of increasing their psychophysiological responses to appear more like PTSD veterans. For instance, when the non-PTSD veterans were asked to "fake bad," they showed a mean heart rate increase of close to 6 bpm during the combat sounds.

With the use of discriminant function analyses, Gerardi and colleagues (1989) developed a classification rule that used the single largest heart rate response, or the largest heart rate increase from music to combat sounds on any trial, and determined that a cutoff score of +7 bpm correctly classified 70.2% of the PTSD veterans and 88.2% of the non-PTSD veterans, for a total hit rate of 76.9%. In order to discern faking from nonfaking veterans, a decision rule was developed that considered both baseline heart rate (≤ 67 bpm) and heart rate response (≤ 10 bpm) on any trial simultaneously. This rule correctly classified 66.7% of the veterans attempting to fake PTSD and 83.3% of the total sample.

In a large study designed to determine the merit of psychophysiological responses in PTSD assessment, Blanchard, Kolb, and Prins (1991) studied a total sample of 200 veterans who served in Southeast Asia. The first subsample consisted of 104 veterans, 69 of whom were diagnosed with PTSD. The remaining 96 subjects, 52 of whom were diagnosed with PTSD, served as a cross-validation sample. The experimental procedures were the same as those reported above (Blanchard et al., 1986), and the psychophysiological measures were heart rate, blood pressure, and frontalis EMG.

Blanchard, Kolb, and Prins (1991) reported that the major purpose of this study was to use discriminant function analyses to determine the incremental degree of assessment accuracy by adding physiological variables from different response sites. Possibly because of this focus, descriptive statistics were only presented for basal heart rate and basal blood pressure for the initial sample. The PTSD veterans had a mean heart rate of 74.8 bpm compared to 67.1 bpm for the non-PTSD combat veterans, a mean systolic blood pressure of 122.8 mm Hg compared to 115.3 mm Hg, and a mean diastolic blood pressure of 72.3 mm Hg compared to 65.6 mm Hg. For the cross-validation sample, only basal heart rate was presented; the PTSD veterans had a mean heart rate of 76.9 bpm, and the non-PTSD veterans had a mean heart rate of 67.7 bpm.

The results of the discriminant function analyses, performed in a stepwise manner and designed to determine the incremental value of adding additional physiological data, revealed that HR alone correctly classified 75% of the overall sample. The addition of blood pressure parameters led to an incremental increase of 5%, or a total of 79.8%, whereas the addition of variables from frontal EMG led to no increment in correct classification. Analyses of HR data on the cross-validation sample resulted in a correct discrimination of 83% of the sample.

PSYCHOPHYSIOLOGICAL INVESTIGATIONS OF PTSD: NONCOMBAT POPULATIONS

Because most psychophysiological assessment of PTSD has focused on combat-related trauma, the advancements in strategies and procedures used in this domain should serve as a guide for furthering the sophistication of multimodal assessment in other trauma-related areas. For example, although the literature on rape-related PTSD is fairly comprehensive in assessing the psychological impact of the traumatic event, it is currently lacking in thoroughly assessing the psychophysiological responses of groups of rape victims (Resnick, Kilpatrick, & Lipovsky, 1991).

Blanchard and Abel (1976) reported a case study in which biofeedback was used to help treat a 30-year-old woman who had a 15-year history of a rape-induced psychophysiological cardiovascular disorder. After undergoing four baseline sessions, she received treatment sessions that lasted 40 minutes (15 minutes of adaptation, 5 minutes of baseline, and two 10-minute experimental trials). The trials initially involved counterbalanced exposure to one of two neutral audiotapes (e.g., descriptions of fixing a meal or going on a ride) or to one of three rape audiotapes (one recounting the actual episode, the other two describing the resulting trauma). She subsequently received biofeedback training, which she utilized during initial exposure to the neutral tapes and then to the rape accounts.

Although the mean heart rates during the different phases of treatment were not presented, the authors reported that the patient's heart rate reached levels over 150 bpm during exposure to the rape-related audiotapes. They did report the change in average heart rate, which was calculated by subtracting the average heart rate during baseline from the average heart rate during the audiotapes. As deduced from the figure presented, the results revealed an average increase of about 0.5 bpm during the four sessions of initial baseline, and an average increase of around 7.3 bpm during the four sessions in which she heard the aversive rape-related audiotape prior to receiving biofeedback training. After receiving eight sessions of feedback training while listening to a neutral tape, she evidenced a decrease in average heart rate of about 2.9 bpm. She subsequently showed an average heart rate decrease of about 3.9 bpm during the 25 sessions in which she received feedback training while listening to the aversive rape-related audiotape. These results evidenced good generalization and maintenance at 4 months' follow-up.

In another single case study of rape-related PTSD, Rychtarik, Silverman, Van Landingham, and Prue (1984) described the use of implosive therapy in the treatment of a 22-year-old woman who was an incest victim from ages 12 to 15. The patient received five 80- to 90-minute sessions on five consecutive days, during which time repeated exposure through imagery to the incest scene and related traumatic events were presented and behavioral, physiological, and self-report measures were recorded. The physiological indices included frequency of skin conductance responses (SCR), defined as any .20 micromhos or greater increase in conductivity occurring within 5 seconds, and change in skin conductance level (SCL) from baseline to scene presentation, determined by computing the mean of the lowest point across four 15-second intervals per minute, then averaging these mean scores across the relaxation period (5 minutes) and the scene presentations (three 5-minute intervals).

The graphs presented by the researchers show that the patient evidenced within-session changes in SCL from baseline to scene presentation ranging from about 15.7 micromhos during the first session to around 3.8 micromhos during the fourth session. The average change for the five sessions was estimated to be 7.3 micromhos and was close to 2.5 micromhos at 6 weeks' follow-up, evidencing synchronous reduction from previous levels. SCR data were presented in graphic form for the generalization probes (defined as a 5-minute imagery scene that was preceded and followed by 5-minute relaxation periods) and used to determine the extent to which extinction of arousal in the implosive scene generalized to other real-life stressors associated with the incest trauma. The number of SCRs across generalization probes ranged from close to 7 during the first session to 0 during the fifth session, with an overall mean of around 4.4. At 6 weeks' follow-up, the number of SCRs remained 0, indicating generalized extinction.

In one of the only studies of psychophysiological assessment of a group of rape victims, Kilpatrick, Best, Amick, and Veronen (1984) monitored the heart rate (bpm) and skin conductance reactions (an increase of .005 micromhos during the assessment phases) of 26 victims (mean age of 24.8 years) who were seeking treatment for significant anxiety at least 2 months after being raped. After an adaptation and habituation period, physiological data collection began with a 2-minute baseline period, followed by the audiorecorded presentation of the following 1-minute scenes: pleasant, neutral, least-feared target, intermediate-feared target, and most-feared target. A 1-minute rest period occurred between each of the scenes.

The results revealed baseline measures of 72.7 bpm for heart rate and 1.62 frequency/min for electrodermal responses. During the five scene presentations (pleasant, neutral, and the three feared-target scenes), average heart rate responses were greatest during the least aversive of the target scenes, with a reading of 77.75 bpm. Although these responses were significantly different from baseline levels, Kilpatrick and colleagues (1984) did not consider them to be clinically relevant. Furthermore, during the most-feared scene, the average heart rate was only 75.98 bpm, which was not significantly different from baseline. Comparable data were observed for electrodermal responses. Although the greatest average electrodermal responses occurred during the most-feared scene (3.92 frequency/min), the average electrodermal responses to the pleasant scene were 3.65 frequency/min.

Kilpatrick and associates (1984) concluded that as a group the rape victims did not display hyperarousal during baseline, and that physiological responses to the target scenes were not significantly greater than baseline levels. Furthermore, after assigning the victims to subgroups of high, moderate, and low responders in terms of cardiovascular and electrodermal responsivity based on a rank ordering, 31% of the victims were classified as both low-heart-rate and low-electrodermal responders, whereas only 11.5% were classified as high responders on both of these measures. Although the authors concluded that these data do not support the hypothesis that rape victims maintain a continuous, unremitting hyperaroused state, they noted a great deal of intersubject variability regarding psychophysiological responsivity. In turn, they suggested that the analogue conditions and choice of stimuli may have lowered physiological arousal.

In another of the first documented studies not employing military veterans, Davidson and Baum (1986) examined the relationship between chronic stress and PTSD symptomatology by comparing 52 randomly selected residents living within 5 miles of Three Mile Island (TMI) with 35 controls living approximately 80 miles away. Demographic information for the two groups was comparable for age, sex, education, and income, and the data were obtained nearly 5 years after the accident at the nuclear power station. Compared to the control subjects, the TMI neighbor residents were found to have significantly higher baseline values for HR (76.4 vs. 68.7 bpm), systolic blood pressure (125.4 vs. 117.7 mm Hg), and diastolic blood pressure (76.5 versus 71.9 mm Hg).

More recently, Blanchard, Hickling, and Taylor (1991) observed that the distinctive pattern of physiological responding documented in combat veterans was also seen in a small sample ($N = 4$) of individuals who received a diagnosis of PTSD subsequent to a motor vehicle accident (MVA). These individuals underwent a comparable laboratory procedure to that described by Pitman et al. (1987), with the image used being an idiosyncratic verbal description of the subject's MVA. The physiological measures were heart rate, blood pressure, and electrodermal activity.

Extrapolations from the graphs and figures presented show that three of the four subjects had a mean resting heart rate of less than 70 bpm, and one (as the authors documented) had a mean basal heart rate of 77 bpm. All four subjects were noted to have 10–15 bpm increases in heart rate to mental arithmetic, and three of the subjects had an average increase of 9.2 bpm in response to reminiscence of the traumatic event.

The authors reported that each subject showed an observable increase in SBP to at least one of the two MVA images, although only one subject showed an increase to both presentations. If one estimates from the graphic data, it appears that the mean SBP for the four subjects was about 124 mm Hg, during initial baseline around 126 mm Hg during the first MVA exposure, and about 127 mm Hg during the second exposure.

Because DBP and skin resistance level (SRL) measures were presented in tabular form, it was not necessary to extrapolate the means for these data. The authors concluded that DBP was overall less responsive to the MVA imagery; however, one subject was noted to increase DBP from 80.5 mm Hg during initial baseline to 110 mm Hg during the first MVA image. The mean initial baseline measure for all four subjects was 78.8 mm Hg, and the mean recording during the first MVA image was 88.7 mm Hg.

The same subject whose DBP responded so notably also evidenced a decrease in SRL from initial baseline to first MVA image of 19.97/1000Ω, to 8.50/1000Ω. Two of the subjects, however, evidenced almost no response at all. The mean initial baseline reading for the four subjects was 20.85/1000Ω, and the mean reading during the first MVA image was 16.2/1000Ω. Based on the overall results, the authors concluded that heart rate yielded the most reliable evidence of arousal to stimulus cues of traumatic events.

SUMMARY

The data from the laboratory studies reviewed above provide compelling evidence that psychophysiological measurement is a valuable implement in the assessment of PTSD. Although the results have generally shown better specificity than sensitivity in PTSD classification (Orr, 1990), the finding of autonomic responsiveness to stimuli reminiscent of combat has been so consistent and distinctive (Blanchard, 1990) that it has been accepted by the Veterans Administration (VA) as a diagnostic marker of PTSD (Gronvall, 1986, study cited in Blanchard, 1990). The results of a major multicenter study initiated nearly 7 years ago (Kolb & Keane, 1988) to discern and clarify these phenomenon are forthcoming (T. Keane, personal communication, August 29, 1994).

Though the majority of studies examining psychophysiological assessment of PTSD have utilized Vietnam veterans, it is clear that future development and validation of these methods needs to be adapted to individuals exposed to other sources of trauma, such as rape, natural disasters, or loss of a child. Given the paucity of current available data, such studies will enable researchers to investigate the similarities and differences of physiological manifestation that disparate victim groups portray across unique traumatic events.

Moreover, research on noncombat populations will provide a better opportunity to examine the potential differences in psychophysiological reactivity and emotional sequelae between men and women diagnosed with PTSD. As evidence of the efficacy of psychophysiological assessment in understanding the phenomenology and assisting in the diagnosis of PTSD continues to accrue, technological and methodological advances in physiological assessment may help discern whether an autonomic nervous system diathesis exists that somehow predisposes individuals to develop PTSD. Nevertheless, for the present it appears that psychophysiological assessment technologies do indeed yield valuable information concerning (a) the arousal dimension of the theorized two-factor constituency of PTSD and (b) the differential diagnosis of PTSD.

REFERENCES

Blanchard, E. B. (1990). Elevated basal levels of cardiovascular responses in Vietnam veterans with PTSD: A health problem in the making? *Journal of Anxiety Disorders, 4,* 233–237.

Blanchard, E. B., & Abel, G. G. (1976). An experimental case study of the biofeedback treatment of a rape-induced psychophysiological cardiovascular disorder. *Behavior Therapy, 7,* 113–119.

Blanchard, E. B., Hickling, E. J., & Taylor, A. E. (1991). The psychophysiology of motor vehicle accident related post-traumatic stress disorder. *Biofeedback and Self-Regulation, 16,* 449–458.

Blanchard, E. B., Kolb, L. C., Gerardi, R. J., Ryan, P., & Pallmeyer, T. P. (1986). Cardiac response to relevant stimuli as an adjunctive tool for diagnosing post-traumatic stress disorder in Vietnam veterans. *Behavior Therapy, 17,* 592–606.

Blanchard, E. B., Kolb, L. C., Pallmeyer, T. P., & Gerardi, R. J. (1982). A psychophysiological study of post-traumatic stress disorder in Vietnam veterans. *Psychiatric Quarterly, 54,* 220–229.

Blanchard, E. B., Kolb, L. C., & Prins, A. (1991). Psychophysiological responses in the diagnosis of post-traumatic stress disorder in Vietnam veterans. *Journal of Nervous and Mental Disease, 179,* 97–101.

Cannon, W. B. (1914). The emergency function of the adrenal medulla in pain and in the major emotions. *American Journal of Physiology, 33,* 356–372.

Davidson, L. M., & Baum, A. (1986). Chronic stress and post-traumatic stress disorders. *Journal of Consulting and Clinical Psychology, 54,* 303–308.

Dobbs, D., & Wilson, W. P. (1960). Observations on persistence of war neurosis. *Diseases of the Nervous System, 21,* 686–691.

Everly, G. S. (1989). *A clinical guide to the treatment of the human stress response.* New York: Plenum.

Gerardi, R. J., Blanchard, E. B., & Kolb, L. C. (1989). Ability of Vietnam veterans to dissimulate a psychophysiological assessment for post-traumatic stress disorder. *Behavior Therapy, 20,* 229–243.

Gillespie, R. D. (1942). *Psychological effects of war on citizen and soldier.* New York: Norton.

Gronvall, J. A. (1986). The vision of *Physician's Guide,* Veterans Administration Department of Medicine, Clinical Affairs, Chapter 20. Psychiatric Sequelae of Military Duty in a War Zone, 20.3(d).

Guyton, A. G. (1987). *Human physiology and mechanisms of disease* (4th ed.). Philadelphia: Saunders.

Kallman, W. M., & Feuerstein, M. J. (1986). Psychophysiological procedures. In A. R. Ciminero, K. S. Calhoun, & H. E. Adams (Eds.), *Handbook of behavioral assessment* (2nd ed., pp. 325–350). New York: Wiley.

Kardiner, A. (1941). The traumatic neuroses of war. *Psychosomatic Medicine Monographs,* 11–111.

Keane, T. M., Fairbank, J. A., Caddell, J. M., Zimering, R. T., & Bender, M. E. (1985). A behavioral approach to assessing and treating post-traumatic stress disorder in Vietnam veterans. In C. R. Figley, (Ed.), *Trauma and its wake* (pp. 257–294, and appendix A). New York: Brunner/Mazel.

Keane, T. M., Zimering, R. T., & Caddell, J. M. (1985). A behavioral formulation of post-traumatic stress disorder in Vietnam veterans. *Behavior Therapist, 8,* 9–12.

Kilpatrick, D. G., Best, C. L., Amick, A. E., & Veronen, L. J. (1984). *Psychophysiological assessment in the treatment of rape-induced anxiety.* Paper presented at the 18th annual convention of the Association for Advancement of Behavior Therapy, Philadelphia.

Kline, N. A., & Rausch, J. L. (1985). Olfactory precipitants of flashbacks in post-traumatic stress disorder: Case reports. *Journal of Clinical Psychiatry, 46,* 383–384.

Kolb, L. C. (1984). The post-traumatic stress disorders of combat: A subgroup with a conditioned emotional response. *Military Medicine, 149,* 237–243.

Kolb, L. C., & Keane, T. M. (1988). "*Physiology study of chronic post-traumatic stress disorder*" (Cooperative Studies Program No. 334). Washington, DC: Veterans Administration.

Lyons, J. A., Gerard, R. J., Wolfe, J., & Keane, T. M. (1988). Multidimensional assessement of combat-related PTSD: Phenomenological, psychometric, and psychophysiological considerations. *Journal of Traumatic Stress, 1,* 373–394.

Malloy, P. F., Fairbank, J. A., & Keane, T. M. (1983). Validation of a multimethod assessment of post-traumatic stress disorders in Vietnam veterans. *Journal of Consulting and Clinical Psychology, 51,* 488–494.

Mower, O. H. (1960). *Learning theory and behavior.* New York: Wiley.

Orr, S. P. (1990). Psychophysiologic studies of post-traumatic stress disorder. In E. L. Giller (Ed.), *Biological assessment and treatment of post-traumatic stress disorder* (pp. 137–157). Washington, DC: American Psychiatric Press.

Pallmeyer, T. P., Blanchard, E. B., & Kolb, L. C. (1986). The psychophysiology of combat-induced post-traumatic stress disorder in Vietnam veterans. *Behavior Research Therapy, 24,* 645–652.

Pitman, R. K., Orr, S. P., Forgue, D. F., de Jong, J. B., Claiborn, J. M. (1987). Psychophysiologic assessment of post-traumatic stress disorder imagery in Vietnam combat veterans. *Archives of General Psychiatry, 44,* 970–975.

Resnick, H. S., Kilpatrick, D. G., & Lipovsky, J. A. (1991). Assessment of rape-related post-traumatic stress disorder: Stressor and symptom dimensions. *Psychological Assessment: A Journal of Consulting and Clinical Psychology, 3,* 561–572.

Rychtarik, R. G., Silverman, W. K., Van Landingham, W. P., & Prue, D. M. (1984). Treatment of an incest victim with implosive therapy: A case study. *Behavioral Therapy, 15,* 410–420.

van der Kolk, B. A., & Greenberg, M. S. (1987). The psychobiology of the trauma response: Hyperarousal, constriction, and addiction to traumatic reexposure. In B. A. van der Kolk (Ed.), *Psychological trauma* (pp. 63–87). Washington, DC: American Psychiatric Press.

Wenger, M. A. (1948). Studies of autonomic balance in Army Air Forces personnel. *Comparative Psychology Monographs, 19*(Series No. 101), 1–111.

Wolfe, J., Keane, T. M., Lyons, J. A., & Gerardi, R. J. (1987). Current trends and issues in the assessment of combat-related post-traumatic stress disorder. *Behavior Therapist, 10,* 27–32.

9

Neuropsychology of PTSD

Problems, Prospects, and Promises

A. MacNEILL HORTON, JR.

Perhaps one of the most interesting descriptions of post-traumatic stress disorder (PTSD) was that presented in the short story "Soldiers Home," which was written by Ernest Hemingway following his return to the United States after serving in the Italian army during World War I. It is also intriguing, if not too speculative, to imagine that Hemingway's traumatic experiences during World War I may have played a major role in much of his later work. For example, such novels as *A Farewell to Arms* and *For Whom the Bell Tolls* both deal with war-related traumatic experiences. When one reflects that post-traumatic stress disorder can last for decades, the possibilities become particularly interesting.

Of course, although PTSD as a syndrome has been recognized since the time of Freud (1921), most empirical work only dates from the time of World War II (Everly, 1989). There is an interesting story (which may or may not be true) that General Douglas MacArthur first became cognizant of the problem when it was reported to him that he was losing more soldiers to "battle fatigue" than he was to the Japanese during the Pacific campaign. In the last decade, more recent work has attempted to formulate a definition of PTSD.

> The essential nature of this disorder is the development of characteristic symptoms following a psychologically distressing event that is outside the range of usual human experience (i.e., outside the range of such common

---

A. MacNEILL HORTON, JR. • Psych Associates, Towson, Maryland 21204.

Psychotraumatology, edited by George S. Everly, Jr. and Jeffrey M. Lating. Plenum Press, New York, 1995.

experiences as simply bereavement, chronic illness, business losses, and marital conflict). (APA 1987, p. 247)

This is the third and final chapter within the portion of this text dedicated to the assessment of post-traumatic stress (Part II). Chapter 7 addressed the assessment of the psychological domain, whereas Chapter 8 addressed the assessment of the psychophysiological arousal domain. Yet both chapters argued in support of a multidimensional assessment battery. In order to achieve this goal, the neuropsychological domain cannot be overlooked.

It is important to realize, as noted in Chapter 7, that there are a plethora of other psychiatric conditions that may parallel or exist phenomenologically subsequent to PTSD. For example, anxiety and depression may be associated with PTSD to such a degree that concomitant diagnoses may be made. In addition, there may be symptoms that are suggestive of an organic mental disorder or an adjustment disorder (APA, 1987); in an adjustment disorder, however, the stressor usually is within the range of common experience. There may also be alcohol or drug abuse to the point that psychoactive substance abuse disorder could be diagnosed (Keane, Gerardi, Lyons, & Wolfe, 1988). In addition, social problems such as marital instability and difficulties with work behaviors can be noted (APA, 1987). Others have suggested that there may be a biological or neuropsychological foundation of PTSD (Kolb, 1987). Indeed, some workers in this area have postulated that PTSD is a disorder of arousal (Everly, 1990). Should neuropsychological factors be involved in PTSD, than careful assessment should be able to identify them in a reliable fashion.

The purpose of this chapter is to discuss the use of neuropsychological assessment in PTSD. As noted by others (Wolfe, Keane, Lyons, & Gerardi, 1987), PTSD is a particularly complex problem that will require the use of comprehensive evaluation procedures to assess it. In addition, a number of workers in this field (Everly & Horton, 1989; Wolfe & Charney, 1991) believe that it is important to assess neuropsychological status in PTSD. Though perhaps the most popular and helpful models of PTSD have been based on behavioral conceptualizations (Keane, Zimering, & Caddell, 1985), other workers have suggested that information processing, physiological, and psychobiological perspectives could be quite helpful in terms of unraveling PTSD (Wolfe & Charney, 1991). The perspective of this chapter in some ways follows the earlier conceptualization of Wolfe and Charney (1991) who identify three major issues that need to be considered in discussing the use of neuropsychological assessment in PTSD. This particular chapter will perhaps, however, treat these three areas with a somewhat different emphasis. In a very oversimplified manner, it might be said that the three perspectives reflect the hypothesized relationships between PTSD and neuropsychological impairment.

Simply put, patterns of causation or relationship between PTSD and neuropsychological impairment are the building blocks around which this chapter has been constructed. Three possible relationships are proposed. The first postulate would be that PTSD can cause neuropsychological impairment; this might be reflected in a simple equation of PTSD = NPI. The second postulate is the null version of the first; that is, PTSD does not cause neuropsychological impairment, or PTSD ≠ NPI. Nonetheless this postulate suggests that an information processing perspective could be useful in terms of understanding PTSD (see Wolfe & Charney, 1991). The third postulate simply proposes that the two conditions may coexist in a noninteracting fashion—that PTSD can coexist with neuropsychological impairment, or PTSD + NPI. A motor vehicle accident, for example, could result in a significant degree of head trauma (and thus concentration, memory, and concept formation/abstraction difficulties directly related to the head trauma) as well as PTSD (Horton, 1993).

POSTULATE 1: POST-TRAUMATIC STRESS DISORDER CAUSES NEUROPSYCHOLOGICAL IMPAIRMENT

Perhaps the most well-articulated rationale for a neuropsychological hypothesis for PTSD was that advanced by Kolb (1987). Kolb noted that the conditioned fear symptoms and hyperactivity noted in animals that had been uncontrollably shocked were remarkably similar to the physiological and behavioral symptoms of combat veterans with chronic PTSD. The suggestion, then, was that PTSD was a result of a classical conditioning paradigm. Kolb (1987) was particularly concerned with the fact that environmental experiences may provide sensory stimulation that influences the functional and anatomical development of the brain. He noted a number of conditions where the failure to provide certain sensory input would result in a developmentally impaired state in lower animals.

Indeed, Kolb went to the point of suggesting that excessive external stimulation might actually have effects at the neuronal level. He used the relatively straightforward example of the extreme stimulation of the auditory system at rock concerts, where individuals who sit close to the amplified speakers may suffer measurable hearing loss. If the sound intensity is too high or too frequent, then the hearing loss may be permanent. Similarly, individuals are warned that looking into the sun for long periods of time could cause deterioration of the optic system.

> The primary result of excessive emotional stimulation is its effect on the function and perhaps the structure of the cortical neuronal barrier, particularly as it concerns control of aggressivity. Such stimulus overload occurs when the human organism's capacity to process information signaling threat

> to life overwhelms the cortical defensive structural processes concerned with perceptual discrimination and effective adaptive responses for survival. (Kolb, 1987, p. 993)

Kolb (1987) goes on to suggest that this emotional stimulation, if continued at high intensity and repeated multiple times, may lead to the depression of synaptic processes and thus impair perception and learning. Moreover, he postulates that "the neuronal synaptic structures affected are probably located in the temporal-amygdaloid complex concerned with agonistic behavior; these structures are stressed by recurrent intense stimulation. They may recover, be temporarily impaired, or undergo permanent change, which is known to occur in the peripheral (acoustic) sensory system" (p. 993). Kolb also notes a possible role for lower brain stem structures, such as the medial hypothalamic nuclei and the locus coeruleus. He goes on to suggest that

> the hypothesis presented here of functional change in neuronal and synaptic cortical processing of intense memories of aversive stimulation allows an understanding of the variegated symptom expressions of the condition. We may define the symptoms of PTSD as 1) impaired perceptual, cognitive, and affective functions; 2) release of functions; 3) reactive affective states and avoidant behaviors; and 4) restitutive symptoms and behaviors. (p. 994)

Wolfe and Charney (1991) cover a similar train of thought in terms of outlining a model of the psychobiology of PTSD. Like Kolb, they suggest that severe uncontrollable stress triggers a primary emotional response that is followed by rapid classical conditioning. Also, neuronal changes are postulated to impair ability to learn and to self-regulate emotions. Wolfe and Charney (1991) further suggest that a number of neurotransmitter and neuropeptide systems can be implicated; these pathways may include the noradrenergic, dopaminergic, serotonergic, benzodiazepine, opioid, and hypothalamic-pituitary-adrenal systems. Rather straightforwardly, it is hypothesized that certain symptoms of PTSD may be related to changes in specific neurotransmitter systems. For example, certain types of symptoms may be related to serotonin functions, and the use of a medication that works on the serotonergic system (e.g., Prozac) might be particularly efficacious.

A reformulation of Kolb's viewpoint has been advanced by Everly (1989), whose view of a "neurological hypersensitivity phenomenon" suggests a different perspective. Everly (1990) postulates that high-intensity neural stimulation leads to a subsequent hypersensitivity for neurological excitation within the limbic circuitry, and that this heightened sensitivity can cause a variety of types of psychological disturbance. One of these types, obviously, would include PTSD.

Everly's hypothesis would be consistent with dysfunction of brain structures that play a major role in memory (i.e., the hippocampus). Thus it may be suggested that PTSD may represent a classic "physioneurosis" consisting of anatomical and physiological neuronal transformations that serve as a basis for hypersensitivity and subsequent extraordinary neuronal excitivity. Everly (1989) similarly suggests that the condition of neuronal excitability might be found in the locus-coeruleus-born noradrenergic projections of the septal-hippocampal-amygdalar regions of the limbic system.

A logical extension of Everly's hypothesis would be that PTSD patients may show memory impairment, although clinical experience and other data (Dalton, Pederson & Ryan, 1988) have not provided evidence for widespread neuropsychological dysfunction over a number of cognitive domains in PTSD patients. Everly and Horton (1989) conducted a study to address this issue. They administered the four-word short-term memory test (Ryan & Butters, 1980)—a modification of the Peterson paradigm, which is well known in experimental psychology—to 14 patients who had been diagnosed as having PTSD. Everly and Horton (1989) note that

> the four-word short-term memory test requires the examiner to read four unrelated words and then say a three-digit number. The patient counts backwards by 3's from the three-digit number for an interval of 15 or 30 seconds. At the end of the interval, the patient repeats the to-be-remembered material. Typically, five trials equally divided between the two time intervals are administered. The score is a percentage of total words correctly recalled. (p. 808)

The results suggested possible neuropsychological impairment; 12 out of 14 patients were impaired on one of two criteria utilized in the investigation. As noted by Everly and Horton (1989), these data essentially support the hypothesis that PTSD patients may possess a cognitive deficit that is manifested as an impairment in short-term memory functioning. (long-term memory functioning in these patients appeared to be unimpaired). Other studies have suggested that memory dysfunction and concentration difficulties may be associated with PTSD (Brett, Spitzer, & Williams, 1988; Fairbank, Keane, & Malloy, 1983; Silver & Iacono, 1984). Sutker, Galina, West, and Allain (1990) tested a number of former prisoners of war from the Korean conflict and World War II on a selective battery of neuropsychological measures of intelligence and memory; they found that even when the possible effect of malnutrition was controlled for, prisoners of war differed from control subjects on measures of immediate memory recall.

Although available data are admittedly preliminary and do not clearly confirm the hypotheses, as noted by Everly and Horton (1989), neither do the data disconfirm the hypotheses. Thus it will be necessary to develop additional research to address the question of PTSD producing neuropsychological impairment. Because the best evidence available suggests that neuropsychological impairment in PTSD is not widespread, and very specialized neuropsychological measures may be necessary to elucidate the subtle memory dysfunction that has been postulated to exist in PTSD patients (Everly & Horton, 1989).

POSTULATE 2: PTSD DOES NOT CAUSE NEUROPSYCHOLOGICAL IMPAIRMENT, BUT NEUROPSYCHOLOGICAL ASSESSMENT CAN BE HELPFUL

This particular suggestion rests for the most part on very elaborate models of information processing that have recently entered neuropsychology from cognitive psychology. To a large extent, this information-processing perspective is largely drawn from the experimental psychology literature. Wolfe and Charney (1991) suggest that information processing may provide conceptual models for PTSD and will help elucidate cognitive processes in the initiation and continuance of PTSD symptoms. They note that "one cornerstone of the information processing model in anxiety disorders is the establishment of affectively-charged semantic memory network that preferentially processes trauma or threat-related stimuli and may directly contribute to the persistence of symptomatology" (p. 576).

Wolfe and Charney go on to say that the type and quality of information processing may determine the functional presentation of PTSD symptoms. They argue that although classical conditioning can account for the general physiological responding to PTSD, the exact timing and character of response to specific stimuli is better explained by information-processing models. For example, although it is understandable that a patient might be sensitized to stimuli directly related to combat, it is less clear when they will present symptoms to objects or stimuli that are fairly far removed from the specific situation within which they were classically conditioned. The information-processing model provides a way of understanding the nature and quality of informational representations in the cerebral cortex that would explain the riddles of the precise frequency and duration of PTSD symptoms. Also, Wolfe and Charney (1991) feel that both the enduring nature of some PTSD symptoms and the function of memory in PTSD may be best explained through an information-processing model.

As has been well articulated (Tulving, 1983), there are multiple memory systems in the human brain. Traditional dichotomies of short-term and long-term memory have since given way to suggestions of episodic/semantic and procedural/implicit memory dichotomies. Perhaps one of the most exciting recent developments, however, has been that of the theoretical understanding of implicit memory (Schacter, 1992). Whereas explicit memory involves intentional and conscious recollection and retention of information, implicit memory is an unintentional, unconscious form of recollection; simply put, it does not depend on the awareness of the subject that he or she has stores of memory. Indeed, tests of implicit memory require special conditions that do not rely on the subjects' awareness of the to-be-recalled information. Experiments in the future may more fully elucidate where and which types of symptoms of PTSD lie in explicit memory, as well as which symptoms or understandings or types of information processing may be subserved by implicit memory. Interestingly, Wolfe and Charney (1991) suggest that studies of such "higher order" tests as the Stroop Color and Word Test (Golden, 1976) have demonstrated "subtle cognitive processing change in traumatized patients in a manner that differentiates from the performance of normal inpatients with general anxiety disorders" (p. 577).

POSTULATE 3: PTSD MAY COEXIST WITH NEUROPSYCHOLOGICAL IMPAIRMENT

As also noted by Wolfe and Charney (1991), there may be interactions between psychological and physical components of trauma that are of particular interest. Simply put, it is entirely possible that a patient may have had a minor head injury (Davidoff, Kessler, Laidstain, & Mark, 1988) or a toxic disorder (Silverman, Hart, Stockman, & Hammer, 1989) whereby both PTSD and clear neurological insult coexist. The study by Sutker, Galina, West, and Allain (1990) mentioned earlier—wherein prisoners of war from the Korean conflict and World War II were assessed—is an example of a situation where central nervous system impairment in patients with PTSD could have been attributable to a physical cause (in this case, malnutrition). Neurological insult that may coexist with PTSD may come from a variety of causes: traumatic brain injury, toxic disorders, malnutrition, and possibly others. The challenge is to sort out the specific parameters of the patient's problem.

It might be noted, however, that some clinicians have asserted that it is not possible for a patient both to have PTSD and to suffer head trauma (Sbordone, 1991). Rather, it is suggested that if a person has lost consciousness, then PTSD is not possible; but if there is no loss of consciousness, then the person would not have had head trauma. Put another way, if a person has loss of consciousness or amnesia, it is not possible for the PTSD to develop from that single event. At the same time, however, other traumatic events associated with a motor vehicle accident (or head trauma that results from such an accident) could produce PTSD; for example, finding out that a loved one had died in the accident (Sbordone, 1991). A condition for the PTSD to develop, of course, is that the traumatic event would fall outside the range of retrograde or anterograde amnesia.

A contrary viewpoint (Horton, 1993) is that conditions of PTSD and head trauma could coexist because each involves different brain areas. Head trauma would most likely involve cortical structures, whereas PTSD would be hypothesized to involve subcortical structures (Everly & Horton, 1989). Indeed, a case documented in England (McMillan, 1991) appeared to suggest that there was both severe head trauma and PTSD in a motor vehicle accident. Similarly, in a recent case in the United States, a patient was found to have both mild head injury and PTSD (Horton, 1993). In the American case, the patient was referred for treatment of PTSD; only after behavior-therapy techniques had caused the PTSD symptoms to abate was the neuropsychological impairment identified. The neuropsychological deficits improved over a 2-year follow-up period, but PTSD symptoms did not return (Horton, 1993).

NEUROPSYCHOLOGICAL ASSESSMENT OF PTSD

It might be suggested that given the likelihood of overlooking mild head trauma or other organic conditions (Bennett & Curiel, 1988), neuropsychological assessment is indicated in all cases of PTSD where there is even a remote possibility of concurrent psychiatric or neurological conditions. There are a number of important issues to consider in terms of planning for neuropsychological assessment of patients who may have PTSD. Some of these relate to general assessment issues in PTSD (Wolfe et al., 1987); at this point in time, it is well accepted that PTSD requires a comprehensive multiaxial approach to assessment (Keane, Wolfe, & Taylor, 1987).

It has been averred that the comprehensive assessment of PTSD is twofold: that is, it involves both the assessment of symptoms and experiences related to PTSD and the assessment of possible coexisting psychological disorders (Keane et al., 1987). Perhaps the most frequently used approaches have included (a) structured clinical interviews, (b) behavioral and psychophysiological assessment, (c) psychometric assessment (MMPI, etc.), (d) therapist ratings and the use of reports from significant others and available files and records (i.e., military duties and accident reports; Keane et al., 1987). Such a comprehensive multiaxial approach is necessary because there are a number of factors that can cloud or mimic the picture of PTSD symptoms. Among these variables are premorbid adjustment, developmental history, and the existence of concurrent clinical syndromes (Wolfe et al., 1987).

It might be suggested that neuropsychological assessment contributes to the comprehensive multiaxial assessment of PTSD by both identifying concentration and memory problems caused by PTSD and assessing neuropathology and its neuropsychological effects (which may not be attributable to PTSD). First and foremost there is the concern that the patient may have associated neurological conditions that may or may not be related to the stressor experience (e.g., head trauma from a motor vehicle accident).

As suggested by Wolfe and Charney (1991), such assessments might include the Wisconsin Card Sorting Test (Lezak, 1983), the Stroop Color and Word Test (Golden, 1976), or the Trail Making Test (Reitan, 1958). The Wisconsin Card Sorting Test is often used as a measure of nonverbal concept formation (Horton & Wedding, 1984). The Stroop Color and Word Test is thought of as a measure of cognitive flexibility (Horton & Wedding, 1984).The Trail Making Test assesses visual scanning, motor functioning, perceptual ability, and the ability to rapidly shift psychological sets (Horton & Wedding, 1984). As a group, they form a fairly effective neuropsychological screening battery. These tests should be used, of course, in the context of a comprehensive multiaxial assessment approach, as outlined earlier (Keane et al., 1987; Wolfe et al., 1987).

In addition, if one accepts the notion that PTSD is likely to have a subcortical locus in the brain, the use of specialized memory testing using the Peterson paradigm (Everly & Horton, 1989; Ryan & Butters, 1980) would appear warranted. Very sensitive measurement of attention and concentration skills could also be accomplished with the Paced Auditory Serial Addition Task (Gronwall, 1977). Indeed, in some very complex cases where there is the clear possibility of psychiatric and/or neurological complications, the use of an entire Halstead-Reitan Neuropsychological Test Battery (Reitan & Wolfson, 1993) with supplemental memory, attention, and concentration testing could well be justified.

SUMMARY

This chapter has discussed the role of neuropsychological testing in PTSD. After a brief review of the symptoms of PTSD, three perspectives or models of PTSD and neuropsychological impairment were outlined. The first postulate is that PTSD can cause neuropsychological impairment, or PTSD = NPI. The second postulate is the null version of the first; that is, PTSD does not cause neuropsychological impairment, or PTSD ≠ NPI. The third postulate simply proposes that the two conditions may coexist in a noninteracting fashion, an idea that can be symbolically represented as PTSD + NPI. Each of these perspectives was discussed in turn. In addition, some suggestions for neuropsychological assessment of PTSD were briefly outlined. It is thought that a neuropsychological perspective will prove to be quite valuable as researchers and clinicians attempt to understand further the complex nature of PTSD and to devise more effective diagnostic strategies and treatment procedures. The hope and expectation is that this chapter will be of some aid in these very difficult tasks.

REFERENCES

American Psychiatric Association. (1987). *Diagnostic and statistical manual of mental disorders (rev. 3rd ed.).* Washington, DC: Author.

Bennett, T. L., & Curiel, M. P. (1988). Complex partial seizures presenting as psychiatric illness: A case study. *International Journal of Clinical Neuropsychology, 10,* 41–44.

Brett, E. A., Spitzer, R. L., & Williams, J. B. W. (1988). DSM-III-R criteria for post-traumatic stress disorder. *American Journal of Psychiatry, 145,* 1232–1236.

Dalton, J. E., Pederson, S. L., & Ryan, J. J. (1988). Effects of PTSD on neuropsychological test performance. *Bulletin of the National Academy of Neuropsychologists, 5,* 44–45.

Davidoff, D. A., Kessler, H. R., & Laidstain, D. F., & Mark, V. H. (1988). Neurobehavioral sequelae of minor head injuries: A consideration of post-traumatic syndrome versus post-traumatic stress disorder. *Cognitive Rehabilitation, 6,* 8–13.

Everly, G. S. (1989). *A clinical guide to the treatment of the human stress response.* New York: Plenum.

Everly, G. S. (1990). Post-traumatic stress disorder as a disorder of arousal. *Psychology and Health, 4,* 135–145.

Everly, G. S., & Horton, A. M., Jr. (1989). Neuropsychology of post-traumatic stress disorder: A pilot study. *Perceptual and Motor Skills, 68,* 807–810.

Fairbank, J. A., Keane, T. M., & Malloy, P. F. (1983). Some preliminary data on psychological characteristics of Vietnam veterans with post-traumatic stress disorder. *Journal of Consulting and Clinical Psychology, 51,* 912–919.

Freud, S. (1921). Foreword. In S. Ferenczi et al. (Eds.), *Psychoanalysis war neurosis.* New York: International Psychoanalytic Press.

Golden, C. J. (1976). Identification of brain disorders by the Stroop Color and Word Test. *Journal of Clinical Psychology, 32,* 621–626.

Gronwall, D. (1977). Paced auditory serial addition task: A measure of recovery from concussion. *Perceptual and Motor Skills, 44,* 367–373.

Horton, A. M., Jr. (1993). Post-traumatic stress disorder and mild head trauma: Follow-up of a case study. *Perceptual and Motor Skills, 76,* 243–246.

Horton, A. M., Jr., & Wedding, D. (1984). *Clinical and behavioral neuropsychology.* New York: Praeger.

Keane, T. M., Gerardi, R. J., Lyons, J. A., & Wolfe, J. (1988). The interrelationship of substance abuse and PTSD: Epidemiological and clinical considerations. In M. Galanter (Ed.), *Recent developments in alcoholism* (Vol. 6). New York: Plenum.

Keane, T. M., Wolfe, J., & Taylor, K. L. (1987). Post-traumatic stress disorder: Evidence for diagnostic validity and methods of psychological assessment. *Journal of Clinical Psychology, 43*(1), 32–43.

Keane, T. M., Zimering, R. T., & Caddell, J. M. (1985). A behavioral formulation of the post-traumatic stress disorder in Vietnam veterans. *Behavior Therapist, 8,* 9–12.

Kolb, L. C. (1987). A neuropsychological hypothesis explaining post-traumatic stress disorder. *American Journal of Psychiatry, 114,* 989–995.

Lezak, M. D. (1983). *Neuropsychological assessment* (2nd ed.). New York: Oxford University Press.

McMillan, T. M. (1991). Post-traumatic stress disorder and severe head injury. *British Journal of Psychiatry, 159,* 431–433.

Reitan, R. M. (1958). Validity of the Trail Making Test as an indicator of organic brain damage. *Perceptual and Motor Skills, 8,* 271–276.

Reitan, R. M., & Wolfson, D. (1993). *The Halstead-Reitan Neuropsychological Test Battery: Theory and clinical interpretation* (2nd ed.). Tucson, AZ: Neuropsychology Press.

Ryan, C., & Butters, N. (1980). Learning and memory impairment in young and old alcoholics: Evidence for the premature aging hypothesis. *Alcoholism, 4,* 190–198.

Sbordone, R. J. (1991). *Neuropsychology for the attorney.* Orlando, FL: Deutsch.

Schacter, D. L. (1992). Understanding implicit memory: A cognitive neuroscience approach. *American Psychologist, 47,* 559–569.

Silver, S. M., & Iacono, C. U. (1984). Factor analytic support for DSM-III's post-traumatic stress disorder for Vietnam veterans. *Journal of Clinical Psychology, 44,* 5–14.

Silverman, J. J., Hart, R. P., Stockman, S. J., & Hammer, R. M. (1989). 18-month follow-up on neuropsychiatric effects of pentaborane intoxication. *Journal of Traumatic Stress, 2,* 463–476.

Sutker, P. B., Galina, Z. H., West, J. A., & Allain, A. N. (1990). Trauma-induced weight loss and cognitive deficits among former prisoners of war. *Journal of Consulting and Clinical Psychology, 58,* 323–328.

Tulving, E. (1983). *Elements of episodic memory.* Oxford, England: Oxford University Press.

Wolfe, J., & Charney, D. S. (1991). Use of neuropsychological assessment in post-traumatic stress disorder. *Psychological Assessment, 3,* 573–580.

Wolfe, J., Keane, T. M., Lyons, J. A., & Gerardi, R. J. (1987). Current trends and issues in assessment of PTSD. *Behavior Therapist, 10,* 27–32.

III

Treatment of Post-Traumatic Stress

In addressing the phenomenology of post-traumatic stress and its epiphenomenon PTSD, this text has attempted to provide not only an amalgam of microanalyses but also an overarching construct, or macroanalytic perspective, on the nature of post-traumatic stress within which more detailed microanalyses may derive greater coherency. Part III will follow the same tack as it addresses the issue of the treatment of post-traumatic stress.

In Chapter 10, Everly embraces the posited two-factor model of post-traumatic stress introduced in Chapter 3 and employs it, once again, as a potentially unifying construct within which to view virtually all forms of post-traumatic therapy. The chapter introduces neurocognitive therapy as an integrating *metatherapeutic strategy* within which various diverse and specific therapeutic tactics may be marshalled for consideration and subsequent employment. The neurocognitive framework may then be used to gain further insight into subsequent chapters.

In Chapter 11, Friedman reviews biological therapeutic interventions and, in doing so, addresses the neurological-hypersensitivity aspect of the two-factor neurocognitive model. In Chapter 12, van der Hart et al. provide an elegant review of the work of pioneer psychotraumatologist Pierre Janet, as well as rich insight into the psychological-hypersensitivity concept. Brende in Chapter 13 presents a therapeutic process anchored in the legacy of the 12-step models but applied to post-traumatic stress; it also introduces the spiritual aspects of healing.

In Chapter 14, Horowitz and Kaltreider describe how brief therapy principles may be applied to post-traumatic stress. This chapter, though originally published in 1979, represents a classic therapeutic formulation heralding two important forthcoming events in psychiatry: the formal recognition of post-traumatic stress disorder and the rise in popularity of brief psychotherapeutic interventions. Finally, Chapter 15, by Ochberg, represents a well-constructed integrative and multidimensional approach to the treatment of post-traumatic stress. Ochberg's post-traumatic therapy implicitly embraces some of the tenets of the holistic health movement of the late 1970s, but it applies them within a post-traumatic framework.

10

The Neurocognitive Therapy of Post-Traumatic Stress

A Strategic Metatherapeutic Approach

GEORGE S. EVERLY, JR.

It was Kurt Lewin who said, "There is nothing so practical as a good theory." The present instance provides the opportunity for the value of theory to be demonstrated. The two-factor phenomenological formulation of post-traumatic stress introduced in Chapter 3 yields a natural corollary: a two-factor therapeutic approach to the treatment of post-traumatic stress. The purpose of this chapter is to introduce such a two-factor metatherapy.

A TWO-FACTOR NEUROCOGNITIVE THERAPY

It has been proposed that post-traumatic stress and its epiphenomenon post-traumatic stress disorder (PTSD) have as their foundational phenomenological base a core two-factor constituency (Everly, 1992, 1993). That constituency consists of (a) a neurological hypersensitivity (i.e., a pathognomonic status of and/or propensity for excessive subcortical CNS, autonomic, and neuroendocrine neurological arousal; Everly, 1990), and (b) a psychological hypersensitivity (i.e., a trauma-initiated contradiction to the individual's worldview pertaining to safety, security, and/or the perception of self, and

---

GEORGE S. EVERLY, JR. • International Critical Incident Stress Foundation, Ellicott City, Maryland 21042; Union Memorial Hospital, Baltimore, Maryland 21218; Department of Psychology, Loyola College, Baltimore, Maryland 21210.

Psychotraumatology, edited by George S. Everly, Jr. and Jeffrey M. Lating. Plenum Press, New York, 1995.

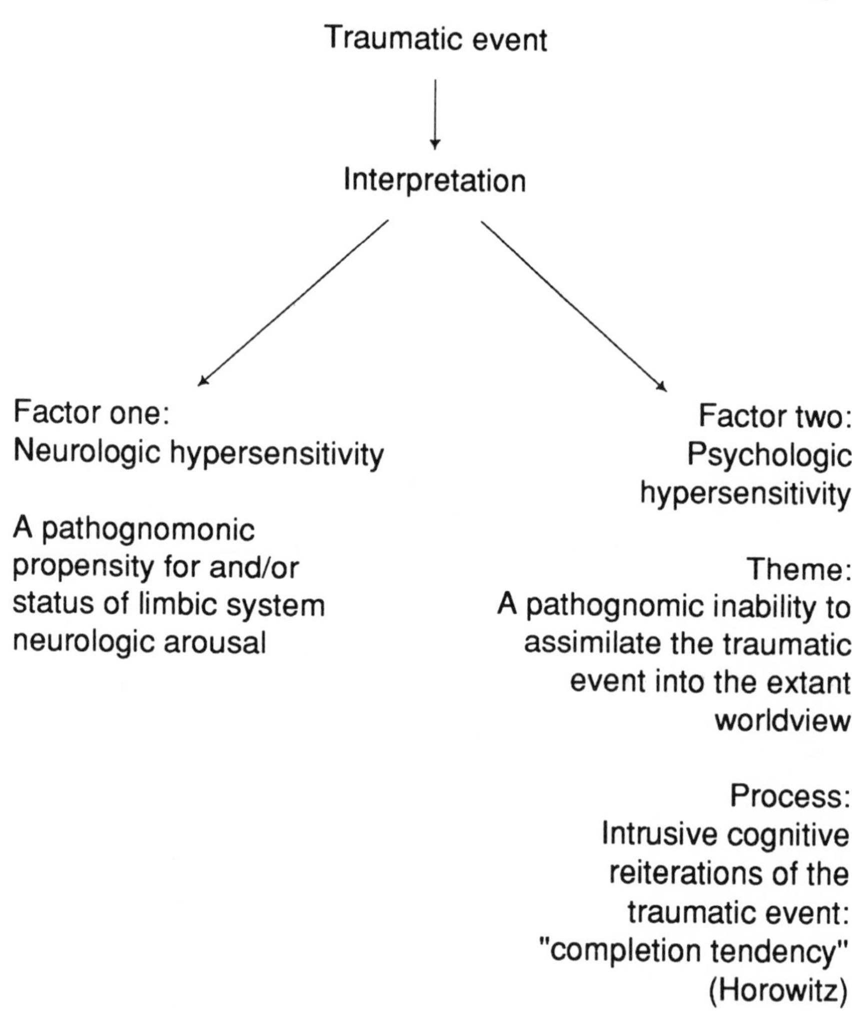

Figure 10.1 A two-factor formulation of post-traumatic stress

the inability of the individual to assimilate that trauma into the extant worldview despite a natural reiterative cognitive propensity to gain convergence) (see Horowitz, 1986). This phenomenological model is shown in Figure 10.1. If, indeed, therapy is the natural corollary of phenomenology, then it seems reasonable that a two-factor therapeutic formulation might also emerge.

Neurocognitive therapy is a therapeutic approach based on a recognition of the two pathognomonic factors at work in post-traumatic stress syndromes and on the notion that both factors need to be explicitly or implicitly addressed in successful therapy (*neuro-* referring to factor one, and *cognitive-* to factor two).

NEUROCOGNITIVE THERAPY AS A METATHERAPY

As used in the present context, *metatherapy* refers to an overarching, amalgamating therapeutic construct. I use the term here to indicate that neurocognitive therapy represents a strategic therapy formulation as opposed to a tactical set of specific therapeutic guidelines. The essence of neurocognitive therapy is simply that the most effective therapeutic formulations will be those that strategically address both of the pathognomonic factors of post-traumatic stress. Yet because neurocognitive therapy stops short of dictating specific therapeutic tactics, it remains a strategic formulation process (i.e., a metatherapy). The specific tactical therapeutic interventions may vary from patient to patient, depending upon the idiosyncratic needs of the patient and the preference/orientation of the therapist. Such an approach to therapy is consonant with the extant integrative-psychotherapy movement (Norcross & Goldfried, 1992).

TREATMENT OF NEUROLOGICAL HYPERSENSITIVITY: NEUROLOGICAL DESENSITIZATION

Everly (1990) has argued that PTSD and post-traumatic stress in general should be considered "disorders of arousal," and van der Kolk (1988) has viewed PTSD as a pathological manifestation of an inability to modulate arousal. It seems clear that post-traumatic stress represents a pathognomonic hypersensitivity residing within the subcortical limbic circuitry. This hypersensitivity may be conceived of as a lowered functional threshold for depolarization of neurons within the limbic system and its immediate neurological and neuroendocrine effector mechanisms. The natural corollary of this recognition would be that successful treatment of post--traumatic stress depends on a first step of neurological desensitization—that is, reducing the pathognomonic status of neurological hypersensitivity.

Numerous therapeutic interventions are available to achieve neurological desensitization. Several are reviewed below:

1. Removing the individual from stressful, overstimulating conditions is an important first step in therapy. Occupationally, this might mean "light duty" or "leave" status for a brief period of time if the trauma is related to (or if recollections of the trauma are engendered by) the work environment. Reduction or elimination of sympathomimetic substances (e.g., caffeine, theobromine, and related stimulants) is highly recommended.

2. Catharsis is initially encouraged. Clearly, there are few if any emotional disorders that do not benefit from catharsis (Heider, 1974). There is evidence that catharsis not only serves as a cognitive purging technique (Bettleheim, 1984) but initiates autonomic nervous system recovery after

excitation (Kahn, 1966; Pennebaker & Susman, 1988). Catharsis should not be seen as an end unto itself, however, lest it resensitize the individual.

3. Behavioral interventions that engender a "relaxation response" may prove highly useful in reducing neurological hypersensitivity.

Weil (1974) and Gellhorn (1958, 1964, 1965) both argue from a physiological perspective on psychiatric disorders that although the brain's neurology can be behaviorally altered into a dysfunctional, pathogenic status (see Chapter 3), it can also be altered so as to correct pathognomonic status. Weil (1974) discusses four mechanisms by which the brain's "tranquilizing system" (primarily the limbic system) may be facilitated and relaxation/restoration experienced:

- Reduction of the intensity of stimulus (exteroceptive, interoceptive, and proprioceptive) bombardment (e.g., via relaxation techniques)
- Reduction of the rate of stimulus bombardment (e.g., selective/focused attention)
- A shift from stimulus specificity to stimulus nonspecificity (e.g., sensory deprivation)
- Deep tactile pressure (e.g., massage)

Weil argues that these mechanisms act primarily through reticular, hypothalamic, and upper limbic structures and processes.

Gellhorn appears in agreement with Weil but is far more specific in his analyses. Gellhorn (1964) states "that states of abnormal emotional tension are alleviated in various 'relaxation' therapies through reducing proprioceptive impulses which impinge on the posterior hypothalamus and maintain the cerebral cortex in an abnormal state of excitation" (p. 457). More specifically, Gellhorn (1958) cogently argues that neuromuscular relaxation techniques (those designed to reduce skeletal muscle tension) can be effective methods of reducing the ergotropic tone of the limbic and hypothalamic nuclei. In other words, neuromuscular relaxation training techniques can be used effectively to lower hypothalamic excitability.

Herbert Benson (1983) has written extensively on what he calls the "relaxation response"—a hypometabolic response capable of being engendered by a wide and diverse variety of relaxation techniques. The relaxation response appears to gain its therapeutic effectiveness from several factors: (a) its ability to reduce catecholaminergic reactivity, (b) its ability to reduce neuromuscular tone, (c) its ability to interrupt cognitive ruminations, and (d) its ability to engender a sense of self-efficacy/self-control (see Everly & Benson, 1989, for a review).

It should be noted that according to Wilson (1989), PTSD has as key elements of its pathological constituency increased catecholaminergic reactivity, increased neuromuscular tension, cognitive ruminations, and a diminished sense of self-control. Thus we see, at least theoretically, that the use of the relaxation response should prove to be an almost ideal strategy for the treatment of PTSD.

Evidence has failed to demonstrate that there is one best technique to engender the relaxation response; therefore, therapists should employ the techniques that are most likely to be of value on a case-by-case basis. Such techniques as biofeedback may prove of value to individuals who have a high susceptibility to boredom and/or who need to see their therapy "quantified." Imagery and mantra meditation, in contrast, may be quite useful for patients who are more cognitively flexible (without having schizoidal or psychotic propensities) and can more readily harness their own imagination in a positive manner. Special note of the value of breathing techniques in reducing ergotropic tone and manifest arousal (Everly, 1989) should be made here.

Regardless of the relaxation technology employed, Benson (1983) noted that "the relaxation response results in physiological changes which are thought to characterize an integrated hypothalamic function. These physiological changes are consistent with generalized decreased sympathetic nervous system activity" (p. 212). Interestingly, Gellhorn and Loofbourrow (1963) noted more than three decades ago that "if it were possible to alter the autonomic reactivity at the hypothalamic level important therapeutic results might be obtained" (p. 90). It now seems clear that such an effect or its approximation is indeed attainable, and that it is attainable on the basis of behavioral interventions. Hoffman et al. (1982) have generated compelling evidence that regular practice in hypometabolic self-regulatory training (e.g., meditation) works to dampen sympathetic nervous hypersensitivity and hyperfunction at the level of the target organ. It may be that some form of down-regulation of excitatory receptors is engendered by consistent practice of the relaxation response, thus achieving the desired neurological desensitization.

4. Psychotropic medications may serve a valuable function in the neurological desensitization of PTSD. Medications such as benzodiazepines, certain antidepressants, and especially certain anticonvulsants may achieve neurological desensitization (Everly, 1989). A discussion of those agents is not the focus of this chapter; such discussion appears elsewhere in this volume (see Chapter 11). Yet it is worth noting that for some PTSD patients, psychotropic medication may be less than effective or desirable. Similarly, medication does little to engender a sense of self-efficacy. Thus it may be that in some cases the use of behavioral interventions that reduce arousal and foster neurological desensitization can be used to augment the usual course of psychotropic medication, or to facilitate recovery without the aid of psycho-

Table 10.1 Methods for Neurological Desensitization

1. Reducing environmental stimulation
2. Catharsis
3. Relaxation response training
4. Psychotropic medications

tropic medications. Clearly, however, there will be instances where psychotropic medication will be a necessary aspect of the treatment of PTSD, especially in the most severe of cases.

Table 10.1 lists the four interventions discussed above for the achievement of neurological desensitization.

TREATMENT OF PSYCHOLOGICAL HYPERSENSITIVITY: COGNITIVE INTERVENTION AND THE WELTANSCHAUUNG

So far it has been argued that some form of neurological desensitization is a useful first step in the treatment of post-traumatic stress. Neurological desensitization, though, will seldom exert enough of a therapeutic impact to remove all of the patient's symptomatoloy. Consistent with the two-factor model, psychotherapeutic intervention addressing the posited contradiction to the Weltanschauung (worldview) seems required. The pathognomonic contradiction to the worldview may take form in (a) a contradiction to the safety/security assumptions about the world itself (Bowlby, 1969; Everly, 1992; Taylor, 1983; Wilson, 1989) and/or (b) a contradiction of the individual's self-perception (Bowlby, 1969; Everly, 1992; Frankl, 1959; Lifton, 1988; Wilson, 1989).

The reader will recall that according to pioneer psychotraumatologist Pierre Janet, the interpretation of the traumatic event is what ultimately determines psychopathology. Developmentalists and philosophers appear to agree that human beings struggle to make sense out of the world around them. Bowlby (1969) argues that we create world and personal models; beliefs about the world and ourselves that make it safe to venture forth, explore, affiliate. Janoff-Bulman (1992) refers to these formulations as "assumptions." These constructs point out that human beings require an understanding of (as well as safety and security from) the world around them, and therefore, they create assumptive explanatory models that do indeed render the world safe and predictable, at least psychologically. The intricate and artful Greek and Roman mythologies may have been motivated by just such a need. The aggregation of assumptions, ideologies, and related interpretational constructs may collectively be referred to as one's worldview (or weltanschauung).

Abraham Maslow (1970) constructed a theory of human motivation that provides further insight into the interpretation phase of psychotraumatogenesis. Janet explained psychotraumatogenesis as the patient being overwhelmed by the traumatic stressor and being left in a condition of perceived helplessness and a lack of understanding; I have extended that notion here to mean that some aspect of the patient's weltanschauung has been violated or contradicted. Maslow (1970) interpreted trauma as a threat to the second most basic of all human needs, the need for safety and security.

Thus the key aspect of the process of psychotraumatogenesis is the patient's interpretation of the traumatic stressor. Interpretational mechanisms serve to augment or mitigate the negative impact that the traumatic event will ultimately have. Humans construct interpretational worldviews (weltanschauungs) that provide order and safety in an otherwise chaotic world. Trauma, conversely, serves to directly violate or contradict the aspect of the weltanschauung that addresses safety and security. The trauma represents a piece of the puzzle of life that cannot be easily explained nor integrated. It is so extreme that it serves to challenge the entire weltanschauung; the world once again appears chaotic, malevolent, threatening, and insecure. Maslow explains that once challenged or contradicted, this need for safety becomes a consuming quest that fixates the patient at this rudimentary level of human existence—perhaps for a lifetime.

It should be clear at this point that the successful therapy of the post-traumatic stress patient is based upon assisting the individual in assimilating, integrating, or resolving the traumatic event into an ego-syntonic weltanschauung. In the words of Janoff-Bulman (1988), "From a cognitive perspective the key to the victim's recovery process is the reestablishment of an integrated, organized set of basic assumptions. . . . The traumatic event must be assimilated into the victim's assumptive world, or the assumptive world must accommodate the new data" (p. 107).

Strategies Addressing the Worldview

According to Janet (van der Kolk, Brown, & van der Hart, 1989), "Making intellectual sense out of a traumatic event leads to constructive coping and a subjective sense of calm and control." According to Maslow (1970), "Basic need gratification is primary in the dynamics of actual cure or improvement" (p. 68). In the terminology of this chapter, the psychotherapy of post-traumatic stress entails assisting the patient in integrating the traumatic event into the weltanschauung in such a way that the Maslovian need for safety is once again satisfied and the world is once again understandable and safe.

The most basic of initial steps in the psychotherapeutic process becomes listening to the patient's accounts of the trauma with the intention of discovering what it means to the patient. In other words, what specific aspect of the patient's safety Weltanschauung was violated or contradicted by the trauma. This will be revealed as some fundamental and deeply endorsed belief or assumption about the world that, subsequent to the trauma, appears questionable at best and destroyed at worst.

Once the therapist has identified how the traumatic event has been interpreted by the patient as violating a deeply endorsed belief about the world, the key to the successful psychotherapeutic resolution of adult-onset trauma resides not within the specific choice of psychotherapeutic *tactics*, of which there is an awesome array that may prove of value. Rather, the key to successful treatment resides in effectively conceptualizing the most efficient and effective treatment *strategy*, then selecting the tactics guided by the strategic formulation. There are three global strategies that can be employed in order to integrate or otherwise resolve psychological trauma:

1. Integrating the trauma into the patient's existing Weltanschauung
2. Allowing the trauma to be understood as a parallel aspect of the existing Weltanschauung (i.e., an exception to the rule)
3. Using the trauma to demonstrate the invalidity of the extant worldview and the need to create a new worldview wherein the trauma more readily fits (Everly, 1994).

Integrating the trauma into the aspect of the Weltanschauung that deals with safety may be achieved via several approaches, which are summarized below (Everly, 1994):

1. Reinterpreting the trauma itself (success vs. failure)
2. Reinterpreting the valence of the trauma (something positive could be learned, it could have been worse, there is a "silver lining," etc.)
3. Reinterpreting the role the patient specifically played in the etiology of the trauma (disputing overgeneralized self-blame)
4. Reinterpreting the overall importance of the trauma (as less important' than originally assumed)
5. Insight, understanding, control, self-efficacy

Integrating the trauma into the existing Weltanschauung is the most ego-syntonic process the therapist can choose, but it often requires considerable creativity. Allowing the trauma to be understood as a parallel to the existing weltanschauung will often be the second most ego-syntonic and parsimonious of strategic options, especially for patients who were premorbidly inclined to accept "exceptions to the rule." Attempting to replace the extant weltanschauung totally is clearly the most formidable task the therapist faces. It should be attempted only when other options have been exhausted, or the extant weltanschauung is demonstrably self-defeating.

Strategies Addressing Self-Perception

As Lifton (1988), Bowlby (1969), Wilson (1989), and Frankl (1959) have argued, the loss of the sense of personal meaning, personal control, self-perception, and self-efficacy vis-à-vis the trauma are important elements of psychotraumatogenesis. The corollary is that the restoration of a favorable sense of self and a sense of control are important factors in the recovery process. Bandura's concept of self-efficacy is especially useful in the therapy of post-traumatic stress. Enhancing self-efficacy is intrinsically therapeutic for post-traumatic stress because it not only enhances self-esteem but combats the perception of helplessness and conveys the perception that the world is more controllable (i.e., safer).

Bandura (1982) has described four sources that affect the cognitive perception of self-efficacy. They are as follows:

- *Performance.* "Enactive attainments provide the most influential source of efficacy information. . . . Successes raise efficacy appraisals, repeated failures lower them" (Bandura, 1982, pp. 26–27). Bandura has shown perceptions of self-efficacy to influence subsequent performance as well as autonomic nervous system activity. Though enactive attainment appears to be the single most powerful way of influencing perceptions of self-efficacy, it is important to note that attainment is in the eye of the beholder. Objective success shows no favorable impact on self-efficacy if the individual *perceives* that success as "failure."
- *Vicarious experience.* "Self-efficacy appraisals are also partly influenced by vicarious experiences. Seeing or visualizing similar others perform successfully can raise self-percepts of efficacy in observers that they too possess the capabilities to master comparable activities. . . . By the same token, observing others to be of similar competence fail despite high efforts lowers observers' judgments of their own capabilities and undermines their efforts" (Bandura, 1982, p. 27). Such modeling of experience as described may be done in vivo, in vitro, or symbolically.
- *Verbal persuasion.* Verbal persuasion comprises such things such as suggestion, education, and reinterpretation of exogenous, environmental, or interoceptive stimuli so as to improve perceptions of self-efficacy. Such cognitive alterations may be done by one self or by another (e.g., a therapist). In the case of other-directed persuasion, the ethos of the other may affect outcome.
- *Physiological/affective arousal.* "People rely partly on their state of physiological arousal in judging their capabilities and vulnerability to stress. Because high arousal usually debilitates performance, individuals are more likely to expect success when they are not beset by aversive arousal. . . . Fear reactions generate further fear through anticipatory self-arousal. . . . People can rouse themselves to elevated levels of distress that produce the very dysfunctions they fear. Treatments that eliminate emotional arousal . . . heighten perceived efficacy with corresponding improvements in performance" (Bandura, 1982, p. 28). Biofeedback and relaxation training are useful interventions here.

Table 10.2 Methods for Cognitive Change

Worldview:
1. Integrating trauma into the extant weltanschauung
2. Creating a parallel weltanschauung
3. Creating a new weltanschauung

Self-perception via self-efficacy:
1. Enactive attainment
2. Vicarious learning
3. Verbal persuasion
4. Physiological self-regulation

Thus Bandura has provided a useful guide to enhancing the construct of self-efficacy in victims of psychological trauma, as well as other patients. Table 10.2 summarizes the neurocognitive strategies to address the psychological-hypersensitivity factor within post-traumatic stress.

SUMMARY

The purpose of this chapter has been to introduce neurocognitive therapy. Neurocognitive therapy of post-traumatic stress represents a metatherapy—an overarching strategic therapeutic framework within which specific therapeutic tactics may be formulated. The essence of neurocognitive therapy is simply that post-traumatic stress possesses a two-factor constituency: (a) neurological hypersensitivity, and (b) psychological hypersensitivity (via a contradicted worldview). The corollary of this construction is that the therapy of post-traumatic stress should address both phenomenological factors to be maximally effective.

In this chapter I have reviewed strategies for addressing the neurological-hypersensitivity factor through neurological desensitization. Similarly, I have reviewed strategies for addressing the putative contradiction to the worldview regarding safety, security, and/or a sense of self through integrating or resolving the trauma and/or through self-efficacy training.

Specific therapeutic interventions are most likely to be maximally effective when applied in a fashion consistent with the tenets of "psychotherapy integration" (Norcross & Goldfried, 1992). Specific therapeutic tactics for reducing stress are detailed in Everly (1989).

REFERENCES

Bandura, A. (1977). Self-efficacy. *Psychological Review, 84,* 191–215.

Bandura, A. (1982). The self and mechanisms of agency. In J. Suls (Ed.), *Psychological perspectives on the self* (pp. 3–39). Hillsdale, NJ: Erlbaum.

Benson, H. (1983). The relaxation response. *Trends in Neuroscience, 6,* 281–284.

Bettleheim, B. (1984). Afterword. In C. Vegh, *I didn't say goodbye.* New York: Dutton.

Bowlby, J. (1969). *Attachment and loss; Vol. I: Attachment.* New York: Basic Books.

Everly, G. S. (1989). *A clinical guide to the treatment of the human stress response.* New York: Plenum.

Everly, G. S. (1990). PTSD as a disorder of arousal. *Psychology and Health: An International Journal, 4,* 135–145.

Everly, G. S. (1992, Feb.). *Psychotraumatology: A two-factor formulation of post-traumatic stress.* Paper presented at the Fourth Montreux Congress on Stress, Montreux, Switzerland.

Everly, G. S. (1993). Psychotraumatology: A two-factor formulation of posttraumatic stress. *Integrative Physiological and Behavioral Science, 28,* 270–278.

Everly, G. S. (1994). Short-term psychotherapy of acute adult onset post-traumatic stress. *Stress Medicine, 10,* 191–196.

Everly, G. S. & Benson, H. (1989). Disorders of arousal. *International Journal of Psychosomatics, 36,* 15–22.

Frankl, V. (1959). *Man's search for meaning.* Boston: Beacon.
Gellhorn, E. (1958). The physiological basis of neuromuscular relaxation. *Archives of Internal Medicine, 102,* 392–339.
Gellhorn, E. (1964). Motivation and emotion. *Psychological Review, 71,* 457–472.
Gellhorn, E. (1965). The neurophysiological basis of anxiety. *Perspectives in Biology and Medicine, 8,* 488–515.
Gellhorn, E. & Loofbourrow, G. (1963). *Emotions and emotional disorders.* New York: Harper and Row.
Heider, J. (1974). Catharsis in human potential encounter. *Journal of Humanistic Psychology, 14,* 27–47.
Hoffman, J., Benson, H., Arns, P., Stainbrook, G., Landsberg, L., Young, J., & Gill, A. (1982). Reduced sympathetic nervous system responsivity associated with the relaxation response. *Science, 215,* 190–192.
Horowitz, M. (1986). *Stress Response Syndromes,* 2nd Ed. Northvale, NJ: Aronson.
Janoff-Bulman, R. (1988). Victims of violence. In S. Fisher & J. Reason (Eds.). *Handbook of life stress, cognition, and health* (pp. 101–113). New York: Wiley.
Janoff-Bulman, R. (1992). *Shattered assumptions.* New York: Free Press.
Kahn, M. (1966). The physiology of catharsis. *Journal of Personality and Social Psychology, 3,* 278–286.
Lifton, R. J. (1988). Understanding the traumatized self. In J. P. Wilson, Z. Harel, & B. Kahana (Eds.), *Human Adaptation to Extreme Stress* (pp. 7–31). New York: Plenum.
Maslow, A. H. (1970). Motivation and Personality. New York: Harper and Row.
Norcross, J., & Goldfried, M. (1992). *Handbook of psychotherapy integration.* New York: Basic Books.
Pennebaker, J. W. & Susman, J. (1988). Disclosure of traumas and psychosomatic processes. *Society, Science, and Medicine, 26,* 327–332.
Taylor, S. (1983). Adjustment to threatening events. *American Psychologist, 38,* 1161–1173.
Weil, J. (1974). *A neurophysiological model of emotional and intentional behavior.* Springfield, IL: Charles C Thomas.
Wilson, J. P. (1989). *Trauma, transformation, and healing.* New York: Brunner/Mazel.
van der Kolk, B. (1988). The trauma spectrum. *Journal of Traumatic Stress, 1,* 273–290.
van der Kolk, B., Brown, P., & van der Hart, O. (1989). Pierre Janet on posttraumatic stress. *Journal of Traumatic Stress, 2,* 365–378.

11

Biological Approaches to the Diagnosis and Treatment of Post-Traumatic Stress Disorder

MATTHEW J. FRIEDMAN

Biological approaches to the diagnosis and treatment of PTSD are receiving increasing attention from scientists and clinicians. Research findings appear to suggest that patients with PTSD display marked abnormalities in sympathetic nervous system arousal, in hypothalamic-pituitary-adrenocortical function, in the endogenous opioid system, and in the physiology of sleep and dreaming. Such results enable us to expand our theoretical understanding of PTSD from a purely psychological context to a bio-psycho-social model in which many different factors contribute to the pathology of PTSD.

In this chapter I will review current advances in biological research on PTSD, and I will demonstrate how a biological perspective may complement psychological diagnostic techniques to achieve greater precision in identifying PTSD. This is especially pertinent in distinguishing PTSD from either major depressive disorder (MDD) or panic disorder (PD), because PTSD exhibits many of the same symptoms as each of these other psychiatric illnesses.

I will also review current knowledge on pharmacotherapy of PTSD in the context of our present understanding of the unique pathophysiology of

---

MATTHEW J. FRIEDMAN • National Center for PTSD, Department of Veterans Affairs Medical and Regional Office Center, White River Junction, Vermont 05009; and Dartmouth College Medical School, Hanover, New Hampshire 03756. Reprinted from *Journal of Traumatic Stress,* Vol. 4, No. 1.

Psychotraumatology, edited by George S. Everly, Jr. and Jeffrey M. Lating. Plenum Press, New York, 1994.

this disorder. Neurobiological models also suggest why patients with PTSD may be particularly susceptible to alcohol and other chemical abuse/dependency. Such theoretical considerations will be reviewed in the context of treatment implications of patients with the dual diagnosis of PTSD and chemical abuse/dependency.

HISTORICAL PERSPECTIVE

Abraham Kardiner's research on World War I veterans during the 1940s has proved to be highly influential in stimulating modern biological approaches to PTSD (Kardiner, 1941; Kardiner & Spiegel, 1947). Theorizing from the psychological perspective of stress and adaptation, Kardiner stated that (what is now called) PTSD was a "physioneurosis" in which the patient's adaptive capacity was "smashed." He believed that PTSD was both a psychological and a physiological disorder with its own unique pathophysiology. To underscore this biological orientation Kardiner labeled the dissociative episodes now called flashbacks as an "epileptic symptom complex," implying that they were caused by some disorder of brain function.

A few years later Cohen and others investigated neurocirculatory asthenia (NCA) on a clinical population consisting mostly of combat veterans (Cohen et al., 1948; Cohen & White, 1950). Placing their work in a historical context of physiological and medical research on combat survivors dating back to the Civil War (Beard, 1869; DaCosta, 1871; Hartshorne, 1864; Lewis, 1917; Wood, 1941), they recognized that NCA had previously had many other names, including soldier's heart, anxiety neurosis, nervous exhaustion, DaCosta's syndrome, irritable heart, and effort syndrome. Cohen and associates elegantly showed that combat veterans with NCA had many abnormalities that could be readily detected when they were asked to perform muscular work on a treadmill. Patients with NCA (a) could not work as long as controls, (b) had a metabolic defect evidenced by less efficient oxygen consumption and higher blood lactate concentration, (c) had reduced pulmonary ventilatory efficiency, (d) had excessively high pulse rates during work, and (e) showed abnormal reactivity to painful stimuli.

Because most of their subjects were World War II veterans, Cohen and associates speculated about the possible impact of military experience on their experimental observations. They noted that many of their subjects had been in good health before the onset of NCA. They also noted that the vast majority of their subjects "blamed the army for their difficulties" and that "a high percentage of patients . . . reported a harrowing experience in combat" (Cohen et al., 1948, p. 278). Other subjects suggested that family violence, death, and illness preceded the onset of NCA. Cohen et al. never went beyond such preliminary observations to explore the possibility that exposure to trauma was the common denominator for many of their subjects.

They were apparently unaware of Kardiner's work on the impact of combat trauma and concluded that the cause of NCA was "unknown."

These important early investigations by Cohen et al. have recently been rediscovered by researchers studying the pathophysiology of panic disorder. Perhaps Cohen et al.'s, assertion that NCA had no known etiology accounts for the fact that their work is seen as a pioneering effort in the field of panic disorder rather than PTSD. Recent findings with PTSD patients by biologically oriented investigators, however, suggest that the work of Cohen et al. is also relevant to PTSD. With regard to cardiovascular function, Israeli combat veterans with PTSD exhibit low effort tolerance and decreased cardiac reserve in comparison with controls (Shalev et al., 1990). Burn patients with PTSD have significantly lower pain thresholds than burn patients without PTSD (Perry et al., 1987). Reports of a possible link between chronic pain and PTSD (Benedikt & Kolb, 1986; Rapaport, 1987) are also consistent with these observations of hyperalgesia among PTSD patients. Finally, reports of higher rates of somatic complaints among Israeli combat veterans with PTSD (Solomon & Mikulincer, 1987) update similar observations by Cohen et al. (1948) among World War II veterans with NCA.

These clinical observations indicate how exposure to trauma may alter the body's normal physiology and health. At face value, such findings suggest that the port of entry into our health care system for some PTSD patients may be via cardiac, pain, or other medical clinics. At another level, of course, such findings suggest that PTSD is associated with a number of biological alterations that may be expressed somatically as well as psychiatrically.

BIOLOGICAL ALTERATIONS ASSOCIATED WITH PTSD

Sympathetic Nervous System

Dysregulation of the sympathetic nervous system has been demonstrated by monitoring the psychophysiological response of combat veterans upon exposure to traumagenic stimuli, by measuring urinary catecholamine levels, and by determination of peripheral alpha-2 and beta-adrenergic receptor binding in patients with PTSD (Table 11.1).

A thorough discussion of this research is beyond the scope of this chapter, and the reader is referred to Kolb's (1987) elegant recent review for more information. Briefly, uncontrolled findings on combat veterans with PTSD include increased muscle tension (Gillespie, 1942) and increased heart rate, respiration rate, and EEG alpha rhythm (Dobbs & Wilson, 1960). A major methodological breakthrough occurred when Blanchard et al. (1982) recognized that the hallmark of PTSD is a conditioned emotional response to meaningful stimuli that trigger thoughts, memories, and feel-

Table 11.1 Biological Alterations Associated with PTSD

1. Sympathetic nervous system hyperarousal
   a. Elevated baseline sympathetic physiological indices
   b. Sympathetic psychophysiological response upon exposure to traumagenic stimuli
   c. Elevated urinary catecholamine levels
   d. Reduced platelet MAO activity
   e. Down-regulation of adrenergic receptors
2. Hypofunction of hypothalamic-pituitary-adrenocortical axis
   a. Decreased urinary cortisol levels
   b. HPA suppression following dexamethasone
   c. Unique elevation of urinary catecholamine/cortisol ratio
3. Abnormalities of the endogenous spioid system
   a. Stress induced analgesia by traumagenic stimuli
   b. General lowering of the pain threshold at rest
4. Sleep abnormalities
   a. Initiating and maintaining sleep: increased sleep latency, decreased total sleep time, decreased sleep efficiency, increased number of awakenings, increased body movements
   b. Sleep architecture: changes are controversial
   c. Traumatic nightmares are unique

ings uniquely associated to the trauma itself. They have shown that at baseline, Vietnam combat veterans with PTSD exhibit higher heart rate, systolic blood pressure, and forehead EMG than controls. More importantly, PTSD patients exhibit dramatic physiological arousal after exposure to an audiotape of combat sounds played at gradually increasing volume levels. The heart rate, systolic blood pressure, and EMG responses of PTSD patients were so much greater than those of controls that blind raters correctly classified them 95.5% of the time. Similar results have been obtained in other laboratories (Brende, 1982; Malloy et al., 1983). Psychophysiological arousal in Vietnam combat veterans with PTSD has also been elicited by other traumagenic stimuli (Pitman et al., 1987, 1990).

One would predict that sympathetic psychophysiological hyperreactivity would be associated with elevated catecholamine levels. Indeed, elevated urinary norepinephrine (Kosten et al., 1987; Mason et al., 1985) and epinephrine levels (Kosten & Krystal, 1988; Kosten et al., 1988) have been found in Vietnam combat veterans with PTSD. Kosten et al. (1987) reported that 24-hour urinary norepinephrine and epinephrine levels in PTSD patients were significantly higher than those of normals and of patients with panic disorder, major depressive disorder, undifferentiated schizophrenia, paranoid schizophrenia, and manic-type bipolar disorders. Mason and associates (1985) had previously reported that PTSD patients have a higher urinary norepinephrine/cortisol ratio. This ratio results both from elevated urinary norepinephrine levels and from the reduced urinary cortisol levels that are uniquely found in PTSD patients (Mason et al., 1986; see below).

Whereas elevated catecholamine levels may be biochemical markers for the sympathetic dysregulation association with PTSD, they may also reflect another abnormality, reduced monoamine oxidase (MAO) activity in combat veterans with PTSD. MAO is a major degradative enzyme in catecholamine metabolism, so reduced MAO activity could lead to higher systemic norepinephrine and epinephrine levels. In this regard, Davidson and associates (1985) reported a significant reduction in platelet MAO activity among combat veterans with PTSD. As discussed by Kosten and Krystal (1988), interpretations of these findings must be cautious because of the simultaneous occurrence of depression and/or alcoholism in many of these patients.

Finally, three studies on adrenergic receptor binding are consistent with all of the above results, suggesting that PTSD is associated with higher sympathetic nervous function. One would predict that increased adrenergic synaptic activity should desensitize or down-regulate adrenergic receptors. Consistent with this prediction, Perry et al. (1987) observed fewer total platelet alpha-2 receptor binding sites in 12 Vietnam veterans with PTSD as compared with 13 age-matched controls. In addition to down-regulation, Perry et al. (1988) showed in a more recent report that the alpha-2 receptor complex is uncoupled and therefore functions less efficiently in the platelets of patients with PTSD. Similarly, Lerer and associates (1987) studied beta-adrenergic receptor binding in both intact lymphocytes and platelet membrane preparations. They found that PTSD patients exhibited abnormally low beta-adrenergic receptor-mediated cAMP signal transduction.

Hypothalamic-Pituitary-Adrenocortical (HPA) Axis

Turning from the sympathetic nervous system to the hypothalamic-pituitary-adrenocortical (HPA) axis, data on urinary cortisol levels and the dexamethasone suppression test (DST) suggest that hypofunction of the HPA axis is associated with PTSD. Mason and associates (1986) have shown that 24-hour urinary free-cortisol levels are significantly lower among PTSD patients than in most other psychiatric disorders. Furthermore, normal suppression of the HPA axis by dexamethasone has been shown in PTSD patients (Kudler et al., 1987). Two theoretical explanations have been proposed to explain HPA axis hypofunction in PTSD. Mason et al. (1986) have cited older psychosomatic research suggesting that denial and psychological defenses can exert a strong suppressive effect upon urinary corticosteroid levels. A more parsimonious hypothesis postulates that biological rather than psychological mechanisms may account for HPA axis hypofunction. This argument is based on the previously discussed possibility that PTSD is associated with increased central noradrenergic activity. Because norepinephrine inhibits the release of corticotropin-releasing hormone (CRH; Price et al., 1986), the postulated increased central sympathetic activity of PTSD would be expected to inhibit the entire HPA system.

Endogenous Opioid System

Kosten and Krystal (1988) have suggested that adrenergic inhibition of CRH may also account for a disturbance in the endogenous opioid system associated with PTSD. CRH promotes release of ACTH from the pituitary; ACTH is coreleased with beta endorphin, which influences the activity level of the endogenous opioid system. Kosten and Krystal postulate that inhibition of CRH by excessive sympathetic arousal therefore will also produce an endogenous opioid deficiency in patients with PTSD. This prediction is consistent with previously mentioned clinical reports of lowered pain thresholds in PTSD patients (Perry et al., 1987) and of a possible link between chronic pain and PTSD (Benedikt & Kolb, 1986; Rapaport, 1987). Finally, Pitman and associates (1990) have recently shown that exposing Vietnam veterans with PTSD to combat scenes from the movie *Platoon* produces a naloxone-reversible 30% decrease in pain responses. This important finding of stress-induced analgesia suggests not only that PTSD is associated with dysregulation of the endogenous opioid system but also that a possible baseline opioid deficiency might be dramatically reversed when PTSD patients are exposed to traumagenic stimuli.

Sleep and Dreaming

Abnormalities in sleep and dreaming also appear to be associated with PTSD. Patients often have difficulty initiating and maintaining sleep (Table 11.1). In addition, several studies show marked disruption of sleep architecture in PTSD exemplified by increased stage 1, increased stage 2, decreased delta sleep, decreased REM latency, and increased total REM percentage (Kramer & Kinney, 1985, 1988; Kramer et al., 1982; Lavie et al., 1979; Schlossberg & Benjamin, 1978). These results are controversial, however, especially with regard to REM latency and total REM percent (Greenberg et al., 1972; Van Kammen et al., 1987). An excellent review by Ross et al. (1989) clarifies methodological problems and substantive contradictions on the emerging literature on sleep in PTSD.

In addition to alterations in physiological sleep, disturbed dreaming is a prominent abnormality in chronic PTSD (Kramer, 1979; van der Kolk et al., 1984). Traumatic nightmares may arise out of REM or non-REM (NREM) sleep (van der Kolk et al., 1984). As noted earlier (Friedman, 1981), these nightmares appear to be unique to PTSD because they are neither REM dream anxiety attacks nor NREM night terror/nightmares (Kramer, 1979).

Ross et al. (1989), however, suggest that PTSD nightmares may actually be a newly identified phenomenon called REM sleep without atonia. The signifying characteristic of the PTSD nightmare is an "instant replay" of the traumatic event, often accompanied by nocturnal muscle movements that are consonant with the events of the nightmare.

Neurobiological Models of PTSD

A number of models have been proposed to integrate the biological abnormalities and clinical symptoms associated with PTSD. Discussion of these models is beyond the scope of this article and the reader is referred to recent reviews for more details (Friedman, 1988; Kolb, 1987; Kosten & Krystal, 1988; van der Kolk, 1987; van der Kolk et al., 1985). All of these models presuppose hyperarousal of the central noradrenergic system and focus especially on the locus coeruleus because it is instrumental in the neurobiology of arousal and panic.

Kolb (1987) has postulated that the excessive and prolonged high-intensity stimulation from traumatic exposure produces cortical neuronal and synaptic changes in patients with chronic PTSD. He hypothesizes that the conditioned fear response of PTSD therefore is associated with alteration in brain functions that control aggressive expression and the sleep-dream cycle. This model accounts for the dramatic psychophysiological response in PTSD patients following exposure to traumagenic stimuli.

Van der Kolk and associates (1985) have proposed that the animal model of learned helplessness in response to inescapable shock may be directly applicable to PTSD. They hypothesize that long-term potentiation of locus coeruleus pathways to the hippocampus and amygdala may produce the hyperarousal, traumatic nightmares, and flashbacks that characterize PTSD. Such a theory also suggests that fluctuations in endogenous opioid levels will affect the response to traumagenic stimuli, because the locus coeruleus is inhibited by opioids. The inescapable shock theory offers a neurobiological rationale for stress-induced analgesia and for the "action junkie" behavior that is sometimes considered secondary to PTSD. It also has implications for opiate addiction that will be discussed later.

Van der Kolk (1987) and Friedman (1988) have independently suggested that kindling is a neurobiological model that may be as applicable to PTSD as it is to a cocaine model of psychosis (Post & Kopanda, 1976). Kindling is a process by which neuroanatomic structures, especially those in the limbic system, become increasingly sensitized following repeated exposure to electrical stimulation or cocaine-like drugs. Kindling can lead progressively to profound neurophysiological abnormalities such as grand mal seizures or to the progressive development of aberrant behavior. According to this model, chronic central sympathetic arousal in PTSD, mediated by the locus coeruleus, kindles limbic nuclei, thereby producing a stable neurobiological abnormality. Kindling would explain the stability of PTSD—if untreated, it can persist for decades (Archibald & Tuddenham, 1965). This model also suggests that an antikindling drug such as carbamazepine might be pharmacologically efficacious in PTSD.

BIOLOGICAL APPROACHES TO DIAGNOSIS

Among biological diagnostic techniques that have been tested are psychophysiological assessment, the dexamethasone suppression test (DST), the sleep EEG, sodium lactate infusion, and the sodium amytal interview. In this section I will review the applicability of these diagnostic techniques to PTSD and evaluate their potential for distinguishing PTSD from major depressive disorder (MDD) and panic disorder (PD; see Table 11.2).

Psychophysiological Assessment

Currently the best and most specific biological diagnostic test for PTSD is psychophysiological assessment. This diagnostic technique is based on the fact that traumagenic stimuli elicit sympathetic hyperarousal, as discussed earlier (Blanchard et al., 1982; Kolb, 1987; Malloy et al., 1983; Pitman et al.,

Table 11.2 Biological Diagnostic Tests for PTSD

	PTSD	MDD	PD
I. Psychophysiological responses to traumagenic stimuli			
Sympathetic arousal	+	−	−
Stress-induced analgesia	+	−	−
II. HPA axis abnormalities			
DST	−	+	−
Urinary cortisol	↓	↑	?
III. Sleep EEG abnormalities			
Initiating and maintaining sleep	↓	↓	↓
Movements during sleep	↑	0	↑
Stage 1 and stage 2	↑	0	0
Delta	↓	↓	0
REM	↑/↓	↑/0	0
REM latency	↑/↓	↓	0
IV. Sodium lactate infusion			
Panic attacks	?	−	+
Flashbacks	?	−	−
V. Sodium amytal interview	+	−	−

Note: + = proven diagnostic value, − = no apparent diagnostic value, ? = unknown diagnostic value, ↓ = reduced, 0 = no change, ↑ = increased.

1987). This technique is both sensitive and powerful when one uses a general stimulus such as an audiotape of combat sounds or a visual excerpt from a movie such as *Platoon*. It is even more discriminatory when the provocative stimulus is an individualized autobiographical traumatic anecdote (Pitman et al., 1987).

Exposure to traumagenic stimuli may also have practical applicability as a clinical paradigm for testing biological markers other than sympathetic arousal, such as HPA axis function or stress-induced analgesia. In the development of standard diagnostic approaches, however, biological markers in PTSD patients should be assessed both at baseline and immediately after provocation by traumagenic stimuli.

Dexamethasone Suppression Test

The dexamethasone suppression test (DST; Carroll et al., 1981) has enjoyed wide use in diagnosing major depressive disorder (MDD). It is based on the fact that MDD is a disorder that is associated with hyperfunctioning of the HPA system. For this reason, dexamethasone, which normally suppresses HPA activity, cannot do so in patients with MDD. Depressed patients therefore are often "nonsuppressors" when challenged by the DST. In an earlier article (Friedman, 1988), I suggested that DST might be useful for distinguishing PTSD from MDD. After all, PTSD appears to be associated with hypofunctioning of the HPA system, whereas MDD seems to be just the opposite. Therefore I predicted that PTSD patients would have a normal DST; they would be suppressors, whereas patients with MDD would be nonsuppressors. The work of Kudler et al. (1987) was consistent with this prediction. Patients with PTSD alone were suppressors, whereas those with *both* PTSD and MDD were nonsuppressors following a dexamethasone challenge. Subsequently, Halbreich and associates (1988) confused the issue when they compared DST responses of patients with MDD alone with a second group that had *both* MDD and PTSD. This time the MDD + PTSD patients were suppressors, in contrast to MDD-alone patients, who were nonsuppressors. These results indicate that when PTSD and MDD coexist in the same patients, PTSD-induced HPA hypofunction may neutralize MDD-induced HPA hyperfunction. From the practical standpoint of clinical diagnosis, Halbreich et al.'s results have two implications. First of all, they suggest that the DST may have limited value in distinguishing PTSD from MDD. Second, and more importantly, these results suggest that when both PTSD and MDD occur simultaneously, each may alter the biological expression of the other.

Sleep EEG

Investigations on the sleep EEG of depressed patients have shown that MDD is reliably associated with alterations in sleep architecture. Specifically, depressed patients exhibit reduced REM latency and reduced delta sleep, and the duration of the first REM period is prolonged in MDD (Akiskal, 1983; Dube et al., 1986; Kupfer & Thase, 1983; Ross et al., 1988). As discussed earlier and shown in Table 11.2, it would appear that there might be enough differences between MDD and PTSD to predict that the sleep EEG will play an important role in the differential diagnosis of MDD versus PTSD. There is a problem with such a prediction. First of all, if (as suggested above with regard to the DST) the simultaneous occurrence of MDD and PTSD alters the unique biological expression of each disorder, then the sleep EEG may also lose its specificity in patients who have both depression and PTSD. Indeed, such a possibility may explain some controversies in the literature and especially why some investigations have observed sleep EEG findings in PTSD patients that look more like expected results in depression (Greenberg et al., 1972; Kauffman et al., 1987, Van Kammen et al., 1987).

To summarize, the potential usefulness of the sleep EEG in distinguishing MDD from PTSD has not been adequately tested. Perhaps it will be more useful for future studies to focus primarily on the length of the first REM period rather than the total nocturnal percentage of REM sleep (Ross et al., 1988). Undoubtedly future studies will have to state quite explicitly whether their clinical populations meet diagnostic criteria for MDD, PTSD, or both.

The sleep EEG, however, should easily distinguish PTSD from PD. There is apparently no disturbance of the sleep architecture in PD, although panic patients do exhibit difficulty initiating and maintaining sleep and, like PTSD patients, show increased body movements while asleep (Dube et al., 1986; Hauri et al., 1989).

Sodium Lactate Infusion

One of the most definitive diagnostic tests for PD is the sodium lactate infusion. Pitts and McClure's (1967) original observation that intravenous administration of sodium lactate can precipitate panic attacks in patients with PD has been replicated by many investigators. PD and PTSD share many characteristics in common. Both disorders may be associated with locus coeruleus dysregulation, because both exhibit sympathetic hyperarousal and sudden surges of anxiety. In addition, PTSD flashbacks may meet DSM-III-R diagnostic criteria for panic attacks (Mellman & Davis, 1985). For these reasons, it would be very interesting to learn whether sodium lactate can induce PTSD symptoms as it can panic attacks. To date, the only report on this subject is quite confusing (Rainey et al., 1987). Although the authors report that lactate infusion precipitated flashbacks in all seven subjects, only one such "flashback" was a reexperiencing of combat trauma. All other "flashbacks" occurred in a hospital setting more comparable to the laboratory experimental situation than to the combat trauma responsible for the later development of PTSD. Furthermore, because all patients met DSM-III-R criteria for PD as well as PTSD, their susceptibility to sodium lactate may differ considerably from the responsivity of PTSD patients who do not simultaneously meet DSM-III-R criteria for PD. In my opinion, it is still unclear whether PTSD patients will respond to a lactate infusion. It is an important question that needs to be investigated systematically. Furthermore, other established provocative tests for PD, such as carbon dioxide inhalation (Fryer et al., 1987) and yohimbine challenge (Charney et al., 1987), also need to be explored with PTSD patients.

Sodium Amytal Interview

PTSD has revived interest in narcosynthetic exploration of repressed traumatic experiences or dissociative episodes triggered by traumagenic stimuli (Kolb, 1985). After decades of neglect, the sodium amytal interview is proving to be a useful clinical tool for identifying catastrophic stressors that are too terrifying for discussion in the normal state of consciousness. Clearly this diagnostic technique has a unique applicability to PTSD, in contrast to MDD or PD.

As defined by Kolb (1985), narcosynthesis is drug-induced recall of repressed material through an abreactive experience. Through this procedure, repressed material becomes consciously available for later integration and synthesis by the personality. The amytal interview is not an end in itself but rather a technique for exposing material through narcosynthetic abreaction that must be worked through in subsequent psychotherapy. Candidates for this approach are individuals who have complete or partial amnesia for recurrent episodes of abnormal behavior in which they may become aggressively threatening or violent. Such dissociative episodes are often precipitated by traumagenic stimuli and seem more likely to occur if the patient has been drinking beforehand.

The key to the narcosynthetic approach is videotaping the entire session. After full recovery of consciousness, the patient reviews the entire tape with his or her therapist so that recently repressed information can be incorporated into ongoing psychotherapy. The reader is referred to Kolb (1985) for further details on indications, contraindications, and the specific technique for the amytal interview.

Differential Diagnosis: PTSD, MDD, and PD

Because PTSD shares many symptoms in common with MDD and PD, it is useful to review current knowledge on biological diagnostic tests to clarify their distinguishing features as well as their similarities. PTSD and MDD are both associated with symptoms such as dysphoria, guilt, grief, anhedonia, irritability, social withdrawal, and insomnia. In addition, both disorders respond to some of the same medications (shown in Table 11.3 and discussed below). Likewise, PTSD and PD are anxiety disorders marked by sympathet-

Table 11.3 Response to Medication: PTSD, MDD, and PD

	PTSD	MDD	PD
Tricyclic antidepressants	+	+	+
MAO inhibitors	+	+	+
Carbamazepine	(+)	?	0
Lithium	(+)	+	0
Benzodiazepines	(+)	−	+
Alprazolom	(+)	+	+
Propranolol	(+)	−	+
Clonidine	(+)	−	(+)
Neuroleptics	±	±	0

Note: + = proven therapeutic efficacy, (+) = promising uncontrolled trials, 0 = ineffective, − = worsens condition.

ic hyperarousal, an association with depressive symptoms, panic attacks, responsivity to similar medications (see Table 11.3), and a hypothesized locus coeruleus dysregulation.

In my opinion, the observations tabulated in Table 11.3 are consistent with the hypothesis that each of these three disorders has a unique biological profile that can be detected by appropriate diagnostic techniques. It is necessary to sound two cautionary notes about the data summarized in the table. First of all, it is premature to be dogmatic about any of these findings on PTSD, given the general paucity of studies. Second, because DST results (Halbreich et al., 1988) suggest that when PTSD and MDD occur simultaneously, each may alter the biological expression of the other, further research is needed in which PTSD, MDD, and PD are compared systematically in the same experimental protocol.

To summarize, as shown in Table 11.3, the psychophysiological response to traumagenic stimuli is the hallmark of PTSD with regard to hyperarousal of the sympathetic nervous system and as manifested by the endogenous opioid mobilization associated with stress-induced analgesia. Although PD is also marked by hyperarousal of the adrenergic system, panic attacks are spontaneous events (rather than a response to emotionally charged stimuli) and are essentially a physiological event devoid of the psychological meaning associated with PTSD episodes. The distinctive HPA hyperactivity of MDD contrasts with HPA hypoactivity in PTSD. For practical purposes, because the DST is normal in PTSD and urinary cortisol levels are not routinely obtained, testing the HPA axis may have limited value in the clinical diagnosis of PTSD. All three disorders show sleep EEG abnormalities, and all three exhibit difficulties initiating and maintaining sleep. Only PTSD and MDD appear to exhibit alterations in the sleep architecture, as discussed previously. The sodium lactate infusion has not been adequately tested in PTSD, as also noted above. Finally, the sodium amytal interview is uniquely applicable to PTSD.

CLINICAL PSYCHOPHARMACOLOGY

From our current understanding it appears that any drug that can reduce excessive noradrenergic activity will be beneficial in PTSD. This might be accomplished by direct antagonism of sympathetic nervous system arousal (propranolol and other beta-adrenergic blocking agents), or by reduction of brain locus coeruleus activity via inhibiting alpha-2 adrenergic receptors (clonidine, tricyclic antidepressants). If PTSD results from limbic kindling (Friedman, 1988; van der Kolk, 1987) an antikindling agent such as carbamazepine might also be effective.

Most of the information on pharmacotherapy comes from open trials and case reports. A number of double-blind investigations are currently in process, and a few preliminary reports have been presented. Given the current paucity of data from controlled clinical trials, it should come as no surprise that prescribing practices may differ widely from one place to another. For example, at one VA hospital 59% of all PTSD patients received tricyclic antidepressants either exclusively (38%) or in combination with other psychotropic agents (Embry & Callahan, 1988). At another VA hospital, 71% of PTSD patients received benzodiazepines either exclusively (36%) or in combination with other drugs (Ciccone et al., 1990).

Tricyclic Antidepressants

Several clinical reports indicate that tricyclic antidepressants (TCAs) may be effective drugs for PTSD. Published observations suggest that TCAs reduce such specific PTSD symptoms as hyperarousal, intrusive recollections, flashbacks, and traumatic nightmares. Although the antidepressant action of TCAs is often useful against depressive symptoms that may be associated with PTSD, the primary therapeutic target symptoms under discussion here are PTSD and not MDD symptoms. Anecdotal reports and open trials using rating scales have generally reported that TCAs reduce DSM-III-R intrusive recollection and hyperarousal symptoms but have little effect on avoidant symptomatology (Blake, 1986; Bohnlein et al., 1985; Burstein, 1982; Embry & Callahan, 1988; Falcon et al., 1985; Friedman, 1981, 1988; Marshall, 1975; van der Kolk, 1987). Similar results have been obtained with different traumatized cohorts such as accident victims, burn patients, combat veterans, and Cambodian concentration camp survivors. Davidson et al. (1988) conducted an 8-week double-blind randomized trial of amitriptyline versus placebo. They found that amitriptyline was most effective in patients who had depressive symptoms and that this drug did not appear to have specific effects on either intrusive or avoidant PTSD symptoms. In contrast, Frank et al. (1988), conducting a randomized double-blind trial of imipramine, phenelzine (an MAO inhibitor), and placebo observed moderate reduction in both intrusive ad avoidant PTSD symptoms with greater effects on intrusive symptoms. Their observation that improvement in PTSD symptoms was independent of the antidepressant response to imipramine conflicts directly with Davidson et al.'s conclusions. Clearly there is need for additional research, as these results cannot be reconciled.

MAO Inhibitors

MAO inhibitors (MAOIs) have received attention since Hogben and Cornfield (1981) reported that they reduced panic, anxiety, insomnia, and intrusive symptoms in 5 combat veterans with PTSD. MAOIs are attractive agents to consider because of their proven efficacy against the sympathetic dysregulation of panic disorder, their antidepressant activity, and their inhibition of REM sleep. Phenelzine is the only MAOI that has been studied, and most reports describe open-trial case reports on very few patients (Milanes et al., 1984; Shen & Park, 1983). In two larger studies, Davidson et al. (1987) and Lerer et al. (1987) conducted open trials on 11 and 22 combat veterans, respectively. Both groups observed that phenelzine's primary PTSD effect was on intrusive rather than avoidant symptoms, although reductions in general anxiety and depressive symptoms were also prominent. The only randomized double-blind trial has been Frank et al.'s comparison of imipramine, phenelzine, and placebo discussed above. These investigators reported that phenelzine was even more effective than imipramine against intrusive symptoms; it produced little improvement in avoidant symptoms. The therapeutic efficacy of MAOIs (like imipramine) in this study was completely independent of its antidepressant effect.

The decision to prescribe phenelzine will have to take into consideration a realistic expectation of patient compliance with regard to dietary restrictions and abstention from alcohol, opiates, and other drugs. Therefore high rates of alcoholism and chemical abuse/dependency in combat veterans with PTSD (Branchy et al., 1984; Keane et al., 1988) may preclude extensive use of phenelzine, efficacy notwithstanding.

Carbamazepine

Carbamazepine is an anticonvulsant that was first introduced into psychiatry by Post and Kopanda (1976), who suggested that it be prescribed in lithium-refractory bipolar affective disorder. They based this suggestion on a kindling model of endogenous psychosis.

As noted above, kindling is a neurobiological model that may also be applicable to PTSD (Friedman, 1988; van der Kolk, 1987). For this reason, two investigations have monitored the efficacy of carbamazepine in 10 PTSD patients. Seven patients showed marked reductions in intensity and frequency of the intrusive or "reexperiencing" symptoms of PTSD, such as recurrent nightmares, flashbacks, and intrusive recollections (Lipper et al.,

1986). A second open-trial study by Wolf et al. (1988) showed alleviation of impulsivity, violent behavior, and angry outbursts in 10 Vietnam combat veterans with PTSD. Because there has been speculation that complex partial seizures may cause a syndrome similar to PTSD (Greenstein et al., 1986; Stewart & Bartucci, 1986), Wolf et al.'s results are especially notable as all of their carbamazepine patients had normal EEGs and had no symptoms of temporal lobe epilepsy.

Finally, it should be noted that despite the many similarities between PTSD and PD with respect to sympathetic hyperarousal, kindling may not be an appropriate model for PD. Uhde et al. (1988) recently reported on a 3-week double-blind trial of carbamazepine versus placebo in 14 patients with PD. In contrast to its therapeutic value in PTSD, carbamazepine was not effective in PD.

Propranolol

Propranolol is an adrenergic beta-blocker that has documented efficacy in anxiety (Suzman, 1971; Tanna et al., 1977; Tyrer & Lader, 1974) and in panic disorder (Ravaris et al., 1986). As noted above, it is an attractive drug to consider because it would be expected to antagonize the peripheral and (probably the) central sympathetic hyperarousal associated with PTSD. Another advantage of propranolol is that it is a nonbenzodiazepine anxiolytic that can be prescribed without fear of fostering addiction or chemical abuse/dependence in susceptible PTSD patients. In an open trial of propranolol with 14 Vietnam veterans who received 120–160 mg daily for 6 months, most patients reported improvement with specific reductions in nightmares, intrusive recollections, hypervigilençe, insomnia, startle responses, and angry outbursts (Kolb et al., 1984). A controlled trial of up to 2.5 mg/kg/day propranolol in 11 sexually or physically abused children with acute PTSD (Famularo et al., 1988) demonstrated significant reduction of intrusive and arousal symptoms. When placebo was substituted for propranolol, the children's symptoms returned to predrug intensity.

Clonidine

Clonidine is an alpha-2 adrenergic agonist currently used in hypertension and opiate withdrawal. It reduces central adrenergic activity by reducing locus coeruleus activity. For that reason it holds out promise as an effective antidote to the adrenergic hyperactivity associated with anxiety disorders. The only information on clonidine in PTSD comes from an open trial with 9 Vietnam veterans who received a daily dose of 0.2–0.4 mg (Kolb et al., 1984). Eight patients had a favorable response marked by lessened explosiveness, reduced nightmares, improved sleep, lessened startle, reduced intrusive thinking, and less hyperalertness. As with propranolol, the authors were careful not to overstate their findings and urged others to conduct systematic controlled trials of both propranolol and clonidine to establish their usefulness in PTSD.

Benzodiazepines

Benzodiazepines are potent anxiolytics that have been prescribed widely for PTSD despite their lack of proven efficacy in controlled trials. Use of benzodiazepines in PTSD, of course, carries with it the risk of addiction and chemical abuse/dependency in susceptible patients (Friedman, 1981, 1988; van der Kolk, 1987). Practical clinical concerns about addiction notwithstanding, the kindling model of PTSD indicates that there may be a neurobiological rationale for prescribing these drugs. Several studies have shown that benzodiazepine receptor binding is increased significantly during the development of limbic kindling (McNamara et al., 1985; Morita et al., 1985; Tietz et al., 1985). This suggests that benzodiazepines and other GABA agonists or synergists might be particularly efficacious in PTSD.

Alprazolam

Alprazolam is a triazolo-benzodiazepine that apparently differs from other benzodiazepines because of its demonstrated antipanic and antidepressant properties (Feighner et al., 1983; Sheehan, 1982). It is currently used widely in PTSD, although there presently are no double-blind studies demonstrating its efficacy. In addition to concerns about addiction and dependence (mentioned previously with regard to all benzodiazepines), alprazolam's pharmacokinetic properties have raised additional concerns. Specifically, its short half-life makes the risk of rebound anxiety and serious withdrawal symptoms greater for alprazolam than for other benzodiazepines that are eliminated more slowly (Higgitt et al., 1985; Noyes et al., 1985).

Lithium

Lithium has been suggested as an effective treatment for PTSD even in patients with no personal or family history of bipolar or cyclothymic illness (Kitchner & Greenstein, 1985; van der Kolk, 1983). Van der Kolk (1987) reported that 14 out of 22 PTSD patients tried on lithium reported markedly diminished autonomic hyperarousal, a decreased tendency to react to stress as if it were a recurrence of their original trauma, and a marked decrease in alcohol intake. Van der Kolk stated that the therapeutic response to lithium in his patients was "clinically indistinguishable" from the aforementioned results with carbamazepine reported by Lipper et al. (1986). As with most other drugs reviewed in this section, there are no systematic double-blind trials of lithium in PTSD.

Neuroleptics

The last drugs to consider are the neuroleptics or antipsychotic agents. When disturbed Vietnam combat veterans first appeared in VA hospitals in the late 1960s and in the 1970s, many of them were prescribed neuroleptics. Psychiatrists impressed by the agitation, bizarre and explosive behavior, rage, anti-authoritarian beliefs merging into paranoia, and brief psychotic episodes that we now call flashbacks often chose a neuroleptic as the drug of first choice. Since that time, we have learned that adrenergic hyperarousal rather than psychotic thinking is the primary target in pharmacotherapy of PTSD. Reduction of DSM-III-R intrusive recollections and arousal symptoms by TCAs, MAOIs, or other drugs is often sufficient to reduce or eliminate psychotic-appearing manifestations of PTSD in most patients. Having learned after almost two decades of misuse and overuse of antipsychotic agents we can now state that neuroleptics have no place in the *routine* treatment of PTSD.

I am not saying that neuroleptics have no value in pharmacotherapy for this disorder, but that they should be used judiciously as a second or third choice following clinical trials of TCAs or other potential first-line drugs. Indications for neuroleptics include aggressive psychotic symptoms (frequently paranoid), overwhelming anger, fragmented ego boundaries, self-destructive behavior, and frequent flashback episodes characterized by visual and auditory hallucinations of traumatic events (Atri & Gilliam, 1989; Friedman, 1981, 1988; Walker, 1982). Mueser and Butler's (1987) report on 5 Vietnam veterans with combat-related PTSD who had auditory hallucinations suggests that there may be a subgroup among PTSD patients for whom neuroleptics are specifically indicated.

Comparative Pharmacotherapy: PTSD, MDD, and PD

Although numerous psychotropic agents have been used for PTSD, there is only one double-blind investigation suggesting that both imipramine and phenelzine have specific efficacy against both intrusive and avoidant symptoms (Frank et al., 1988). A second double-blind trial of amitriptyline versus placebo must be considered equivocal because amitriptyline was most effective in depressed PTSD patients and showed little therapeutic specificity against the symptoms of PTSD (Davidson et al., 1988). With the exception of one study with propranolol in traumatized children, promising claims for the effectiveness of other drugs have not been validated in double-blind clinical trials.

Table 11.3 shows similarities and differences in the psychopharmacological spectrum of action for PTSD, MDD, and PD. All three disorders appear to respond to TCAs, MAOIs, and probably alprazolam. Carbamazepine and lithium, which may be effective in PTSD and MDD, are without potency in PD. Although both drugs are efficacious in bipolar affective disorder, only lithium has proven therapeutic value in MDD. Benzodiazepines and antiadrenergic agents such as propranolol and clonidine (which may be useful in PTSD and PD) can worsen the symptoms of MDD. Finally, neuroleptics (which may be useful in a carefully selected minority of PTSD cases) have limited usefulness in psychotic MDD and are of no value in PD. To summarize, it can be seen from Tables 11.2 and 11.3 that despite considerable overlap in diagnostic abnormalities and responsivity to pharmacological agents, PTSD, MDD, and PD appear each to have unique biological characteristics.

PTSD AND CHEMICAL ABUSE/DEPENDENCY

Most clinicians who treat combat-related PTSD readily acknowledge that therapy is often complicated by coexisting symptoms of alcohol or other chemical abuse/dependency. This clinical impression is confirmed by published reports indicating that 60% to 80% of patients seeking treatment for PTSD have concurrent diagnoses of substance abuse or dependence (Branchey et al., 1984; Keane et al., 1988). Some have argued that such high rates of substance abuse are attributable to the fact that alcohol and other drugs were extremely available to military personnel stationed in Vietnam during the war (Sapol & Roffman, 1969; Wedding, 1987). This cannot explain, however, why veterans with higher levels of combat exposure are more likely to abuse alcohol than those who saw considerably less combat (Keane et al., 1988). Indeed, the latter finding suggests that neurobiological alterations associated with PTSD make affected individuals more susceptible to alcohol and illicit drug use.

Among the biological abnormalities occurring in PTSD, sympathetic nervous system hyperarousal and chronic lowering of endogenous opioid levels are most likely to generate susceptibility to chemical abuse/dependency. Any drug that can suppress central adrenergic activity—such as alcohol, central depressants, marijuana, or opiates—will produce temporary relief in the person suffering from PTSD. Furthermore, the possibility of a chronic opioid deficiency (indicated by lowered pain thresholds) suggests that PTSD patients might successfully ameliorate intolerable symptoms with heroin, methadone, and other opiates. Kosten and Krystal (1988) have elegantly reviewed the biological basis for PTSD symptoms and substance abuse. Arguing theoretically from van der Kolk's inescapable shock model of PTSD, they speculate that "use of ethanol or other drugs such as heroin in acute stress settings of war is an active adaptive style" and that "individuals with a history of recreational substance abuse may be more prone to 'self-medicate'" (Kosten & Krystal, 1988, p. 60). They also point out that during the vicious addiction-withdrawal cycle, the adrenergic arousal associated either with alcohol or opiate withdrawal will trigger a conditioned emotional response associated with PTSD symptoms. In other words, the normal difficulties of treating chemical dependency are multiplied by the complex risk of exacerbating PTSD symptoms. This may be an even greater problem in cases of opiate dependence, because heroin not only dampens adrenergic hyperarousal but may also serve to replenish an endogenous opioid system that has been depleted because of the pathophysiology of PTSD.

Although it is possible that central stimulants effectively relieve the dysphoria of PTSD, especially when depression is also present, one might predict on neurobiological grounds that the incidence of cocaine and amphetamine abuse among PTSD patients will be lower than expected. This is because central stimulants will facilitate sympathetic hyperarousal, thereby exacerbating PTSD symptoms. To my knowledge this has not been studied systematically. In my own clinical experience, however, PTSD patients do not like the heightened emotional state produced by cocaine, amphetamines, and other stimulants. They generally prefer alcohol, marijuana, central depressants, or opiates. Furthermore, cocaine and stimulant users with PTSD are usually also dependent on alcohol, marijuana, opiates, and the like.

When PTSD and chemical abuse/dependency occur simultaneously, they must be treated simultaneously. Rigid adherence to the generic treatment formulas found in many alcohol and drug rehabilitation programs is a prescription for failure. This is because the complex interrelationships between intrapsychic, behavioral, and biological aspects of PTSD and concurrent chemical abuse/dependency demand a comprehensive approach. A detailed description of treatment strategies for patients who carry the dual diagnosis of PTSD and chemical abuse/dependency is beyond the scope of this chapter. Psychopharmacological strategies to be integrated in such an approach may include disulfram (Antabuse) for alcohol dependence and the opiate antagonist naltrexone. Kosten and Krystal (1988) have suggested that the mixed opiate agonist-antagonist buprenorphine may be uniquely suited to "suppress conditioned noradrenergic activation and maintain antagonist self-administration" (p. 62) in PTSD patients undergoing opiate withdrawal. The bottom line, as noted by Stone (1988), is a therapeutic approach that respects both the psychological and neurobiological implications of autopharmacotherapy in patients who suffer from PTSD and chemical abuse/dependency.

CONCLUSION

1. The unique pattern of biological abnormalities associated with PTSD appear to differentiate this disorder from MDD and PD.

2. Provocative laboratory tests that probe PTSD-induced alterations in

noradrenergic activity, the HPA axis, the endogenous opioid system, and the sleep cycle should enable us to achieve greater precision in diagnosing PTSD.

3. Almost every conceivable psychotropic agent has been reported to have efficacy in PTSD. Almost all of these claims are based on clinical anecdotes or open drug trials except for two double-blind investigations on imipramine, phenelzine, and amitriptyline and one controlled study with propranolol.

4. Neurobiological alterations associated with PTSD may make affected individuals more susceptible to alcohol, opiate, and other illicit drug use. The complex interrelationships between intrapsychic, behavioral, and biological aspects of PTSD and concurrent chemical abuse/dependency demand a comprehensive approach to both problems simultaneously.

5. Successful pharmacotherapy for PTSD has generally provided alleviation of DSM-III-R intrusive recollections and arousal symptoms. Avoidant symptoms, impacted grief, guilt, rage, problems with intimacy, and moral pain do not appear to respond to medication. Therefore, it should be understood that drug treatment alone can never alleviate the suffering in PTSD. Pharmacotherapy is primarily useful as an adjunct to psychological (intrapsychic and/or behavioral) treatment of PTSD.

REFERENCES

Akiskal, H. S. (1983). Diagnosis and classification of affective disorders: New insights from clinical and laboratory approaches. *Psychiatr. Dev., 2,* 123–160.

Archibald, H. C. & Tuddenham, R. D. (1965). Persistent stress reaction after combat: A 20 year follow-up. *Arch. Gen. Psychiat., 12,* 475–481.

Atri, P. B., & Gilliam, J. H. (1989). Letter. *Am. J. Psychiat., 146,* 128.

Beard, G. M. (1869). Neurasthenia or nervous exhaustion. *Bost. Med. Surg. J., 3,* 3–217.

Blake, D. J. (1986). Treatment of acute post-traumatic stress disorder with tricyclic antidepressants. *South. Med. J., 79,* 201–204.

Benedikt, R. A., & Kolb, L. C. (1986). Preliminary findings on chronic pain and post-traumatic stress disorder. *Am. J. Psychiat., 143,* 908–910.

Blanchard, E. G., Kolb, L. C., Pallmeyer, B. A., & Gerardi, R. J. (1982). A psychophysiological study of post-traumatic stress disorder in Vietnam veterans. *Psychiat. Quart., 54,* 220–229.

Boehnlein, J. K., Kinzie, J. D., Ben, R., et al. 1985). One-year follow-up study of post-traumatic stress disorder among survivors of Cambodian concentration camps. *Am. J. Psychiat, 142,* 956–959.

Branchey, L., Davis, W. & Lieber, C. S. (1984). Alcoholism in Vietnam and Korea veterans: A long term follow-up. *Alcoholism: Clin. Exp. Res., 8,* 572–757.

Brende, J. O. (1982). Electrodermal responses in post-traumatic syndromes. *J. Nerv. Ment. Dis., 170,* 352–361.

Burstein, A. (1982). Treatment of post-traumatic stress disorder with imipramine. *Psychosomatics, 25,* 681–687.

Carroll, B. J., Feinberg, M., Greden, J. F., et al. (1981). A specific laboratory test for the diagnosis of melancholia. *Arch. Gen. Psychiat., 38,* 15–22.

Charney, D. S., Woods, S. W., Goodman, W. K., & Heninger, G. K. (1987). Neurobiological

mechanisms of panic anxiety: biochemical and behavioral correlates of yohimbine-induced panic attacks. *Am. J. Psychiat., 144,* 1030–1036.
Ciccone, P. E., Mazarek, A., Weisbrot, M., et al. (1990). Letter. *Am. J. Psychiat., 146,* 812.
Cohen, M. E., White, P. D., and Johnson, R. E. (1948). Neurocirculatory asthenia, anxiety neurosis or the effort syndrome. *Arch. Int. Med., 81,* 260–281.
Cohen, M. E., & White, P. D. (1950). Life situations, emotions and neurocirculatory asthenia (anxiety neurosis, neurasthenia, effort syndrome). *Res. Publ. Assoc. Res. Nerv. Ment. Dis., 29,* 832–864.
DaCosta, J. M. (1871). On irritable heart: A clinical study of a form of functional cardiac disorder and its consequences. *Am. J. Med. Sci., 61,* 17–52.
Davidson, J., Lipper, S., Kilts, C. D., et al. (1985). Platelet MAO activity in posttraumatic stress disorder. *Am. J. Psychiat., 142,* 1341–1343.
Davidson, J., Walker, J. I., & Kilts, C. (1987). A pilot study of phenelzine in the treatment of post-traumatic stress disorder. *Brit. J. Psychiat., 150,* 252–255.
Davidson, J., Kudler, H., Smith, R., et al. (1988, May). *Amitriptyline treatment of PTSD.* Presented at 141st annual meeting of the American Psychiatric Association, Montreal.
Dobbs, O., & Wilson, W. P. (1960). Observations on persistence of war neurosis. *Dis. Nerv. Sys., 21,* 686–691.
Dube, S., Jones, D. A., & Bell, J. (1986). Interface of panic and depression: Clinical and sleep EEG correlates. *Psychiat. Res., 119,* 119–133.
Embry, C. K., & Callahan, B. (1988). Effective pharmacotherapy for post-traumatic stress disorder. *VA Pract., 5,* 57–66.
Falcon, S., Ryan, C., Chamberlain, K., & Curtis, G. (1985). Tricyclics: Possible treatment for posttraumatic stress disorder. *J. Clin. Psychiat., 46,* 385–389.
Famularo, R., Kinscherff, R., & Fenton, T. (1988). Propranolol treatment for childhood posttraumatic stress disorder, acute type: A pilot study. *Am. J. Dis. Child., 142,* 1244–1247.
Feighner, J. P., Aden, G. C., Fabre, L. F., Rickels, K., & Smith, W. T. (1983). Comparison of alprazolam, imipramine and placebo in the treatment of depression. *J. Am. Med. Assoc., 249,* 3057–3064.
Frank, J. B., Kosten, T. R., Dan, E., et al. (1988, May). *Imipramine and phenelzine treatment of PTSD.* Presented at 141st annual meeting of the Am. Psychiat. Assoc., Montreal.
Friedman, M. J. (1981). Post-Vietnam syndrome: recognition and management. *Psychosomatics, 22,* 931–943.
Friedman, M. J. (1988). Towards rational pharmacotherapy for post-traumatic stress disorder. *Am. J. Psychiat., 145,* 281–285.
Fryer, M. R., Uy, J., Martinez, J., et al. (1987). CO_2 challenge of patients with panic disorder. *Am. J. Psychiat., 144,* 1080–1082.
Gillespie, R. D. (1942). *Psychological effects of war on citizen and soldier.* New York: Norton.
Greenberg, R., Pearlman, C. A., & Gampel, D. (1972). War neuroses and the adaptive function of REM sleep. *Brit. J. Med. Psychol., 45,* 27–33.
Greenstein, R. A., Kitchner, I., & Olsen, K. (1986). Post-traumatic stress disorder, partial complex seizures, and alcoholism. *Am. J. Psychiat., 142,* 1203.
Halbreich, U., Olympia, J., Glogowski, J., et al. (1988). The importance of past psychological trauma and pathophysiologic process as determinants of current biologic abnormalities. *Arch. Gen. Psychiat., 45,* 293–294.
Hartshorne, H. (1864). On heart disease in the army. *Am. J. Med. Sci., 47,* 89–92.
Hauri, P. J., Friedman, M. J., & Ravaris, C. L. (1989). Sleep in patients with spontaneous panic attacks. *Sleep, 12,* 323–337.
Higgitt, A. C., Lader, M. H., & Fonagy, P. (1985). Clinical management of benzodiazepine dependence. *Brit. Med. J., 291,* 688–690.
Hogben, G. L., & Cornfield, R. B. (1981). Treatment of traumatic war neurosis with phenelzine. *Arch. Gen. Psychiat., 38,* 440–445.
Kardiner, A. (1941). The traumatic neuroses of war. *Psychosomatic Medicine Monographs,* 11–111.
Kardiner, A., & Speigel, H. (1947). *The traumatic neuroses of war.* New York: Hoeber.

Kauffman, C. D., Reist, C., Djenderedjian, A., et al. (1987). Biological markers of affective disorders and posttraumatic stress disorder. A pilot study with desipramine. *J. Clin. Psychiat., 48,* 366–367.

Keane, T. M., Zimering, R. T., & Caddell, J. M. (1985). A behavioral formulation of posttraumatic stress disorder in Vietnam veterans. *Behav. Ther., 8,* 9–12.

Keane, T. M., Gerardi, R. J., Lyons, J. A., et al. (1988). The interrelationship of substance abuse and posttraumatic stress disorder: Epidemiological and clinical considerations. *Rec. Dev. Alcohol., 6,* 27–48.

Kitchner, L., & Greenstein, R. (1985). Low dose lithium carbonate in the treatment of posttraumatic stress disorder: Brief communication. *Milit. Med., 150,* 378–381.

Kolb, L. C. (1985). The place of narcosynthesis in the treatment of chronic and delayed stress reactions of war. In Sonnenberg, S. M., Blank, A. S., & Talbott, J. A. (eds.), *The trauma of war stress and recovery in Vietnam veterans* (pp. 211–226). Washington, DC: American Psychiatric Press.

Kolb, L. C. (1987). A neuropsychological hypothesis explaining post-traumatic stress disorders. *Am. J. Psychiat., 144,* 989–995.

Kolb, L. C., Burris, B. C., Griffiths, S. (1984). Propranolol and clonidine in the treatment of the chronic posttraumatic stress disorders of war. In B. A. van der Kolk, (Ed.), *Post-traumatic stress disorder: Psychological and biological sequelae.* Washington, DC: American Psychiatric Press.

Kosten, T. R., & Krystal, J. (1988). Biological mechanisms in post-traumatic stress disorder: Relevance for substance abuse. *Rec. Dev. Alcohol, 6,* 49–68.

Kosten, T. R., Mason, J. W., Giller, E. L., et al. (1987). Sustained urinary norepinephrine elevation in post-traumatic stress disorder. *Psychoneuroendocrinology, 12,* 13–30.

Kosten, T. R., Giller, E. L., & Mason, J. W. (1988, May). *Psychoendocrine assessment of PTSD.* Presented at 141st annual meeting, American Psychiatric Association, Montreal.

Kramer, M. (1979). Dream disturbance. *Psychiat. Ann., 9,* 50–60.

Kramer, M., & Kinney, L. (1985). Is sleep a marker of vulnerability to delayed posttraumatic stress disorder? *Sleep Res., 14,* 181.

Kramer, M., & Kinney, L. (1988). Sleep patterns in trauma victims with disturbed dreaming. *Psychiat. J. Univ. Ottawa, 13,* 12–16.

Kramer, M., Kinney, L., & Scharf, M. (1982). Sleep in delayed stress victims. *Sleep Res., 11,* 113.

Kudler, H., Davidson, J., & Meador, K. (1987). The DST and post-traumatic stress disorder. *Am. J. Psychiat., 144,* 1068–1071.

Kupfer, D. J., & Thase, M. E. (1983). The use of the sleep laboratory in the diagnosis of affective disorders. *Psychiat. Clin. North Am., 6,* 3–25.

Lavie, P., Hefez, A., Halperin, G., et al., (1979). Long-term effects of traumatic war-related events on sleep. *Am. J. Psychiat., 136,* 175–178.

Lerer, B., Ebstein, R., Shestatsky, M., et al. (1987). Cyclic AMP signal transduction in post-traumatic stress disorder. *Am. J. Psychiat., 144,* 1324–1327.

Lerer, B., Bleich, A., & Kotler, M. (1987). Post-traumatic stress disorder in Israeli combat veterans: Effect of phenelzine treatment. *Arch. Gen. Psychiat., 44,* 976–981.

Lewis, T. (1917). *Reports upon soldiers returned as cases of disordered action of the heart (DAH) or valvular disease of the heart (VDH).* London: His Majesty's Stationery Office.

Lipper, S., Davidson, J. R. T., Grady, T. A., et al. (1986). Preliminary study of carbamazepine in posttraumatic stress disorder. *Psychosomatics, 27,* 849–854.

Malloy, P. F., Fairbank, J. A., & Keane, T. M. (1983). Validation of a multimethod assessment of post-traumatic stress disorders in Vietnam veterans. *J. Consult. Clin. Psychol., 51,* 488–494.

Marshall, J. R. (1975). The treatment of night terrors associated with the post-traumatic syndrome. *Am. J. Psychiat., 132,* 293–295.

Mason, J. W., Giller, E. L., Kosten, T. R., et al. (1985). *Elevation of urinary norepinephrine/cortisol ratio in post-traumatic stress disorder,* Paper presented at "New Research Program and Abstracts," 138th annual meeting of the American Psychiatric Association, Washington, DC.

Mason, J. W., Giller, E. I., Kosten, T. R., Ostroff, R., & Harkness, L. (1986). Urinary free-cortisol in post-traumatic stress disorder. *J. Nerv. Ment. Dis., 174,* 145–149.

McNamara, J. O., Bonhaus, D. W., Shin, C., Crain, B. J., Gellman, R. L., & Giacchino, J. L. (1985). The kindling model of epilepsy: A critical review. *CRC Crit. Rev. Clin. Neurobiol., 1,* 341–391.

Mellman, T. A., & Davis, G. C. (1985). Combat-related flashbacks in post-traumatic stress disorder: Phenomenology and similarity to panic attacks. *J. Clin. Psychiat., 46,* 379–382.

Milanes, F. S., Mack, C. N., & Dennison, J. (1984). Phenelzine treatment of post-Vietnam stress syndrome. *VA Practit.,* 40–49.

Morita, K., Okamoto, M., Seki, K., & Wada, J. A. (1985). Suppression of amygdala-kindled seizures in cats by enhanced GABAergic transmission in the substantia innominata. *Exp. Neurol., 89,* 225–236.

Mueser, K. T., & Butler, R. W. (1987). Auditory hallucinations in combat-related chronic post-traumatic stress disorder. *Am. J. Psychiat., 144,* 299–302.

Noyes, R., Clancy, J., Coryell, W. H., Crowe, R. R., Chaudhry, D. R., & Domingo, D. V. (1985). A withdrawal syndrome after abrupt discontinuation of alprazolam. *Am. J. Psychiat., 142,* 114–116.

Perry, B. D., Giller, E. L., & Southwick, S. M. (1987). Altered platelet alpha 2 adrenergic binding sites in post-traumatic stress disorder. *Am. J. Psychiat., 144,* 1511–1512.

Perry, B. D., Southwick, S. M., & Giller, E. L. (1988, May). *Adrenergic receptor regulation in PTSD.* Paper presented at 141st annual meeting of the American Psychiatric Association, Montreal.

Perry, S. W., Cella, D. F., Falkenberg, J., et al. (1987). Pain perception in burn patients with stress disorders. *J. Pain Sympt. Manag., 2,* 29–33.

Pitman, R. K., Orr, S. P., Forgue, D. F., et al. (1987). Psychophysiologic assessment of post-traumatic stress disorder imagery in Vietnam combat veterans. *Arch. Gen. Psychiat., 44,* 970–975.

Pitman, R. K., van der Kolk, B., Orr, S. P., et al. (1990). Naloxone-reversible analgesic response to combat-related stimuli in post-traumatic stress disorder. *Arch. Gen. Psychiat., 47,* 541–544.

Pitts, F. N., Jr., & McClure, J. N., Jr. (1967). Lactate metabolism in anxiety neurosis. *N. Eng. J. Med., 277,* 1329–1336.

Post, R. M., & Kopanda, R. T. (1976). Cocaine, kindling and psychosis. *Am. J Psychiat., 133,* 627–634.

Price, L. H., Charney, I. D. S., Rubin, A. L., & Heninger, G. R. (1986). Alpha-2 adrenergic receptor function in depression: The cortisol response to yohimbine. *Arch. Gen. Psychiat., 43,* 849–858.

Rainey, J. M., Aleem, A., Ortiz, A., et al. (1987). A laboratory procedure for the induction of flashbacks. *Am. J. Psychiat., 144,* 1317–1319.

Rapaport, M. H. (1987). Chronic pain and post-traumatic stress disorder. *Am. J. Psychiat., 144,* 120.

Ravaris, C. L., Friedman, M. J., & Hauri, P. (1986, May). *A controlled study of alprazolam and propranolol in panic disorder and agoraphobic patients.* Paper presented at 139th annual meeting, American Psychiatric Association, Washington, DC.

Ross, R. J., Ball, W., & Morrison, A. (1990). Letter. *Am. J. Psychiat., 147,* 374.

Ross, R. J., Ball, W. A., Sullivan, K. A. & Caroff, S. N. (1989). Sleep disturbance as the hallmark of post-traumatic stress disorder. *Am. J. Psychiat, 146,* 697–707.

Sapol, E., & Roffman, R. A. (1969). Marijuana in Vietnam. *Journal of the American Pharmaceutical Association,* NS9, 615–630.

Schlossberg, A., & Benjamin, M. (1978). Sleep patterns in three acute combat fatigue cases. *J. Clin. Psychiat., 39,* 546–549.

Shalev, A. Y., Bleich, A. & Ursano, R. J. (1990). Posttraumatic stress disorder: somatic comorbidity and effort tolerance. *Psychosomatics, 31,* 197–203.

Sheehan, D. V. (1982). Current perspectives in the treatment of panic and phobic disorders. *Drug Ther., 7,* 179–193.

Shen, W. W., & Park, S. (1983). The use of monoamine oxidase inhibitors in the treatment of traumatic war neurosis: Case report. *Milit. Med., 148,* 430–431.

Solomon, Z., & Mikulincer, M. (1987). Combat stress reaction, post-traumatic stress disorder and somatic complaints among Israeli soldiers. *J. Psychosom. Res., 31,* 131–137.

Stewart, J. R., & Bartucci, R. J. (1986). Post-traumatic stress disorder and partial complex seizures. *Am. J. Psychiat., 143,* 113–114.

Stone, A. (1988). Letter. *Am. J. Psychiat., 145,* 1485.

Suzman, M. M. (1971). The use of beta-adrenergic blockade with propranolol in anxiety syndrome. *Postgrad. Med. J., 47,* 104–108.

Tanna, V. T., Penningroth, R. P., & Woolson, R. F. (1977). Propranolol in the treatment of anxiety neurosis. *Comp. Psychiat., 18,* 319–326.

Tietz, E. I., Gomaz, F., & Berman, R. F. (1985). Amygdala kindled seizure stage is related to altered benzodiazepine binding site density. *Life Sci., 36,* 183–190.

Tyrer, P. J., & Lader, M. H. (1974). Response to propranolol and diazepam in somatic anxiety. *Brit. Med. J., 2,* 14–16.

Uhde, T. W., Stein, M. B., & Post, R. M. (1988). Lack of efficacy of carbamazepine in the treatment of panic disorder. *Am. J. Psychiat., 145,* 1104–1109.

van der Kolk, B. A. (1983). Psychopharmacological issues in post-traumatic stress disorder. *Hosp. Commun. Psychiat., 34,* 683–691.

van der Kolk, B. A. (1987). The drug treatment of post-traumatic stress disorder. *J. Affect. Dis., 13,* 203–213.

van der Kolk, B. A., Blitz, R., Burr, W., Sherry, S., & Hartmann, E. (1984). Nightmares and trauma: A comparison of nightmares after combat with lifelong nightmares in veterans. *Am. J. Psychiat., 141,* 187–190.

van der Kolk, B. A., Greenberg, M., Boyd, H., & Krystal, J. (1985). Inescapable shock, neurotransmitters, and addiction to trauma: Toward a psychobiology of post-traumatic stress. *Biol. Psychiat., 20,* 314–325.

Van Kammen, W., Christiansen, C., Van Kammen, D., et al. (1987). Sleep and the POW experience: 40 years later. *Sleep Res., 16,* 291.

Walker, J. I. (1982). Chemotherapy of traumatic war stress. *Milit. Med., 147,* 1029–1033.

Wedding, D. (1987). Substance abuse in the Vietnam veteran. *AAOHN J., 35,* 74–76.

Wolf, M. E., Alavi, A., & Mosnaim, A. D. (1988). Post-traumatic stress disorder in Vietnam veterans clinical and EEG findings; possible therapeutic effects of carbamazepine. *Biol. Psychiat., 23,* 642–644.

Wood, P. (1941). DaCosta's syndrome or effort syndrome. *Brit. Med. J., 1,* 767, 805, 845.

12

Pierre Janet's Treatment of Post-Traumatic Stress

ONNO VAN DER HART, PAUL BROWN, and BESSEL A. VAN DER KOLK

Pierre Janet was probably the first psychologist to formulate a systematic therapeutic approach to post-traumatic psychopathology and to recognize that treatment needs to be adapted to the different stages of the evolution of post-traumatic stress reactions. Starting in the early 1880s, Janet developed an eclectic treatment approach based on his clinical experience with many severely traumatized patients with either hysterical (dissociative) or psychasthenic (obsessive-compulsive) post-traumatic features. Our review of Janet's psychotherapy of post-traumatic syndromes covers publications written over a period of 50 years (Janet, 1886, 1889, 1898a, b, 1903, 1904, 1911, 1919/1976, 1923/1925, 1932, 1935). Throughout this chapter, however, we shall refer mainly to his magnum opus on psychotherapy, *Psychological Healing* (PH) (Janet, 1919/1976).

STAGES OF POST-TRAUMATIC ADAPTATION

Janet considered the inability to integrate traumatic memories as the core issue in post-traumatic syndromes: Treatment of psychological trauma

ONNO VAN DER HART • Department of Clinical and Health Psychology, University of Utrecht, Utrecht, The Netherlands; and Dissociation Team, Regional Institute for Ambulatory Mental Health Care, Amsterdam South/New West, Amsterdam, The Netherlands. **PAUL BROWN** • Northpark Hospital Centre, Bundoora, Melbourne, Victoria, Australia. **BESSEL A. VAN DER KOLK** • Trauma Clinic, Massachusetts General Hospital, Harvard Medical School, Boston, Massachusetts 02114. Reprinted from *Journal of Traumatic Stress*, Vol. 2, No. 4.

Psychotraumatology, edited by George S. Everly, Jr. and Jeffrey M. Lating. Plenum Press, New York, 1995.

always entailed an attempt to recover and integrate the memories of the trauma into the totality of people's identities. He never developed a nosology for a post-traumatic stress disorder as such, but he clearly recognized the fundamental biphasic nature of the trauma response, and he described all the contemporary DSM-III criteria for PTSD in great detail in both his case histories and in his theoretical works (see van der Kolk et al., 1989).

He divided the trauma response into three stages: The first one consists of a mixture of dissociative (hysterical) reactions, obsessional ruminations, and generalized agitation precipitated by a traumatic event. The second stage of delayed post-traumatic symptomatology consists of a blend of hysterical, obsessional, and anxiety symptoms in which it often is difficult to recognize the traumatic etiology of the symptoms. The third and last stage is characterized by what modern authors call post-traumatic decline (Titchener, 1986) and includes somatization disorders, depersonalization, and melancholia, ending in apathy and social withdrawal. Like modern writers, Janet recognized that in chronic cases complete recovery is rare, even when the patient is capable of recounting the trauma in detail.

Therapeutic Rapport and Moral Guidance

Janet was very much aware of the need to establish a special, safe patient-therapist relationship before attempting to deal with traumatic memories. He considered "rapport" between patient and therapist indispensible for resolution of the trauma, but recognized that severely traumatized patients are prone to idealization, which can develop into intense "somnambulistic passion" (Janet, 1897, 1935). "Rapport" was not only what we would today call a therapeutic alliance but also a specific method for reducing symptoms and increasing mental energy. True to his times, Janet thought that moral guidance was an essential element of the doctor-patient relationship at all stages of treatment (PH, p. 1112). This was based on the notion of the late 18th-century hypnotists (the *magnétiseurs)* of *rapport magnétique;* the notion of "rapport" also was the ancestor of the psychoanalytic concept of transference. Like Freud (1911/1959), who later declared that "transference is a resistance," Janet considered rapport both a symptom of illness in its own right and a vehicle for cure (Haule, 1986; Janet, 1897). In the hypnotic rapport, the traumatized patient was prone to develop a pathological fixation on the therapist which Janet (1897) called "the somnambulistic influence." He thought that "this strange illusion" (PH, p. 1156) was related to post-traumatic dissociation, narrowing of consciousness, and feelings of helplessness. The intensity of this somnambulistic influence bore no apparent relationship to the therapist's competence. The pathological need for guidance built up between treatment sessions and reached a crescendo—the somnambulistic passion—early in the therapy. Janet claimed that it usually was a transient phenomenon that decreased when patients became ashamed about the intensity of their dependence. The real motivation for therapy came from the patients' despair and their hope for improvement. Janet called their settling down to talk seriously about what troubled them "the act of adoption" (PH, p. 1154; Janet, 1929).

Personality characteristics of the therapist also played an important role in the nature of the therapeutic relationship: He was to position himself not as a parent surrogate or omnipotent protector but as a skilled agent of therapeutic change (PH, p. 1112). Janet advocated two apparently contradictory attitudes for the therapist: On the one hand, the patient must accept his authority and guidance, on the other, the therapist needs to minimize his control over the patient (Janet, 1897; cf. Haule, 1986). Relying too much on the doctor's authority would lead to only temporary cures (Freud, 1914/1958 was to warn later also about the danger of transference cures); ignoring the need to keep patients fundamentally in control over their own lives led to excessive "somnambulistic influence" (today we would call this transference psychosis), which made treatment impossible. Like many contemporary therapists, Janet learned the hard way that if one neglects the dimension of control, passion is likely to get out of hand. In several case reports he tried to demonstrate how "rapport" could be used even with severely disturbed patients to foster independent action rather than excessive dependency and misdirected passion.

"Psychological Force" and "Psychological Tension"

Although most of Janet's concepts are readily understandable in contemporary terms, his notions of psychological force and psychological tension (van der Hart & Friedman, 1989) are not easily translated into contemporary concepts. *Psychological force* referred to the total amount of psychic energy available, *psychological tension* to the level of organization of this energy and the capacity for competent, creative, and reflective action. Janet thought that a person's psychological tension largely determined whether he or she could deal with potentially traumatizing experiences. Once the person was traumatized, the degree of remaining psychological tension also influenced the severity of the patient's impairment and determined what treatment would work. The patient's mental resources must be carefully assessed: In acute and simple post-traumatic reactions, there usually are enough mental energy reserves to do the work of integrating the traumatic memories successfully. Chronic and complex traumatization decreases psychological tension, however, causing mental energy to be wasted on compulsive repetitions, psychosomatic symptoms, wasteful agitations and crises, and impulsive and purposeless acts. The end result is mental exhaustion and disorganization: "The subject is unable to recite the events as they occurred and yet, he remains confronted with a painful situation in which he was unable to play a satisfactory role and make a successful adaptation. The struggle to repeat continually this situation leads to fatigue and exhaustion which have a considerable impact on his emotions" (PH, p. 663).

Janet organized the treatment of this mental exhaustion around three economic principles: increase psychological income by promoting sleep and diet; reduce expenses by curing coexisting medical conditions and relieving crises and agitation; and liquidate debts by resolving traumatic memories. Janet advocated two strategies for treating mental disorganization: channeling energies that would otherwise be wasted on agitations constructively, and stimulating the mental energy level by such methods as performing progressively more difficult tasks (Ellenberger, 1950; Schwartz, 1951).

JANET'S MODEL FOR THE TREATMENT OF POST-TRAUMATIC STRESS

Janet's psychotherapeutic approach to post-traumatic stress consisted of the following stages:

1. Stabilization, symptom-oriented treatment, and preparation for liquidation of traumatic memories
2. Identification, exploration, and modification of traumatic memories
3. Relapse prevention, relief of residual symptomatology, personality reintegration, and rehabilitation

In all phases retrieval, exploration, and modification of traumatic memories were indicated. Taking charge of one's life also needs to be fostered during all stages of post-traumatic stress, within the limits of the patient's capacity. Janet's stage model is very similar to modern models of treatment for post-traumatic stress disorder (PTSD) and dissociative disorders (Braun, 1986; Brown & Fromm, 1986; Parson, 1984; Kluft, 1987; Sachs et al., 1988). Brown and Fromm (1986) identified five stages: (1) stabilization; (2) integration, with the substages of controlled uncovering, integrating introjects, and new personality states; (3) development of self; (4) drive integration; and (5) dealing with enduring biological sensitivity. Each of these stages requires different therapeutic techniques. Similarly, in multiple personality disorder (MPD), a condition with a well-established childhood traumatic etiology, Sachs et al. (1988) have identified five phases: (1) making and sharing the diagnosis, (2) identifying the various personality states and understanding their purpose and function, (3) sharing with the therapist and other personality states the specific traumata associated with each personality state, (4) integrating the various personality states into a single functioning whole, and (5) learning new coping mechanisms that will enable functioning of the unified personality and prevent future splitting of the personality.

Stage models such as these can only provide broad therapeutic guidelines; they must be modified to fit individual cases. Janet varied the sequence and methods according to the stage of the disorder and the status of the patient's mental economy. Certain issues, such as working through the traumatic memories, must be addressed over and over again during the course of treatment. Janet was well aware that systematized treatment approaches without solid scientific verification had serious limitations (PH, p. 1210). He therefore offered his stage model only as an heuristic approach.

STAGE 1: STABILIZATION AND SYMPTOM REDUCTION

People with acute post-traumatic reactions, or with exacerbations of chronic pathology, first of all needed stabilization of symptoms. This consisted mostly of rest (including hospitalization), simplification of lifestyle, and forming a therapeutic relationship. In uncomplicated, generally acute cases these procedures usually were sufficient to allow for retrieval and working through (liquidation) of the traumatic memories. Because of their low level of psychological tension, chronic and complex cases first required mental stimulation and reeducation in preparation for liquidation of the traumatic memories.

Rest, Isolation, and Simplification of Lifestyle

Rest was meant to restore energy and build up reserves and was particularly suitable for patients who were too exhausted by repeated failures to overcome the vicissitudes of the trauma (PH, p. 466). Traumatized patients often had great difficulty achieving a modicum of calm: Acute patients often were delirious, and chronic patients sometimes were so agitated that they could not even lie down. Janet did not have much faith in sedatives such as bromides (PH, p. 693). Hence, even in these agitated, energy-wasting conditions and in depletion states, Janet advocated more active remedies.

In many cases, a simplification of lifestyle was necessary to get treatment under way (PH, p. 473). Janet believed in protecting patients from their social obligations and family pressures. He regularly utilized hospitalization and called this "isolation" (PH, p. 485). Initially, little was expected of the patient beyond automatic (as opposed to complex) activity: The therapist made all the decisions, solved the problems, and made the necessary changes in the environment. Hospitalization was used as an opportunity to effect changes in family organization (PH, p. 587). Janet thought that younger patients with recent trauma histories benefited most from hospitalization, but it often was beneficial for more chronic cases as well. He recognized that institutionalization had serious drawbacks, but he felt that when there was too much disruption in the patient's life, short-term asylum allowed for a more specific focus on the treatment of the psychological trauma (PH, p. 581). For example, his patient Irène twice attempted suicide and became progressively worse until she was hospitalized at the Salpêtrière (Janet, 1904). Sometimes readmission was necessary; for example, Irène returned 3 months after discharge, following the death of her father (Janet, 1904).

Stimulation and Reeducation

For patients suffering from low psychological energy Janet prescribed stimulation in order to get treatment going (PH, p. 942). This included education to enable patients with post-traumatic reactions to perform elementary daily functions, such as eating and sleeping, and to make social contact—particularly in the doctor-patient relationship, where they could begin to face traumatic issues. These methods, to be described more fully under Stage 3, ranged from simple focused self-disclosure (PH, p. 969) to awareness exercises (PH, p. 972). The risks of these treatments, including agitation and fatigue, could be balanced by varying the exercises (PH, p. 982ff) or by stopping them altogether.

Hypnosis for the Stabilization Stage

Hypnosis for symptom relief was commonly used at the end of the 19th century. Janet used hypnosis in the stabilization phase to produce relaxation, to modify symptoms, and to alleviate life-threatening conditions (Janet, 1898a). In some post-traumatic psychasthenias, it could increase the patient's energy level and strengthen the therapeutic rapport. Sometimes Janet used extended hypnosis, for days or even weeks, without offering any specific suggestions (Wetterstrand, 1892). Hypnosis could provide relief from insomnia, conversion reactions, and amnestic states; intractable motor paralyses or life-threatening anorexia could be approached directly; patients could exercise their limbs, eat, or drink and thereby protect their physical well-being (PH, p. 457). Success at this stage improved the rapport and facilitated later hypnotic retrieval of traumatic memories (Barrucand, 1967).

Symptom-oriented suggestions during this stage might address such minor symptoms as headaches, or such debilitating conditions as epileptic pseudoseizures. Janet recognized the limitations of this approach. Sometimes patients were able to accept suggestions unrelated to the trauma, whereas trauma-related material met with stiff resistance. In some cases, this produced an exacerbation of symptoms or the development of new complaints. Janet felt that these failures were the result of emotional states related to subconscious trauma-related fixed ideas that could only be resolved when the underlying traumatic memories were successfully liquidated (van der Hart & Horst, 1989; van der Kolk et al., 1989).

STAGE 2: MODIFICATION OF TRAUMATIC MEMORIES

For Janet, liquidation of traumatic memories was the key to resolution of post-traumatic stress. Dissociated traumatic memories continued as subconscious fixed ideas and emerged periodically out of personal and conscious control as behaviors, feelings states, somatic sensations, and dreams without relevance to current experience but appropriate to the original trauma (Janet, 1893). The lack of integration of the traumatic memories led to arrested personality development. "Unable to integrate the traumatic memories, they seem to have lost their capacity to assimilate new experiences as well. It is . . . as if their personality which definitely stopped at a certain point cannot enlarge any more by the addition or assimilation of new elements: all [traumatized] patients seem to have had the evolution of their lives checked; they are attached to an unsurmountable obstacle" (PH, p. 660). In uncomplicated cases, traumatic memories and the psychological charge associated with them were "near the surface" and often available to nontrance interventions. Simply discussing their experiences and sometimes sharing a diary with the therapist could lead to resolution. Usually post-traumatic patients were more complicated, requiring technical modifications for trance induction, uncovering traumatic memories, and transforming them. Controlled emotional expression of traumatic memories was later taken up by Breuer and Freud (1895/1955) as the cathartic method.

Uncovering Traumatic Memories

Janet pioneered the use of hypnosis and automatic writing in the therapy of post-traumatic patients who suffered mainly from dissociative symptoms (Janet, 1886, 1889, 1898a, b, 1904). He believed that even in the most complicated and chronic cases, memories had to be traced back to the first significant traumatic event. Patients frequently expressed surprise and relief to discover that their symptoms were not physical but attributable to psychological trauma. In many patients, trance induction itself was the first obstacle; some took weeks or months before they could successfully enter into a hypnotic state. Janet thought that these patients often were trying to hide traumatic secrets. Modern explanations of this resistance to trance induction would also include a fear of reexperiencing trauma-related emotions (Brown & Fromm, 1986).

Janet employed a variety of visual imaging techniques to uncover traumatic memories, ranging from direct hypnotic suggestions to automatic writing, and fantasy and dream production. In floridly symptomatic or highly resistant patients, suggestion by distraction eased uncovering techniques. Once traumatic memories had been uncovered, Janet drew upon three treatment approaches: (1) direct reduction, using a technique called neutralization; (2) the substitution method, in which traumatic memories were replaced by neutral or even positive images; and (3) therapeutic reframing. Janet frequently used only hypnotic suggestion to transform traumatic memories. An example of this was Zy, a woman who was admitted to the Salpêtrière suffering from depression, insomnia, and night terrors (Janet, 1896). Trance induction revealed that her dreams dealt with her son's death 3 years earlier, and her father's and brother's before that. Through hypnotic suggestion, Janet first transformed the dream contents and then eliminated them completely. In a similar case, the hypnotic suggestion to "dream aloud" uncovered traumatic memories in his patient Co (Janet, 1895). This 33-year-old woman had become ill 4 years earlier. She had experienced a series of psychological shocks which included witnessing her father's economic ruin, a man being crushed by a streetcar, and the death agony of a close friend. Co suffered from insomnia, and she had no conscious recollection of the traumas. After her admission to the Salpêtrière, Janet produced hypnotic sleep and instructed Co to dream aloud. She was thereby able to recover the traumatic dreams of the funeral of her friend.

Janet uncovered Lucie's traumatic memories using automatic writing (Janet, 1886, 1889). Lucie was one of Janet's earliest patients who suffered from multiple personality disorder (MPD). She had hallucinatory episodes consisting of feelings that scary men were hiding nearby. Lucie was unable to recall an earlier experience related to this phenomenon, either awake or under hypnosis. After Janet encouraged her to use automatic writing under hypnosis her alter-personality, Adrienne, described how at age 7 two men had frightened her while playing at her grandmother's home. In this case, post-traumatic dissociation was responsible for the development of a hidden alter-personality based on the primary fixed idea. A modern author, Summit (1987), has called such states "the hidden child phenomenon."

Neutralization of Traumatic Memories

Hypnotic liquidation of traumatic memories was Janet's most direct and venturous treatment approach (PH, p. 670). It consisted of a stepwise process of reexperiencing and verbalizing traumatic memories, starting with the least threatening, and working toward assimilation of the most traumatic events. For many traumatized patients, however, it was too painful and demanding to actually relive and verbalize the trauma. They simply could not manage to transform the traumatic event into a neutral narrative. Putting pressure on them to do so could lead to increased resistance and produce more unbidden intrusions of traumatic memories; this procedure clearly was not without its risks. When it was cautiously applied in suitably prepared patients, however, traumatic memories often could be successfully assimilated. Janet's most famous example of this approach was Irène (Janet, 1904).

Irène was a 20-year-old Parisienne with an intensely dependent relationship on her mother, who had fallen dead from her bed in front of the patient after a long illness that had exhausted them both. She entered a fugue state and was amnestic for the loss. Her post-traumatic symptoms included somnambulistic crises occurring several times per week. During these episodes Irène dramatically reenacted the sequences of her mother's death and funeral. Janet used hypnosis to uncover the traumatic memories and to liquidate them. At first, attempts to induce hypnosis met with resistance. Trance states frequently resulted in delirious crises in which Irène would mimic her mother's death. Over several months, Irène's memories slowly came into consciousness: "After much labor," Janet reported, "I was able to construct a verbal memory of her mother's death. From that moment . . . the assimilated event ceased to be traumatic" (PH, p. 681).

The Substitution Method

For many patients, symptom-oriented hypnotic approaches were too superficial, and neutralization too potentially traumatizing. Sometimes Janet substituted neutral or even positive imagery for the traumatic memories (Janet, 1889, 1894, 1894/1895, 1898a, b). He changed either the cognitive interpretation of the traumatic events or the patients' emotional reactions. Changing the content of the imagery helped Janet's patient Cam to assimilate the memory of the death of her two children. Janet successfully replaced the hallucinated traumatic images with a picture of blossoming flowers (Raymon & Janet, 1898).

Another example of changing traumatic memories is Marie, one of Janet's early patients at the Salpêtrière (Janet, 1889). Marie had severe anxiety attacks, seizures, and spasms during her menses. Under hypnosis, she recovered the memory of her first menstrual period: She had been totally unprepared and was deeply shocked. To stop the blood flow she jumped into a cold tub; after this she fell ill and didn't menstruate for 5 years. Subsequently she experienced her periods as episodes of reliving the original drama, for which she had total amnesia afterward. Janet's initial attempts to influence Marie's traumatic memories were fruitless. Using hypnotic age regression to the time before her menarche, Janet provided suggestions of normal periods that led to cessation of Marie's monthly crises. Her anxiety attacks persisted, however, until their relationships to another trauma were uncovered. At age 16 Marie had seen an old woman fall down the stairs and die. Since then, just hearing the word *blood* was enough to trigger the somatic sensations related to this traumatic event. The anxiety attacks disappeared when Janet suggested the woman had only tripped and not died. Marie had yet another hysterical symptom: she was blind in her left eye. Initially she was opposed to exploration of this blindness and said she was born with it. Hypnotic age regression to 5 years, however, revealed normal vision. At 6, Marie had been forced to share a bed with a child suffering from impetigo on the left side of her face. The hypnotic suggestion that this child had not had impetigo and was really a nice person relieved Marie's blindness. The improvements were maintained at 5 months' follow-up, and Janet thought that Marie had benefited in her physical appearance as well.

Reframing

Although Janet's hypnotic substitution techniques worked fairly well for patients with predominantly hysterical (i.e., dissociative) post-traumatic symptomatology, technical modifications were required for patients with predominantly psychasthenic features. These patients dealt with their traumatic memories with excessive scrupulousity and obsessions (Janet, 1903). They were plagued by guilt, and preoccupied with how they should have behaved differently. Janet thought that these "mental manias of perfection" were attempts to restore their pretraumatic harmony (Janet, 1935).

Under these conditions, Janet focused purely on the verbal memories, rather than on traumatic imagery, and sought to reframe the narrative account in terms acceptable to the patient. Instead of hypnotic substitution of imagery, he used reassurance and restoration of morale. An example was Janet's treatment of Nicole, a 37-year-old married woman whose post-traumatic psychasthenic illness developed over a period of 12 years (Janet, 1935). Nicole was obsessed with the traumatic ending of a love affair several years prior to her marriage. Following this rejection, she became depressed whenever she thought about her former lover; during these times she experienced terrible feelings of anxiety, abandonment, and guilt. Nicole's subsequent recovery barely concealed the continuing lack of resolution of her psychological trauma. She was silent about the affair, but she continued to suffer from agoraphobia and was beset with fears of dying or fears of throwing herself from a window. She married 6 years later and never wondered whether she should tell her husband about the affair. After her third delivery, which coincided with an anniversary reaction, a radical change occurred: There was a recurrence of the post-traumatic psychasthenic reaction, along with all the memories of the affair and its termination. Nicole confessed to her husband, overwhelming him with interminable and insoluble questions; "How come I didn't offer any resistance? How come I didn't feel any shame after I had been thrown out, no regret? Am I thus not worthy to live? Is the past irreparable? Can I continue as if nothing has happened?"

Janet thought that Nicole functioned at a higher mental level during this second crisis than during the first. She was better able to put her unhappy story into words, but was still ill-equipped to deal with the moral issues over which she was brooding. He helped her to reinterpret her past conduct as pathological rather than immoral. Although still difficult to accept, it was easier to see herself as a patient than as a criminal. In modern terms, Janet substituted Nicole's "patient myth" for a "therapeutic myth" (Frank, 1973; van der Hart, 1988), which made the traumatic event acceptable and promoted its assimilation.

STAGE 3: PERSONALITY REINTEGRATION AND REHABILITATION

Assimilation of traumatic fixed ideas was necessary but insufficient for complete resolution of post-traumatic stress. Three further clinical issues had to be addressed: prevention of relapse, reintegration of the personality, and management of the residual symptoms of the post-traumatic pan-neurosis. All three conditions were associated with psychological instability and a lowering of psychological tension. Janet described how continued reliance on dissociation in the face of threat made these patients vulnerable to repeated relapses. He tried to deal with this problem by trying to stabilize the patient and to consolidate the gains made in the first two treatment stages (Janet, 1893). Psychological trauma often had caused not only an arrest in the capacity to integrate new experiences (Janet, 1904), but sometimes to a regression to earlier developmental stages as well (Janet, 1893).

Specific post-traumatic personality defects included poor attention and concentration; suggestibility; inability to initiate, maintain, follow through on, and complete acts; and constricted affect and hypochondria. Each of these personality deficits could coexist with residual symptoms of the post-traumatic pan-neurosis. These might include functional somatic complaints, motor contractures, psychasthenic doubts, ruminations, and scrupulosity. All patients were likely to experience residual apathy, boredom, and depression. Janet addressed his therapy to these symptoms of the pan-neurosis. Treatment for each of these conditions—relapse prevention, symptom relief, and personality reintegration and rehabilitation—included education, stimulation, and moral guidance. Janet tried to integrate these various therapeutic approaches in order to increase patients' mental energy, recover lost functions, and acquire new skills.

Education

Janet's educational approach was based on a learning model and was aimed at reducing symptoms and restoring personality functions (Janet, 1898a, 1903; PH, p. 710). Post-traumatic patients with residual psychasthenic (obsessional) symptoms, for example, were taught techniques similar to contemporary thought-stopping and response prevention (Janet, 1903). Education was used to restore attention and concentration, motor functions, and contact with reality. Aesthesiogeny was a specific technique for recovery of the awareness for physical sensations (Janet, 1893, 1898a;

PH, p. 788). Janet also described behavioral methods for more complex and purposeful acts. The graduated treatment sequence started by performing simple actions; these were first modeled by the therapist and then carried out by the patient. Simple tasks were repeated until they came naturally, and finally the patient was urged to get involved in spontaneous activities without supervision. Janet remarked that it was not always clear how this could be accomplished; often, he met with resistance regardless of whether he coaxed firmly or gently (PH, p. 741). Treatment failures might develop either recurrences of old symptoms or symptom substitution (PH, p. 743, 745).

Excitation

Although educational activities, hypnosis, and psychological treatment were meant to be psychologically stimulating, most post-traumatic patients required further therapeutic excitation to foster positive emotions, motivation, and a sense of mastery (PH, p. 858). Stimulating activities included awareness exercises (PH, p. 972) and graduated performances of familiar but neglected activities (PH, p. 967). Patients were encouraged to work on their social phobias, residual psychological and external conflicts, procrastination, and unresolved problems. Janet thought that repeated courses of stimulating educational treatment had a cumulative beneficial effect (PH, p. 1022). There was an ever-present risk of fatigue or exhaustion, as well as a need to channel agitation into creative pursuits. Janet encouraged patients to take pride in their own successes and urged them to overlook failures (PH, p. 986). He advocated being truthful, however, when patients asked for feedback about the quality of their performance.

Drug Treatment

Janet saw sedatives (e.g., bromides) and the stimulants as a necesary evil (PH, p. 1030). He made the astute observation that psychological symptoms were often less troublesome when the patient's general health was worse (PH, p. 1064). Nevertheless, he did employ pharmacological agents such as tea, coffee, alcohol, opium, and strychnine to increase psychological tension, and he used physiotherapy, hydrotherapy, and electrical stimulation as well. He also experimented with such newly discovered endocrine preparations as adrenaline, pituitary extract, and thyroxine (Janet, 1904).

Termination

Janet used the hypnotic rapport in the second treatment stage to liquidate the traumatic memories, and in the third stage to stimulate growth and assist in rehabilitation. Reduction of the therapeutic influence signaled the beginnings of termination (PH, p. 1194). The patient developed a quieter attitude, he or she was more open to positive influence, and relapses were less severe and of shorter duration. Janet regarded ingratitude as the best sign of recovery: When the patient started to forget appointments, he or she was on the road to recovery (PH, p. 1198–1199). He lengthened the gap between sessions at this stage, and in severe and complicated cases infrequent appointments maintained the therapeutic influence over time; for example, Janet stayed in touch with Irene for 16 years (PH, p. 1202).

DISCUSSION

Janet's treatment model anticipated modern approaches to therapeutic integration. He was well aware that psychotherapy still was at a prescientific stage and that it was less specific than drug treatment in medicine (PH, p. 1208, 1210). His own data, however, showed that his patients improved more by psychotherapy than was predicted by chance or likely to be attributable to spontaneous remission (PH, pp. 340ff, 1211). He advocated the need to define specific treatment techniques for specified conditions (PH, p. 146) and repeatedly warned against therapeutic panaceas (e.g., PH, p. 132, 464, 490). Janet's approach to psychotherapy was a theoretically informed eclecticism applied to both traditional nosological categories and his own unique model of mental economy. It was truly prescriptive in that characteristics of the disorder, its stages, and the vicissitudes of mental economy dictated treatment rather than vice versa. Janet utilized both traditional methods and his own innovations, but he always embedded treatment within the frame of the therapeutic alliance.

Janet was a flexible clinician who viewed the different stages of post-traumatic syndromes as constantly shifting and returning, requiring different treatment approaches at different times. Sometimes restoration of personality functioning was required before all of the traumatic memories could be assimilated; at other times, retrieval of a traumatic memory could stabilize a patient's mental state (Janet, 1894–1895). In patients with dissociative disorders Janet emphasized integration of traumatic memories more than integration of various personality states: He was impressed by how liquidation of traumatic memories could bring about personal integration, and he frequently saw these two processes occurring simultaneously (Janet, 1893). Modern authors such as Braun (1986) and Sachs et al. (1988) are more outspoken about the need to distinguish a separate treatment phase for the integration of personality states.

Traumatic memories were often difficult to resolve completely because they tended to contain multiple layers: Just when the therapist felt that all of the memories had been explored, a new layer might emerge (Janet, 1894). Janet attributed his failure to help some of his patients with pathological dependence to his inability to reach inaccessible traumatic memories. He reported relatively few examples of liquidation of traumatic memories from before age 6. Contemporary studies of patients with MPD have revealed severe physical and sexual abuse in some patients during infancy (Coons & Milstein, 1986; Kluft, 1987; Putnam et al., 1986).

The substitution technique is one of Janet's most original contributions to psychotherapy. The same technique later shows up in the work of Breukink (1923). Erickson (Erickson & Rossi, 1979), and therapists during the 1980s (Eichelman, 1985; Lamb, 1982, 1985; Miller, 1986; Waxman, 1982). In Janet's and Erickson's approaches the therapist was the operator, but some modern clinicians encourage their patients to be self-directive and to construct and enact their own revisions of the original traumatic event. The question whether such approaches lead to further dissociation of traumatic memories—as Janet thought—or to their implicit assimilation remains unanswered. Contemporary authors (Kluft, personal communication) have warned that in patients with a history of incest where the child was denied validation of the trauma because of threats by the perpetrator, the substitution technique could easily be misunderstood by the patient as an extension of the process of negation of the trauma.

One of Janet's pioneering concepts that has fallen in disuse is his model of mental economy. This model proposed that trauma causes an instability in patients' psychological energy levels and always interferes with psychological tension—the capacity to organize energy into focused and creative action. Recent research has again supported the validity of these concepts: van der Kolk and Ducey (1989), analyzing the Rorschachs of people with PTSD, concluded that "the lack of integration of the traumatic experience causes extreme reactivity to environmental stimuli: the initially overwhelming external event, through lack of assimilation, is perpetuated internally and continues to exert disorganizing effects on the psyche." This research concluded that "the effort to keep memories of the trauma at bay interferes with the capacity to sublimate and fantasize, preventing "thought as experimental action." This interferes with the ability to grieve, and to work through ordinary everyday conflict and to accumulate restitutive, gratifying experiences. Hence, they are deprived of precisely those psychological mechanisms which allow people to cope with the injuries of daily life." Janet's recognition of this unfocused and ineffectual psychological energy provided the rationale for his system of psychotherapy, which divided treatment into those methods that encouraged conservation of mental economy (psychological restitution), and methods to economic augmentation (aimed at psychological growth). Concluding a tribute to the broad scope of Janet's vision, Ellenberger (1950, p. 482) remarked that Janet's psychotherapy is not a partial and exclusive method: "Not only does it not exclude other methods, but it often enables us to understand them better and to specify their domain of application. It is less a special therapy than a general economy of psychotherapy."

REFERENCES

Barrucand, D. (1967). *Histoire de l'hypnotisme en France.* Paris: Presses Universitaires de France.

Braun, B. G., (1986). Issues in the psychotherapy of multiple personality disorder. In B. G. Braun, (Ed.), *Treatment of multiple personality disorder.* Washington, DC: American Psychiatric Press.

Breuer, J., & Freud, S. (1845). *Studies of hysteria.* In J. Strachey (Ed. and Trans.), *The standard edition of the complete psychological works of Sigmund Freud* (Vol. 2). London: Hogarth.

Breukink, H. (1923). Over de behandeling van sommige psychosen door middel van een bijzondere vorm der kathartisch-hypnotische methode. *Nederlands Tijdschrift Geneeskunde, 67,* 1321–1328.

Brown, D. P., & Fromm, E. (1986). *Hypnotherapy and hypnoanalysis.* Hillsdale, NJ: Erlbaum.

Coons, P. M., & Milstein, V. (1986). Psychosexual disturbances in multiple personality. *J. Clin Psychiat., 47,* 106–110.

Eichelman, B. (1985). Hypnotic change in combat dreams of two veterans with PTSD. *Am. J. Psychiat., 142,* 112–114.

Ellenberger, H. F. (1950). La psychothérapie de Janet. *L'Evolution Psychologique* [Special Pierre Janet issue], 465–482.

Erickson, M. E., & Kubie, L. S. (1941). The successful treatment of a case of acute hysterical depression by return under hypnosis to a critical phase of childhood. *Psychoanal. Quart., 10,* 593–609.

Erickson, M. E., & Rossi, E. L. (1979). *Hypnotherapy: An exploratory casebook.* New York: Irving.

Frank, J. (1973). *Persuasion and healing.* Baltimore, MD: Johns Hopkins University Press.

Freud, S. (1958). Remembering; repeating; and working through. In J. Strachey (Ed. and Trans.), *The standard edition of the complete psychological works of Sigmund Freud* (Vol. 12, pp. 147–156). London: Hogarth. (Original work published 1914)

Freud, S. (1959). Formulations on the two principles of mental functioning. In J. Strachey (Ed. and Trans.), *The standard edition of the complete psychological works of Sigmund Freud* (Vol. 12, pp. 218–226). London: Hogarth. (Original work published 1911)

Haule, J. R. (1986). Pierre Janet and dissociation: The first transference theory and its origins in hypnosis. *Am. J. Clin. Hypnosis, 29*(2), 86–94.

Janet, P. (1886). Les actes inconscients et la mémoire pendant le somnambulisme. *Rev. Philos, 25*(1), 238–279.

Janet, P. (1889). *L'Automatisme psychologique.* Paris: Félix Alcan. (Reprint: Société Pierre Janet, Paris, 1973)

Janet, P. (1893). L'Amnésie continué. *Rev. Gen. Sci., 4,* 167–179.

Janet, P. (1894). Histoire d'une idée fixe. *Rev. Philos, 37,*(1), 121–163.

Janet, P. (1894/1895). Un cas de possession et l'exorcisme moderne. *Bull. Travaux Univ. Lyon, 8,* 41–57.

Janet, P. (1895). Les idées fixes de forme hystérique. *Presse Med, 3,* 201–203.

Janet, P. (1897). L'Influence somnambulique et le besoin de direction. *Rev. Philos, 43,*(1), 113–143.

Janet, P. (1898a). Le traitement psychologique de l'hystérie. In A. Robin (Ed.), *Traité de thérapeutique appliquée.* Paris: Rueff.

Janet, P. (1898b). *Nevroses et idées fixes* (Vol. 1). Paris: Félix Alcan.

Janet, P. (1903). *Les obsessions et la psychasthénie* (Vol. 2). Paris: Félix Alcan. (Reprint: Hafner, New York 1976)

Janet, P. (1904). L'Amnésie et la dissociation des souvenirs par l'émotion. *J. Psychol. 1,* 417–453.
Janet, P. (1911). *L'Etat mental des hystériques.* Paris: Félix Alcan.
Janet, P. (1976). *Principles of psychotherapy* (Vol. 2). New York: Arno. (Original work published 1919)
Janet, P. (1925). *Principles of psychotherapy.* London: George Allen and Unwin. (Original work published 1923)
Janet, P. (1929). *L'Evolution de la personnalité.* Paris: Chahine. (Reprint: Société Pierre Janet, Paris, 1984)
Janet, P. (1932). *La force et la faiblesse psychologiques.* Paris: Maloine.
Janet, P. (1935). Réalisation et intérpretation. *Ann. Medico-Psychol, 93*(2), 329–366.
Kluft, R. P. (1987). An update on multiple personality disorder. *Hosp. Comm. Psychiat, 38*(4), 363–373.
Lamb, C. S. (1982). Negative hypnotic imagery and fantasy: Application to two cases of "unfinished business." *Am. J. Clin. Hypnosis, 24,* 266–271.
Lamb, C. S. (1985). Hypnotically induced deconditioning: Reconstruction of memories in the treatment of phobias. *Am. J. Clin. Hypnosis, 28,* 56–62.
Miller, A. (1986). Brief reconstructive hypnotherapy for anxiety reactions: Three case reports. *Am. J. Clin. Hypnosis, 28,* 138–146.
Parson, E. R. (1984). The reparation of self: Clinical and theoretical dimensions in the treatment of Vietnam combat veterans. *J. Contemp. Psychother, 14,* 4–56.
Putnam, F. W., Guroff, J. J., Silberman, E. K., Barban, L., & Post, R. M. (1986). The clinical phenomenology of multiple personality disorder. *J. Clin. Psychiat, 47,* 285–293.
Raymond, F., & Janet P. (1898). *Névroses et ideés fixes* (Vol. 2). Paris: Félix Alcan.
Sachs, R. G., Frischholz & Wood, J. I. (1988). Marital and family therapy in the treatment of multiple personality disorder. *J. Marit. Fam. Ther, 14,* 249–259.
Summit, R. (1987). The hidden child phenomenon: An atypical dissociative disorder. In B. G. Braun (Ed.), *Dissociative disorders 1987: Proceedings of the 4th International Conference of Multiple Personality/Dissociative States,* (p. 6). Chicago: Rush-Presbyterian St. Luke's Medical Center.
Schwartz, L. (1951). *Die Neurosen und die dynamische Psychologie von Pierre Janet.* Basel, Switzerland: Benno Schwege.
Titchener, J. L. (1986). Post-traumatic decline: A consequence of unresolved destructive drives. In C. Figley (Ed.), *Trauma and its wake* (Vol. 2). New York: Brunner/Mazel.
van der Hart, O. (1988). Myths and rituals: Their use in psychotherapy. In O. van der Hart (Ed.), *Coping with loss: The therapeutic use of leave-taking rituals.* New York: Irvington.
van der Hart, O., & Horst, R. (1989). The dissociation theory of Pierre Janet. *J. Traum. Stress, 2,* 397–412.
van der Hart, O., & Friedman, B. (1989). A reader's guide to Pierre Janet on dissociation. *Dissociation, 2*(1).
van der Kolk, B. A., & Ducey, C. P. (1989). The psychological processing of traumatic experience: Rorschach patterns in PTSD. *J. Traum. Stress, 2,* 259–274.
Waxman, D. (1982). *Hypnosis: A guide for patients and practitioners,* London: George Allen and Unwin.
Wetterstrand, O. G. (1982). Uber den künstlich verlängerten Schlaf besonders bei der Behandlung der Hysterie. *Zeitschrift Hypnotismus,* 17–23.

13

Twelve Themes and Spiritual Steps

A Recovery Program for Survivors of Traumatic Experiences

JOEL OSLER BRENDE

Destroy, O Lord and divide their tongues, for I have seen violence and strife in the city. Day and night they go around it on its walls; Iniquity and trouble are also in the midst of it. Destruction is in its midst; Oppression and deceit do not depart from its streets. (Psalm 55:9)

TRAUMA IN AMERICAN SOCIETY

Trauma has become too commonplace in America. Violent street crime permeates large cities. Intergang warfare and wanton shootings invade many ghettos. Robberies, assaults, and rapes (Roth & Lebowitz, 1988) occur frequently, hanging like a gray cloud hovering over the vulnerable who venture alone into side streets, parking lots, and parks (*USA Today,* 1989). The rising rate of alcohol and drug addiction breeds destruction and self-destruction. And now there is a frightening increase in the use and abuse of cocaine and associated crime, gang warfare, and hired assassinations.

JOEL OSLER BRENDE • Regional Psychiatric Division, Central State Hospital, Milledgeville, Georgia 31061; and Department of Psychiatry, Mercer University School of Medicine, Macon, Georgia 31207. Reprinted from J. T. Reese, J. M. Horn, & C. Dunning (Eds.), *Critical Incidents in Policing—Revised* (pp. 39–54). Washington, D.C., U.S. Government Printing Office.

Psychotraumatology, edited by George S. Everly, Jr. and Jeffrey M. Lating. Plenum Press, New York, 1995.

Trauma can also be found within homes where wives and children have been battered, assaulted, and sexually violated (Ochberg, 1988) and where children have run away (McCormack, Burgess & Hartman, 1988). There is pornography, both soft- and hard-core, and television violence, both of which reflect and breed societal dehumanization and violence. There are satanic cults whose members violently and ritualistically sacrifice the lives of unsuspecting victims (*USA Today*, 1989). Subviolent trauma is present in every part of American society where individuals complain of feeling dehumanized, alienated, deprived of justice, and victimized (Young, 1988) without purpose.

POST-TRAUMATIC CONSEQUENCES WITHIN AMERICAN SOCIETY

> My heart is severely pained within me, and the terrors of death have fallen upon me. Fearfulness and trembling have come upon me, and horror has overwhelmed me. So I said, "Oh that I had wings like a dove! I would fly away and be at rest. Indeed, I would wander far off and remain in the wilderness. I would hasten my escape from the windy storm and tempest." (Psalm 55:4)

There are consequences to this epidemic of trauma: dehumanization and violence affecting individual victims, families of victims, American society, and the law enforcers called on to respond to the escalation of trauma.

Individual Victims

Victims of severe stress or trauma suffer symptoms of post-traumatic stress disorder that include nightmares, reenactments, and intrusive memories with associated feelings of fear, guilt, and grief. When they are not feeling "out of control" from those symptoms, they feel "overcontrolled" by amnesia, denial, emotional numbing, and detachment, plus other overcontrol symptoms (American Psychiatric Association, 1987; Horowitz, 1976).

Not described in the American Psychiatric Association (APA) diagnostic manual is the frequent observation that severe trauma often causes dissociative symptoms (Brende, 1986; van der Kolk, 1987) and fragmentation. Fragmented personality disorders are an unfortunate consequence of the betrayal and shame associated with severe and protracted trauma; they are often found in sexually abused children, rape victims, incest victims (Herman, 1988; Roth & Lebowitz, 1988); and Vietnam veterans (Brende, 1983, 1986). The fragmentation to self-identity includes dissociation (Brende, 1986; Speigel, 1988) and, in extreme cases, multiple personality disorder (Braun, 1984; van der Kolk & Kadish, 1987). Neglected in the post-traumatic stress literature are descriptions about spiritual alienation in survivors, particularly those who suffer guilt and shame, although these are described in Vietnam veterans (Brende & McDonald, 1988, 1989; Lifton, 1973; Mahedy, 1986; Williams, 1988).

Families and Society as Victims

There are other less obvious but destructive consequences—the epidemic of deaths from accidents and suicides among our children, adolescents, and young adults; the homeless living in city streets; addicts; repeat offenders; prostitutes; and hardened criminals. Those who have been victimized often perpetuate their post-traumatic symptoms in the form of abusive behavior, broken relationships, addiction, repeated arrests, institutionalizations, and chronic medical problems. As victimization continues, the individual consequences mushroom, and the effects on families and society are far-reaching (Hartman & Burgess, 1988; Ochberg, 1988; Stark & Flitcraft, 1988).

The apathy and even antipathy of Americans toward victims perpetuates the problem. Victims in this country are blamed and misunderstood, often becoming outcasts from families and society (Hartman & Burgess, 1988; Stark & Flitcraft, 1988). Thousands of Vietnam veterans describe feelings of alienation (Brende & McDonald, 1989) and often seek isolated places to live (Brende & Parson, 1985). Unfortunately, independent Americans who deny weakness and vulnerability maintain an attitude of denial and emotional detachment about the conditions of the victimized in society.

There are many other examples of cultural detachment and apathy. Americans frequently deny the destructiveness of violent television and pornography. They tend to not believe that easy access to weapons feeds violence. Americans are emotionally detached from the traumatic effects on those who are arrested, jailed, or imprisoned. Most Americans idealistically believe their country will live on forever in spite of the self-destructive lack of attention to pollution of water, air, countryside, and city. They don't want to believe that it is vulnerable to self-destruction or even to destruction, including the threat of terrorists infiltrating and exploding conventional or nuclear devices.

The increasing self-destruction, alienation, and fragmentation caused by repetitive traumatic events within American society seems to be spiraling out of control. The mental health system cannot keep up with the demand to treat trauma victims and never will. Furthermore, traditional therapy is often inadequate. The government, the legal system, and law enforcement officials are asked to respond to the growing manifestations of this national disorder, but they are also vulnerable to victimization by increasing demands and by repeated exposure of law enforcement officers to violence, close calls with death, survivor guilt, and grief from the deaths of fellow officers and American citizens they are expected to protect.

POST-TRAUMATIC RECOVERY IN A TRAUMATIZED SOCIETY

> Give ear to my prayer, oh God, and do not hide yourself from my supplication. Attend to me, and hear me; I am restless in my complaint, and moan

> noisily, because of the voice of the enemy. Because of the oppression of the wicked; for they bring down trouble upon me, and in wrath they hate me. (Psalm 55:1–8)

Much has been written during the past decade about the treatment of survivors suffering post-traumatic symptoms from a variety of traumas (Brende & Parson, 1985; Figley, 1978, 1985; Horowitz, 1976; Ochberg, 1988; van der Kolk, 1987; Wilson, 1989), but little has been written about the demoralizing effect that traumatic experiences can have on self-esteem, spiritual and emotional integrity, or sense of purpose (Brende & McDonald, 1989; Mahedy, 1986). Survivors in healthy support systems recover from their traumatic experiences when they receive support, protection, and the empathic understanding of friends, family, church, God, and society. Victims who receive support are better able to find such commonly used recovery methods as nutrition, exercise, and humor (Merwin & Smith-Kurtz, 1988). They may also, with help, find it possible to reflect on and recall the trauma in order to experience self-healing and a restoration of repressed emotion (Krystal, 1988). For those who seek psychotherapy, there can be excellent results (Danieli, 1988; Horowitz, 1982; Lindy, 1988; Ochberg, 1988; Parson, 1988).

But there are thousands, perhaps millions, of victims who have withdrawn—either directly or indirectly—as their only way to cope with feelings of anger, fear, guilt, and grief. They do it in many ways, including by living in the mountains, woods, or isolated wastelands like thousands of Vietnam veterans have done (Figley & Leventman, 1980). There are others, finding no ways to break through emotional and spiritual alienation, who have learned to cope with their symptoms through isolation. They live in the impersonal trenches of the big cities; they become the homeless, the incarcerated, and the institutionalized.

There are other thousands who find isolation in much less blatant ways by escaping into wealth, power, quasi-military groups, and a variety of impersonal organizations. They may find no purpose other than the "thrill of the adrenaline" that keeps them going, although they remain emotionally and spiritually alienated.

RECOVERY USING RELIGIOUS AND SPIRITUAL MODALITIES

> He comforts us in all our affliction so that we may be able to comfort those who are in any affliction with the comfort with which we ourselves are comforted by God. (II Corinthians 1:4–11)

Healing has frequently been a central focus of religion in various cultures. Historically, societies have used religious rituals to help their traumatized citizenry. For ages, cultures recognized that their warriors needed to have the opportunity for emotional and spiritual "cleansing" before being reintegrated into society, something not provided America's Vietnam veterans (Brende & Parson, 1985; Figley & Leventman, 1980). Native Americans traditionally use the ritual of the sweat lodge ceremony, where survivors of traumatic events meet together in the present of a tribal medicine man for an emotional and spiritual cleansing experience (Wilson, 1988). Traditionally, Americans have helped survivors of traumatic experiences within closely knit families, groups, and churches rather than expect professional mental health services. Church congregations provide support for the bereaved. Groups of people working together will usually find ways to provide mutual support. When law enforcement officers lose one of their "brothers," they turn out as a group for the funeral, help the surviving family, and contribute in concrete ways to cope with the loss. These ways alone may not always be adequate, however, to help survivors resolve the emotional upheaval they continue to feel for some time.

SURRENDER AS A CONCEPT FOR RECOVERY

> Bow down thine ear, O Lord, hear me; for I am poor and need. Preserve my soul . . . . Be merciful unto me, O Lord: for I cry unto thee daily. (Psalm 86:1–3)

> My heart is not haughty, nor mine eyes lofty. (Psalm 131:1)

Recovery from post-traumatic guilt, shame, demoralization, and spiritual alienation is neglected in traditional treatment, which focuses on resolving primary symptoms of intrusive recollections, emotions, and denial/numbing (Horowitz, 1976, 1982). For those survivors with prolonged guilt and shame associated with protracted and repetitive post-traumatic symptoms and personality disorders, recovery cannot proceed without resolution of guilt and shame. Spiritual recovery approaches are best able to help such individuals. These approaches usually emphasize belief and surrender to God and acceptance of forgiveness.

The principle of surrender is a major teaching within most religions of the world. Muhammad, in 610 A.D., preached a message of submission and surrender to the will of God (Allah) and founded Islam, one of the three major religions of the world believing in a single God (Juri, 1946). Within the Eastern religions there is a belief in accepting life as it comes, including traumatic events. Buddhists teach that catastrophe and suffering are a normal part of existence, meant to be accepted and dealt with as gracefully as possible; one is to try to find meaning in them (Lee & Lu, 1989). Christians hold to a similar belief in the importance of surrender to the will of God, exemplified by the total submission unto death by crucifixion by Jesus Christ. Other examples described in the New Testament include a willingness by followers of Jesus to surrender to the will of God in the face of arrests, stoning, imprisonment, and death.

SURRENDER AND 12-STEP PROGRAMS

Alcoholics and addicts recovering through the use of Alcoholics Anonymous (AA) principles learn to "surrender" their addiction and egocentric attitudes to a higher power. This has been called "letting go and letting God" (Keller, 1985). Surrender is a core concept in 12-step recovery programs and comes out of the AA tradition. This concept was found to be effective by recovering alcoholics who failed to stop drinking through traditional treatments. When they "let go and let God"—that is, when they ceased their futile efforts at breaking their self-destructive addiction patterns and turned themselves and their addictions over to God—the self-destructive patterns finally ceased.

AA and similar 12-step programs have helped hundreds of thousands of individuals recover from a variety of self-destructive patterns and addictions, including cravings for alcohol, drugs, cigarettes, food, gambling, and sex. The most important healing aspect of the 12-step AA program has been described as the recognition of a higher power and willingness to "surrender" to that power (or God, as individually understood) as a way of changing self-destructive, destructive, and self-centered behaviors and gaining power in one's life. This is described in the "Big Book" (Alcoholics Anonymous, 1976) as follows:

> Driven by a hundred forms of fear, self-delusion, self-seeking and self-pity, we step on the toes of our fellows and they retaliate. Sometimes they hurt us, seemingly without provocation, but we invariably find that at some time in the past, we have made decisions based on self which later placed us in a position to be hurt. . . .
>
> Above everything, we . . . must be rid of this selfishness. We must, or it kills us. God makes that possible. And there often seems no way of entirely getting rid of self without His aid. Many of us had moral and philosophical convictions galore, but we could not live up to them even though we would have liked to. Neither could we reduce our self-centeredness much by wishing or trying on our own power. We had to have God's help. . . .
>
> Next, we decided that hereafter in this drama of life, God was going to be our Director. He is the Principal; we are His agents. He is the Father, and we are His children. Most good ideas are simple, and this concept was the keystone of the new and triumphant arch through which we passed to freedom. . . .
>
> He provided what we needed, if we kept close to Him and performed His work well. Established on such a footing we became less and less interested in ourselves, our little plans and designs. More and more we became interested

> in seeing what we contribute to life. As we felt new power flow in, as we enjoyed peace of mind, as we discovered we could face life successfully, as we became conscious of His presence, we began to lose our fear of today, tomorrow or the hereafter. We were reborn. (pp. 62–63)

TWELVE THEMES AND SPIRITUAL STEPS FOR TRAUMA VICTIMS

In 1985, with help from the Bay Pines, Florida, VA hospital chaplain, patients, and key staff personnel, I drew from the 12-step recovery program concepts to develop a 12-week program for trauma victims—particularly Vietnam veterans with severe and recurring symptoms of post-traumatic stress disorder. The themes defined were as follows:

1. Power versus victimization
2. Seeking meaning in survival
3. Trust versus shame and doubt
4. Self-inventory
5. Understanding anger and rage
6. Understanding fear
7. Guilt
8. Grief
9. Suicide versus commitment to life
10. Revenge versus forgiveness
11. Finding a purpose
12. Love and meaningful relationships

This psychoeducational program consisted of a didactic, educational, and discussion "theme group" held three times a week that became a focus for the treatment program. Each week, the theme changed in a stepwise progression so that by the end of 12 weeks, each patient was exposed to the entire sequence.

Eventually many of the veterans, particularly the recovering addicts involved in Alcoholics Anonymous, became interested in forming a volunteer 12-step group patterned in some respects after the AA program (Sorenson, 1985). I found that the veterans who benefited from this program accepted the concept of surrendering their self-destructive and self-centered lifestyles to God, as they individually understood him, and sought his help to gain freedom from the bondage of victimization.

Combat veterans found the program very helpful because it helped them break through the addictive nature of their post-traumatic symptoms and destructive lifestyles, described in victims of other kinds of trauma as well (van der Kolk, 1987). Because survivors of other kinds of trauma besides combat found this program helpful, after leaving the VA system I developed a similar program for survivors of a variety of traumatic experiences, using principles similar to other 12-step programs:

- Believing in a Higher Power, or God, as individually understood
- An attitude of surrender appropriate for each of the 12 steps
- Recovering as an ongoing and sometimes lifelong process
- Leadership provided by trained leaders initially and later by rotating leadership among members of self-help groups
- Education about post-traumatic symptoms
- Group sharing and helping one another during and between group meetings
- Regular attendance

The 12-step program, called TRAUMA SURVIVORS ANONYMOUS, includes the following five ministeps:

1. Acknowledging symptoms
2. Seeking help
3. Surrendering to God, as individually understood
4. Taking action
5. Daily prayer and meditation

TWELVE THEMES AND SPIRITUAL STEPS: AN OUTLINE FOR SURVIVORS OF TRAUMATIC EVENTS

Use this outline as a guide to help your own recovery program. All of the steps are important, but certain ones will apply more specifically than others. If you are a group participant or a group leader, focus on any of the 12 steps or proceed through the steps in sequential order as your group meets.

If you have been in other anonymous 12-step programs, these steps are meant to supplement those programs and not replace them. If you are receiving spiritual help, psychotherapy, or counseling, please use the steps as an adjunct to that process.

As you take each of the 12 steps, practice breaking the victimization cycle each time as follows: (1) acknowledge the symptom, (2) seek help, (3) surrender the problem to God, (4) take action, and (5) pray each day.

Step 1: Power versus Victimization

> We admitted we were powerless over victimization and sought the help of a "good higher power" (God, as individually understood) to gain power in our lives.

This step focuses on understanding and finding ways to gain power over victimization from our post-traumatic symptoms—meaninglessness, self-doubt and shame, uncontrollable angry outbursts, recurring memories and dreams, night terrors, panic, violent and suicidal thoughts, and isolation from people—or from individuals, groups, or organizations that have misused their power. As victims, we recognize that the ways we have attempted to protect or defend ourselves from victimization have often been ineffective or self-destructive and include isolation, emotional numbing, avoidance, aggressive retaliation, or abuse of others. Unfortunately, these ways merely perpetuate a cycle of victimization.

We can begin to break our self-destructive victimization cycle in the following ways:

- *Acknowledge:* That we are powerless to control many or all of our post-traumatic symptoms, protect or defend ourselves adequately from abusive or destructive forces that attempt to control our lives, or control our own destructive use of power.
- *Seek:* Help from a good higher power—individuals, organizations, and God, as individually understood.
- *Surrender:* Our symptoms and destructive uses of power to God, as individually understood.
- *Take action:* Ask for help from individuals, organizations, and God to intervene in our destructive behaviors and regain power in our lives.
- *Daily prayer:* "God, help me to accept that I have little or no power over symptoms of victimization and destructive behaviors. Help me to recognize which of these I can begin to change. Grant me the wisdom to know the difference."

Step 2: Seeking Meaning

> Came to believe that a power greater than ourselves could help us find meaning.

This step is focused on beginning to seek meaning after a traumatic experience or after the lives of others have been taken. It is very difficult to imagine that meaning can be found, but to begin the search means sharing our experiences with others, accepting their support and understanding, and listening to those who may have found meaning in their own traumatic experiences.

We can begin to seek meaning in the following ways:

- *Acknowledge:* That it is difficult, if not impossible, to accept what has happened to us and to find meaning in still being alive, particularly if others were injured or lost their lives.

- *Seek:* Support, understanding, and direction from God and others in order to help us begin to find meaning.
- *Surrender:* Despair, confusion, and meaninglessness to God, as individually understood.
- *Take action:* Seek answers from God, friends, and counselors; listen to the stories of other survivors who have survived in spite of their emotional pain and have found meaning.
- *Daily prayer:* "God, help me to seek for meaning out of tragedy; to seek for understanding why I am alive even though others' lives may have been lost. Grant me the courage to seek clarity rather than remain a prisoner of confusion, despair, and self-pity."

Step 3: Trust versus Shame and Doubt

> Burdened with distrust, shame, and doubt, we made a decision to seek the help of God, as we understood Him, in order to learn to trust.

This step focuses on helping us regain our capacity to trust others, organizations, those in authority, those who want to help us, God, and ourselves. As victims, we may have lost our capacity to trust even those who have wanted to help us. We may have been abandoned or betrayed by those who should have protected us. And we may have trusted out of blind faith. We may continue to seek someone we can trust, even if we were repeatedly abused or misused in the past. And we may not trust anyone but ourselves, and eventually we may have found that we cannot even do that.

We can begin to break the cycle of shame, doubt, and distrust in the following ways:

- *Acknowledge:* That we continue to experience shame, doubt, and distrust in ourselves and others.
- *Seek:* To discover gradually that we can truly trust God and others who want to help us resolve shame, doubt, and distrust.
- *Surrender:* Our shame, doubt, and distrust to God.
- *Take action:* Put trust to the test—in God, friends, and counselors.
- *Daily prayer:* "God, grant me an understanding of the shame and doubt that lies behind my false pride. Teach me how to trust. Grant me the courage to take the risks necessary to trust, gain freedom from shame, and overcome self-doubt."

Step 4: Self-Inventory

> Admitted to ourselves, another human being, and to God, our faults, and sought His help to accept our positive traits and change our negative ones.

As survivors, we may have thought of ourselves as worthwhile only if we could master frightening situations, save others, or defeat our enemies. As victims of traumatic experiences, we may repeat victimization patterns and not know why. We may attract abusers or victimizing circumstances and not know why. We may suffer repeated victimization or self-destructive experiences as a means of self-punishment because of hidden traumatic secrets we would be ashamed to reveal to ourselves or others.

A personal inventory can help us discover the truth about ourselves—about hidden destructive or self-destructive lifestyles or ways in which we may hurt others or destroy relationships. If we are open to listening, a group feedback session can provide us with more truth about ourselves, enhance trust and self-esteem, and help us more easily accept our good qualities and change those that are negative.

We can begin a self-inventory in the following ways:

- *Acknowledge:* That we often do not accept our positive qualities and find it difficult to change negative ones; that we are sometimes guilty of doing self-destructive things, hurting others, breaking relationships, punishing ourselves, and keeping shameful secrets.
- *Seek:* To be free from self-destructive or destructive behaviors, shameful secrets, and self-condemning attitudes; to be open to positive and constructive criticism.
- *Surrender:* Our self-destructive and destructive behaviors, our shameful secrets, our resistances to receiving help and constructive criticism from others.
- *Take action:* Be open to change and ask for feedback from God, friends, and counselors in order that we can learn more about ourselves. Then accept what is positive and begin to change what is negative.
- *Daily prayer:* "God, help me to accept my positive qualities, change those that continue to hurt myself or others, and make amends to those I have harmed, when possible. Grant me the courage to accept the truth—both positive and negative—about myself in order that I can begin to grow toward a more accurate self-understanding."

Step 5: Anger

> Sought God's help to understand anger, control its destructiveness, and channel it in constructive ways.

This step focuses on gaining understanding and relief from destructive anger that automatically erupts in response to perceived threatening individuals or situations. As victims, anger and even homicidal rage may have been a normal reaction for us at the time we were victimized. If we continue to be victimized, we will be chronically angry. Anger may be easier to feel than fear, guilt, or grief. In fact, anger may be a cover-up for all other feelings.

But our anger, if not blocked, may now be unmanageable, frightening, ineffective, destructive, and self-destructive—destroying property or hurting others. If it is blocked or suppressed, we may not be able to recognize it or express it normally; consequently, we will not be able to assert ourselves or channel it constructively.

We can begin to break the victimization cycle of anger in the following ways:

- *Acknowledge:* That we are powerless to recognize normal angry emotions, control angry outbursts, or express anger constructively.
- *Seek:* Help from God and others to control anger or express it constructively.
- *Surrender:* Our destructive and self-destructive anger and the blocks that keep us from perceiving it to God.
- *Take action:* When anger is out of control, seek help from God, friends, and counselors. Reduce excessive anger within by exercising and participating in healthy activities. Seek help to recognize blocked anger. Begin to learn to express anger normally, constructively, and directly in a calm manner. Learn to be assertive.
- *Daily prayer:* "God, help me to accept my anger as a normal emotion even though it may be blocked or may erupt in destructive and self-destructive ways. Help me to control it when it is unmanageable and be more aware of it when it is blocked from my awareness. Grant me the wisdom to know the difference between destructive and constructive anger."

Step 6: Fear

> Sought God's help to relinquish "the wall" around our emotions and His protective presence during moments of terror and risk.

This step focuses on helping us understand and cope with fear. Fear is normal, even lifesaving. But the terror that we may experience at times—both day and night—can make it seem as if we are reliving our trauma again and again, and our fear of the unknown may paralyze us from normal functioning.

Our fear may have been so overwhelming that we blocked it from awareness. If so, we may take risks to feel it again—in the form of an "adrenaline high" that can both excite us and provide us with an opportunity to control our fear and danger. But we may also be suffering from the consequences of suppressed fear, particularly if we have erected a "wall" around our emotions. That wall causes our isolation, distrust, emotional numbing, panic attacks, and risk taking.

We can begin to break the fear victimization cycle as follows:

- *Acknowledge:* That fear is either excessively in control of our lives or

completely blocked so that we take dangerous risks and keep a wall around our emotions.
- *Seek:* The help of God and others that we may be able to relinquish the wall around our emotions; to learn to depend on God and others during terrifying emotions, dreams, and memories; and to learn how to take risks in constructive ways.
- *Take action:* Seek help, begin to let down the wall, and learn that fear can be normal again. Discover that depending on God and others is a healthy thing to do. Begin to take risks, but only in positive ways. Face frightening situations with the help of God and others.
- *Daily prayer:* "God, help me to accept the fact that fear is a normal emotion even though at times it controls my life. Help me to relinquish the wall around my emotions. Grant me the wisdom to know the difference between normal fear and risk taking and abnormal fear and risk taking."

Step 7: Guilt

> Sought God's help to face guilt, to make amends when possible, to accept His forgiveness, and to forgive ourselves.

In this theme, we focus on understanding our guilt and to begin to find ways to gain relief from its destructive consequences. Survivor guilt can be pervasive and self-destructive, particularly if we rightly or wrongly believe we were responsible for the deaths or injuries of others. Guilt can be unbearable if we suffer from repetitive horrifying or guilt-ridden thoughts, dreams, and images, or from persistent depression, physical illness, and suicidal feelings.

Conversely, we may have no conscious awareness of guilt. Yet its consequences can be destructive for us and for others if we engage in abusive or perverse behavior or seesaw between excessive guilt and a distorted or absent conscience. We may have been responsible for the deaths, suffering, or injuries to others—enemies, lawbreakers, or the innocent—but blocked our guilt feelings from awareness. We may have been abandoned or betrayed, feel ashamed because we were not in control of our lives, and continue to feel numb or overwhelmed with the guilt and shame. Excessive and unrelieved guilt will continue to reap its consequences, even when there is lack of conscious awareness of it, until we are free from its bondage.

We can begin to find freedom from the guilt victimization cycle as follows:

- *Acknowledge:* That guilt is abnormal when there is not logical reason for it; that it is normal if we were responsible for the suffering or deaths of others; that it is self-destructive if we continue to punish ourselves.
- *Seek:* Freedom from self-destructive or destructive behaviors, guilty

secrets, self-condemning attitudes, self-destructive symptoms, and a distorted or absent conscience.

- *Surrender:* Our self-destructive and destructive behaviors and our guilty secrets to God.
- *Take action:* Ask for help from God, friends, and counselors to find relief from irrational guilt. Accept forgiveness from God; seek the forgiveness of others we have wronged, when appropriate; and forgive ourselves.
- *Daily prayer:* "God, forgive me for things I have done or failed to do, particularly if those things have led to the deaths or injury of others. Help me to regain my sensitivity and to make amends to those I have hurt, when possible. Grant me freedom from guilt, self-punishing symptoms, and destructive action that have kept me in bondage."

Step 8: Grief

> Sought God's help to grieve those we have lost, face our painful memories and emotions, and let our tears heal our sorrows.

In this step we focus on being able to complete the grief process. Grieving is a normal response to loss, but often we may have failed to complete the grieving process and remain victims of not only our losses but our unresolved emotional pain. If so, we may suffer a variety of consequences—withdrawing from people, denying that the loss ever occurred, intellectualizing rather than feeling emotion, deciding not to depend on others any more, or keeping our relationships at an emotional distance.

Conversely, we may not be able to control our emotions. We may have outbursts of tears or anger, severe depression, intrusive emotions and memories that cloud our thinking and block normal functioning, or obsessions about the object of our loss. If we have not completed grieving, we remain victims of blocked emotions, unresolved anger, depression, and emotionally distant relationships.

We can begin to break the grief victimization cycle as follows:

- *Acknowledge:* That we may be emotionally blocked, unable to grieve losses, and fearful about establishing close relationships once again.
- *Seek:* To be free from blocked emotions, blocked relationships, isolation, and persistent unresolved grief.
- *Surrender:* Our memories and painful emotions related to losses to God.
- *Take action:* Say good-bye to those we have lost, let down the barrier, feel anger and sadness and allow the tears to flow. Take the necessary risks to establish closer relationships, with help from God, friends, and counselors.
- *Daily prayer:* "God, help me to become aware of who and what I have lost, to grieve my losses, change those attitudes and behaviors that

keep me from making close relationships, and grant me the wisdom to learn the difference between 'hanging on' from fear of isolation and abandonment and remembering out of reverence and love."

Step 9: Life Versus Death

Revealed to God and someone we trusted all remaining self-destructive wishes, and, with His help, made a commitment to life.

This step focuses on helping us to gain freedom from our self-destructive wishes and behavior and to face the hopelessness, guilt, or self-directed anger that blocks us from embracing life. Fear, guilt, grief, and rage were once normal responses to surviving traumatic events. As they persist, however, these emotions chronically lead to depression, apathy, suicidal thoughts, suicide, or death from indirect methods. If suicidal thoughts begin to provide a source of comfort, the risk of self-destruction is high now or in the future—particularly if we keep a "suicide plan" in the back of our minds.

How can we change this? It may not be easy; in fact, facing death may seem easier than facing life, particularly if we believe that we have a "just cause" that is worth dying for. Remember that if we were to succeed in taking our own lives, we will have made a final decision without a second chance. And those who survive us will live with the guilt and pain of our deaths for the rest of their lives. Is that the legacy we want to leave them?

Breaking the cycle of destructive, self-destructive, and suicidal anger can begin in the following ways:

- *Acknowledge:* That we are powerless to control our self-destructive and suicidal thoughts and feelings; that we may be contemplating suicide without full awareness of the pain that would remain for the survivors.
- *Seek:* Help from God, family, friends, and counselors to resolve self-destructive thoughts and feelings, ways to find life worth living, and courage to make a commitment to life.
- *Surrender:* Self-destructive and suicidal thoughts, feelings, and plans to God.
- *Take action:* Ask for help from God, friends, and counselors and talk about it with someone you trust. Replace your suicidal plans and death wishes with a commitment to life and find positive thoughts, activities, and relationships to focus on.
- *Daily prayer:* "God, help me to surrender my self-destructive and suicidal thoughts to you and to make a commitment to life. Grant me the wisdom to learn the difference between surrendering my life from motives of selflessness and love, and taking my life out of self-centeredness and hatred."

Step 10: Justice versus Revenge

> Sought God's help to pursue the cause of justice, gain freedom from revengeful wishes and plans, and a desire to be channels of God's forgiveness to those we once hated.

This step focuses on helping us gain freedom from our destructive wishes for revenge and face the hatred, bitterness, and relentless anger that victimize us and block us from achieving true justice. As victims, our homicidal rage has been a normal reaction to feeling victimized or betrayed, being abandoned, or losing the health or lives of our friends or family. And it may seem impossible to forgive those who were responsible because hating is easier than living in peace and love, particularly if life has no other purpose beyond achieving vengeance.

There is a difference between achieving justice and getting revenge. Justice is the basis for love, peace, and freedom for ourselves and those we live with. Revenge, although it brings temporary relief, ultimately becomes a basis for repetitive hatred, destruction, and war. Revenge feeds upon itself and causes destructive consequences, further victimization, and bondage. If our hatred persists, we can bring our friends, families, and country into bondage with us. Revenge breeds only destructive consequences that can easily get out of control—an enormous price for ourselves, our friends, and our families to pay. If we have violent thoughts, if those thoughts are buried within our minds, if we have a mental "blueprint" to kill someone, if our hatred has become dangerous to others and to ourselves, we need help.

Breaking the victimization cycle of bitterness, violence, and revenge can begin in the following ways:

- *Acknowledge:* That we are powerless to control our hatred, vengeful thoughts, and bitterness that only victimizes us, our friends, and our families; that bitterness and hatred may lie deep within us, and even though we aren't fully aware, it hurts us and our friends and families.
- *Take action:* Talk to others who can help us discover ourselves. Renew daily a commitment to seek God's purpose in our lives. Renew our spiritual strength through uplifting words, thoughts, readings, friends, and activities.
- *Daily prayer:* "God, renew me as I surrender myself to You and seek Your purpose for my life today. Lead me on a creative and fulfilling path. Grant me the wisdom to know the difference between my seemingly fulfilling but self-centered way and Your way, a path not easily followed, of selflessness, justice, truth, and love."

Step 11: Finding a Purpose

> Sought knowledge and direction from God and surrendered ourselves to His leadership in order to find a renewed purpose for our lives.

This step focuses on helping us find a purpose for our lives. As victims, our lives once seemed meaningless. But as we have progressed through the first 10 steps, we have begun to discover freedom from the victimization of meaninglessness, distrust, shame, rage, terror, guilt, grief, suicidal desires, hatred, and isolation. This freedom, paradoxically, results from acknowledging, seeking, surrendering, and taking action to change old, self-destructive baggage that we've carried with us for years. Now that we have surrendered all of our baggage, there is nothing else to surrender but ourselves, the next step toward finding a purpose for our lives.

- *Acknowledge:* That we periodically slip back into the bondage of meaninglessness, victimization patterns, distrust, shame, rage, terror, guilt, grief, suicidal desires, hatred, and isolation; that when this happens, we find it difficult to believe there is a purpose for our lives.
- *Seek:* To let go of the baggage of post-traumatic symptoms and find a new sense of purpose; to find a new relationship to God.
- *Surrender:* Not only our post-traumatic baggage but also ourselves to God's leadership and purpose for us.
- *Take action:* Talk to others who can help us discover ourselves. Renew daily a commitment to seek God's purpose in our lives. Renew our spiritual strength through uplifting words, thoughts, readings, friends, and activities.
- *Daily prayer:* "God, renew me as I surrender myself to You and seek Your purpose for my life today. Lead me on a creative and fulfilling path. Grant me the wisdom to know the difference between my seemingly fulfilling but self-centered way and Your way, a path not easily followed, of selflessness, justice, truth, and love."

Step 12: Love and Relationships

> Sought God's love in our lives, renewed our commitment to friends and family, loved those we found difficult to love, and helped those who have been victims as we were.

This step focuses on helping us remain free from self-centeredness and tendencies to slip back into meaningless victimization experiences through learning to love and help others. Having had a spiritual awakening as a result of the first 11 steps, we will find that it is important to practice these principles with others. But we may still have some blocks that prevent us from helping others or accepting and giving love. Thus it is important to remove any blocks preventing us from accepting the love of God, friends, and family.

To build a foundation of loving relationships, it is important to understand and open ourselves to God's love; to renew our commitment to those friends and family whose love we have taken for granted; and to renew the vitality of love and friendships that had died from neglect. With this foundation we can be open to building new friendships—practicing what it means to give and receive. With an attitude of love, we can then carry the recovery message to other survivors and victims who are mired in the bondage of their own unique victimization patterns.

We can begin to love by following these steps:

- *Acknowledge:* That it is often difficult for us to be open to accept the love of others, to accept God's love, to love those we had taken for granted in the past, or to love those who we have found difficult to love.
- *Seek:* Openness to receive God's love and the love of others in our lives; the capacity to commit ourselves to friends and family; and the willingness to be channels of God's love to those who are difficult to love.
- *Surrender:* Ourselves to God's love so that it may flow into and through us.
- *Take action:* Commit ourselves to learning how to receive God's love and the love of others. Commit ourselves to our friends and family members. Seek daily to be channels of God's love to those we find difficult to love, and help those who are suffering from victimization in their lives.
- *Daily prayer:* "God, renew Your love in me as I surrender myself to You today. Help me to commit myself to those whose love I have taken for granted and who depend on me. Grant me the wisdom to love those I have not been able to love and to know the difference between my self-centered attempts to 'love' and the selfless love than can flow from You to others."

REFERENCES

Alcoholics Anonymous. (1976). *Big book.*

American Psychiatric Association. (1987). *Diagnostic and statistical manual of mental disorders* (3rd ed.). Washington, DC: Author.

Braun, B. G. (1984). Towards a theory of multiple personality and other dissociative phenomena. *Psychiatric Clinics of North America, 7,* 171–193.

Brende, J. O. (1983). A psychodynamic view of character pathology in Vietnam combat veterans. *Bulletin of the Menninger Clinic, 47,* 193–216.

Brende, J. O. (1986). Dissociative disorders in Vietnam combat veterans. *Journal of Contemporary Psychotherapy, 17*(2), 77–86.

Brende, J. O., & Parson, E. P. (1985). *Vietnam veterans: The road to recovery.* New York: Plenum.

Brende, J. O., & McDonald, E. (1988, October). *A twelve-theme and -step program for Vietnam combat veterans with posttraumatic stress disorder.* Paper presented at the annual meeting of Society for Traumatic Stress Studies, Dallas, TX.

Brende, J. O., & McDonald, E. (1989). Posttraumatic spiritual alienation and recovery in Vietnam combat veterans. *Spirituality Today, 41*(4).

Danieli, Y. (1988). Treating survivors and children of survivors of the Nazi Holocaust. In F. M. Ochberg (Ed.), *Posttraumatic therapy and victims of violence.* New York: Brunner/Mazel.

Figley, C. R. (1978). *Stress disorders among Vietnam veterans.* New York: Brunner/Mazel.
Figley, C. R. (1985). *Trauma and its wake.* New York: Brunner/Mazel.
Figley, C. R., & Leventman, S. (1980). *Strangers at home: Vietnam veterans since the war.* New York: Praeger.
Hartman, C. R., & Burgess, A. W. (1988). Rape trauma and treatment of the victim. In F. M. Ochberg (Ed.), *Posttraumatic therapy and victims of violence.* New York: Brunner/Mazel.
Herman, J. L. (1988). Father–daughter incest. In F. M. Ochberg (Ed.), *Posttraumatic therapy and victims of violence.* New York: Brunner/Mazel.
Horowitz, M. J. (1976). *Stress response syndromes.* New York: Aronson.
Horowitz, M. J. (1982). Stress response syndromes and their treatment. In L. Goldberger & S. Breznitz (Eds.), *Handbook of stress.* New York: Free Press.
Juri, E. J. (1946). *The great religions of the world.* Princeton, NJ: Princeton University Press.
Keller, J. E. (1985). *Let go, let God.* Minneapolis: Augsburg.
Krystal, H. (1988). *Integration and self-healing.* Hillsdale, NJ: Analytic Press/Erlbaum.
Lee, E., & Lu, F. (1989). Assessment and treatment of Asian-American survivors of mass violence. *Journal of Traumatic Stress, 2*(1), 93–120.
Lifton, R. J. (1973). *Home from the war: Vietnam veterans, neither victims nor executioners.* New York: Simon & Schuster.
Lindy, J. D. (1988). *Vietnam: A casebook.* New York: Brunner/Mazel.
Mahedy, S. P. (1986). *Out of the night: The spiritual journey of Vietnam vets.* New York: Ballentine.
Merwin, M. R. & Smith-Kurtz, B. (1988). Healing of the whole person. In F. M. Ochberg (Ed.), *Posttraumatic therapy and victims of violence.* New York: Brunner/Mazel.
McCormack, A., Burgess, A. W. & Hartman, C. (1988). Familial abuse and posttraumatic stress disorder. *Journal of Traumatic Stress, 1* (2), 231–242.
Ochberg, F. M. (Ed.). (1988). *Posttraumatic therapy and victims of violence.* New York: Brunner/Mazel.
Parson, E. R. (1988). Posttraumatic self disorders (PTsfD): Theoretical and practical considerations in psychotherapy of Vietnam war veterans. In J. P. Wilson, Z. Harel, & B. Kahana (Eds.), *Human adaptation to extreme stress* (pp. 246–282). New York: Plenum.
Roth, S. & Lebowitz, L. (1988). The experience of sexual trauma. *Journal of Traumatic Stress, 1*(1), 79–109.
Sorenson, G. (1985). A twelve-step program for combat veterans. *Vietnam Veterans Newsletter.*
Spiegel, D. (1988). Dissociation and hypnosis in posttraumatic stress disorders. *Journal of Traumatic Stress, 1*(1), 7–35.
Stark, E., & Flitcraft, A. (1988). Personal power and institutional victimization: Treating the dual trauma of woman battering. In F. M. Ochberg (Ed.), *Posttraumatic therapy and victims of violence.* New York: Brunner/Mazel.
Time. (1989, April 17), p. 27.
USA Today (1989, April 27).
van der Kolk, B. (1987). *Psychological trauma.* Washington, DC: APA Press.
van der Kolk, B., & Kadish, W. (1987). Amnesia, dissociation, and the return of the repressed. In B. van der Kolk (Ed.), *Psychological trauma.* Washington, DC: APA Press.
Williams, T. (1988). Diagnosis and treatment of survivor guilt. In J. P. Wilson, Z. Harel, & B. Kahana (Eds.), *Human adaptation to extreme stress.* New York: Plenum.
Wilson, J. P. (1988). Treating the Vietnam veteran. In F. M. Ochberg (Ed.), *Posttraumatic therapy and victims of violence.* New York: Brunner/Mazel.
Wilson, J. P. (1989). *Trauma, transformation, and healing.* New York: Brunner/Mazel.
Young, M. A. (1988). The crime victims' movement. In F. M. Ochberg (Ed.), *Posttraumatic therapy and victims of violence.* New York: Brunner/Mazel.

14

Brief Therapy of the Stress Response Syndrome

MARDI J. HOROWITZ and NANCY B. KALTREIDER

The liaison psychiatrist is frequently called upon to assess the psychological response to loss. He may see a patient in consultation who has been in a catastrophic accident, had a surgical loss of a body part, or is coping with the news of a fatal illness. The medical treatment team may ask more general questions about providing support to patients fearfully anticipating surgery or to bereaved relatives. An understanding of the pattern of the stress response syndrome as an organizing conceptual model can help the liaison psychiatrist to suggest appropriate strategies for primary prevention (Caplan, 1961), intervention, and referral. In this chapter we will discuss the nature of response to a sudden traumatic event and then describe a study of young women after hysterectomy to illustrate its applicability to medical practice. We will outline the strategy for brief psychotherapy for stress response syndromes for those patients who are referred for treatment.*

STRESS RESPONSE SYNDROME

One of the great paradoxes of the mind is that it must use existing inner models to interpret new events; models developed in the past must be used

*An up-to-date manual for these treatments is provided in Horowitz, M. (1986). *Stress Response Syndromes* (2nd ed.). New York: Aronson.

MARDI J. HOROWITZ and NANCY B. KALTREIDER • Center for the Study of Neuroses, Langley Porter Institute, University of California, San Francisco, California 94143.
The editorial assistance of Nancy Wilner is gratefully acknowledged. Reprinted from *Psychiatric Clinics of North America, 2,* 365–378. Copyright 1979 by the authors.
Psychotraumatology, edited by George S. Everly, Jr. and Jeffrey M. Lating. Plenum Press, New York, 1995.

to interpret the present and must be revised to meet the future. Growth and development have favored the best balance between retention of earlier models and the acceptance of new stimuli. But the equilibrium between old forms and new information is not easily or quickly balanced when loss constitutes the present event.

The ideal adjustment to loss is to accept it, to replace that which is lost, and to go on living. But there is an important, painful interval between the first pangs of recognition of loss and adaptation to circumstances as they must be. That interval is characterized by both the intrusion of unusual levels of ideas and feelings and the denial of ideas and numbing of emotions. Underlying these shifts in state are changes in inner models of the self, others, and the world—some caused by alterations in dominance among models, and others resulting from the formation of new models. Such changes are based on gradual processing of the new information.

States That Follow Serious Life Events

If one considers the general disparities of psychological research, a relatively remarkable concordance is found in the clinical, field, and experimental studies of response to the stress of serious events or to vicarious

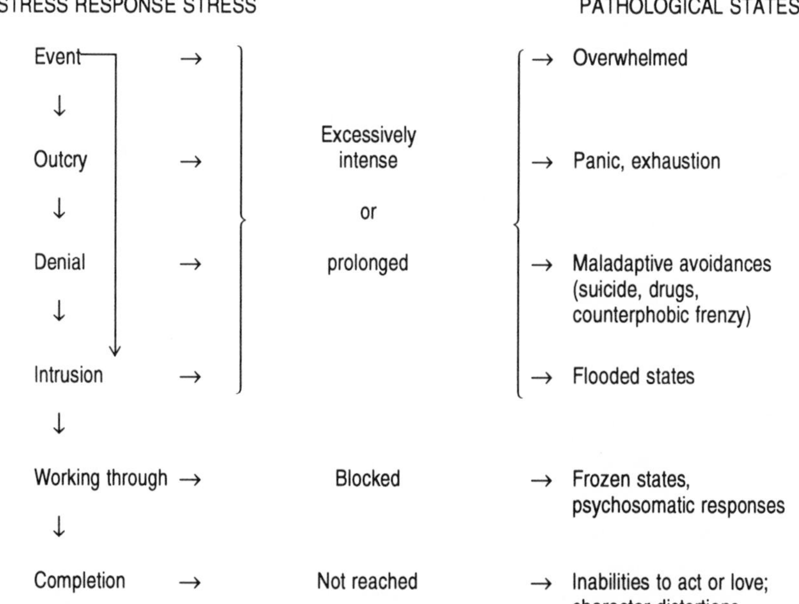

Figure 14.1 Phases of psychological response to stress. After Horowitz, M. J. (1979). Psychological response to serious life events. In V. Hamilton and D. M. Warburton (Eds.), *Human stress and cognition: An information processing approach.* New York: Wiley.

simulations of such events. The frequency of two broadly defined states increases after such occurrences; one is epitomized by intrusive experiences, the other by denial and numbing. These seemingly paradoxical but inextricably interrelated states have been given various names in the extensive literature on stress (Breuer & Freud, 1895/1955; Coehlo, Hamburg, & Adams, 1974; S. Freud, 1920/1955; Janis, 1958; Lazarus, 1966; Parad, Resnik, & Parad, 1976; Parkes, 1972). The contents of these labels of state and phase are usually specific to each individual. The terms, however, point to the general form of the experience, whatever the particular content (Horowitz, 1976).

States of intrusion and of denial or avoidance do not occur in any prescribed pattern; they appear to oscillate in ways particular to each person. Nonetheless, there is a phasic tendency. An initial period of outcry may occur and be followed by either denial or intrusive states, possibly in oscillation with each other. Then, in a period labeled as "working through," the frequency and intensity of each of these states is reduced. When a relative baseline is reached, a period of completion is said to occur. This general sequence and the result of the intensification of these phases are diagrammed in Figure 14.1.

In a special clinic for the evaluation and treatment of persons with stress response syndromes after serious life events (located at the Center for the Study of Neuroses, University of California, San Francisco [UCSF]), we have attempted to clarify these signs and symptoms sequentially. An overview of

Table 14.1 Signs and Symptoms of Denial Phase of Stress Response Syndromes

Perception and attention
Daze
Selective inattention
Inability to appreciate significance of stimuli
Consciousness
Amnesia (complete or partial)
Nonexperience
Ideational processing
Disavowal of meanings of stimuli
Loss of reality appropriateness
Constriction of associational width
Inflexibility of organization of thought
Fantasies to counteract reality
Emotional
Numbness
Somatic
Tension-inhibition type symptoms
Actions
Frantic overactivity to withdrawal

Note: From Horowitz, M. J. (1976). *Stress response syndromes.* New York. Aronson. Reprinted by permission.

Table 14.2 Operational Definitions of Some Important Signs and Symptoms of Denial

Avoidance of associational connections. Inhibiting expectable and fairly obvious personal or general continuations of meaning, implications, contingencies.

Numbness. A present subjective sense of not having feelings, or of feeling "benumbed." Includes a sense that one is not having potential emotions, when it is a sense, however intuitive, rather than a pure intellectualization.

Reduced level of feeling responses to outer stimuli. Includes flatness of expected emotional responses, constriction.

Rigidly role-adherent or stereotyped. Carrying on by playing a part, socially automatic response sets.

Loss of appropriateness of thought to reality by changing attitudes. Going from strong to weak, good to bad, active to passive, liking to disliking, or other changes to the degree that thought about any one meaning or implication is blunted and confused.

Unrealistic narrowing of attention, vagueness, or disavowal of stimuli. Includes flexibility of attention deployment, lack of centering on a focus, and avoidances of certain otherwise likely perceptual information. Includes insensitivity to changes in body.

Inattention, daze. Includes staring off into space, failure to determine significance of stimuli, clouding of alertness.

Inflexibility or constriction of thought. Failure to explore relatively obvious or likely avenues of meaning other than the theme under contemplation.

Loss of train of thought. Temporary or micromomentary lapses in continuation of a communicative experience, or reports of similar inability to concentrate on a line of inner processing of information.

Loss of appropriateness of thought to reality by sliding meanings. Distorting, minimizing, or exaggerating to the point where real meanings are clouded over.

Memory failure. Inability to recall details or sequences of events, amnestic areas, inability to remember in the usually expected manner.

Loss of appropriateness of thought to reality by use of disavowal. Saying to oneself or others that some meanings, that are or would be fairly obvious, are not so.

Warding off trains of reality-oriented thought by use of fantasy. Excessive focus on what might have been, what could be, or imaginative stories as a way of not facing realistic consequences or implications.

Note: From Horowitz, M. J. (1979). Psychological response to serious life events. In V. Hamilton & D. M. Warburton (Eds.), *Human stress and cognition: An information processing approach.* New York. Wiley.

the denial phase is provided in Table 14.1, with operational definitions of some important signs and symptoms of denial in Table 14.2.

Intrusive experiences commonly alternate with denial or avoidance states and are the essential elements of post-traumatic disorders (Freud, 1920/1955). They can be found after every type of serious life event and in laboratory analogies to such events, where a variety of emotional responses are evoked (Horowitz, 1975; Horowitz & Wilner, 1976). In Table 14.3, the overall pattern of such signs and symptoms is organized by the same descriptive sets used in the classification of the denial experiences. The operational definitions for the assessment of intrusive states used by our clinicians to evaluate persons with stress response syndromes are seen in Table 14.4.

We have found that it is very important to query the patient in a particular way after such experiences. Those who are articulate, intelligent, open, and self-confident may, of course, report such experiences spontaneously. But many persons have no experience in communicating the form of ideas and feelings; they usually describe only the contents.

The advantage of the descriptions of state given so far lies in their focus on the form of the experiences, a method for facilitating the examination of response tendencies across a variety of stressful events. There are, however, some contents of response that are also generally prevalent across such events. These contents are the themes that may enter consciousness intrusively or be warded off during periods of denial or avoidance: fear of repetition, fear of merger with victims, discomfort about vulnerability, rage at the source, rage at those exempted, fear of loss of control of aggressive impulses, discomfort about aggressive impulses, guilt or shame about surviving, sadness over losses, guilt or shame about responsibility. These are described in detail elsewhere (Horowitz & Wilner, 1976).

Awareness of the frequency and multiplication of such concerns is particularly useful to those who help others to master these experiences. No person has only one response to an event, and the idea of working through one constellation may be used as a resistance to further assimilation. Some themes are avoided at the same time that others are intrusively present, adding further complexity to the general ordering of response states over time. Working through each concern to a point of completion requires differentiation of reality from fantasy and continued restructuring of the real world and one's place in it.

Table 14.3 Signs and Symptoms of Intrusiveness Phase of Stress Response Syndromes

Perception and attention
Hypervigilance, startle reactions
Sleep and dream disturbances
Consciousness
Intrusive-repetitive thoughts and behaviors (illusions, pseudo hallucinations, nightmares, ruminations and repetitions)
Ideational processing
Overgeneralization
Inability to concentrate on other topics, preoccupation
Confusion and disorganization
Emotional
Emotional attacks or "pangs"
Somatic
Symptomatic sequelae of chronic fight or flight readiness (or of exhaustion)
Actions
Search for lost persons and situations, compulsive repetitions

Note: From Horowitz, M. J. (1976). *Stress response syndromes.* New York. Aronson. Reprinted by permission.

Table 14.4 Operational Definitions of Some Important Signs and Symptoms of Intrusion

Pangs of emotion. A "spell," episode, or wave of feeling that has a quality of increasing and then decreasing, rather than being a prevailing mood or subjective tone.

Rumination or preoccupation. Continuous conscious awareness about the event and associations to the event beyond that involved in ordinary thinking through a problem or situation to a point of decision or completion. It has a sense of uncontrolled repetition to it.

Fear of losing bodily control, or hyperactivity in any bodily system. Includes subjective sensations of urinating, defecating without will; fears of being unable to control vocalization, arm movements; hiding; running; obvious somatic responses such as excessive sweating, diarrhea, tachycardia.

Intrusive ideas in word form. Thoughts that pop into the mind suddenly and unbidden.

Difficulty in dispelling ideas. Once an idea has come to mind, even if thinking about it were deliberate, the person cannot stop awareness of the idea or topic. Emotions and moods that cannot be stopped are included.

Hypervigilance. The person is excessively alert, overly scanning the surrounding environment, too aroused in the sense of perceptual search, tensely expectant, or more driven toward obtaining stimuli than normal.

Reenactments. Any behavior that repeats any aspect of the serious life event, from minor ticlike movements and gestures to acting out in major movements and sequences. Includes enactments of personal responses to the life event, whether or not they were part of the real action surrounding the event.

Bad dreams. Any dream with unpleasant subjective experience, not just the classical nightmare with anxious awakenings.

Intrusive thoughts or images while trying to sleep. (See intrusive ideas and intrusive images.)

Intrusive images. Unbidden sensations in any modality. Any hallucination or pseudohallucination would be scored here as well if it came to mind in a nonvolitional manner. The emphasis here is on sensory quality, which, however similar to that of ordinary thought images, may be more intense and occur as a sudden, unwanted entry into awareness.

Startle reactions. Flinching after noises, unusual orienting reactions, blanching, or otherwise reacting to stimuli that usually do not warrant such responses.

Illusions. A misperception in which a person, object, or scene is misappraised as something else; for example, a bush is seen for a moment as a person, or a person is misrecognized as someone else.

Hallucinations, pseudohallucinations. An imaginary or fantasy-based emotional reaction as if it were real, whether or not the person intellectually thinks it is real. Includes "felt presences" of others in the room. Smell, taste, touch, movement, auditory, and visual sensations are included.

Note: From Horowitz, M. J. (1979). Psychological response to serious life events. In V. Hamilton & D. M. Warburton (Eds.), *Human stress and cognition: An information processing approach.* New York. Wiley.

To summarize, certain common stress response tendencies can be abstracted from clinical, field, and experimental studies among populations reacting to different life events. Simple knowledge of such states helps a person know what to expect and how to assess responses when they occur. Beyond the classification of states of experience, however, understanding why experiences occur may be even more helpful in planning a working-through process.

STRESS RESPONSE SYNDROMES IN A MEDICAL POPULATION

In a study reported in detail elsewhere (Kaltreider, Wallace, & Horowitz, 1979), we selected the experience of loss resulting from a nonelective hysterectomy in women of childbearing age as a relevant model to demonstrate the pattern of response to stress outside a mental health setting. After a chart review, 28 women who represented the spectrum of demographic, medical, and socioeconomic characteristics of patients at the gynecology service of UCSF were seen 1 year after surgery. They participated in extensive psychological interviewing (done by two female clinicians) and filled out experimental rating scales.

We found that the symptomatic pattern characterizing a stress response syndrome, as previously described in a psychiatric outpatient population, was judged by clinical observation of the interviewing psychiatrist to be present at a mild level in 12 (43%) of the posthysterectomy subjects and at a severe level in 5 (18%) others. The remaining 11 subjects (39%) were judged to have responded adaptively to the hysterectomy without presence of the intensity or duration of symptoms that define a stress response syndrome. At 1 year, 8 subjects (29%) were still currently experiencing neurotic symptoms judged by the interviewing psychiatrist to be directly related to the hysterectomy as a stress event. The range of reported symptoms included anxiety, phobias, and obsessive thoughts as well as the depression previously singled out in the literature.

Table 14.5 An Example of Trauma in Brief Psychotherapy

Session	Relationship Issues	Patient Activity	Therapist Activity
1	Initial positive feeling for helper	Patient tells story of event	Preliminary focus discussed
2	Lull as sense of pressure is reduced	Event related to life of patient	Takes psychiatric history
3	Patient tests therapist	Patient adds associations	Realignment of focus
4	Therapeutic alliance deepened		
5		Work on what has been avoided	
6			Time of termination discussed
7–12	Transference reactions interpreted when seen and indicated, and linked to other configurations	Working through central conflicts and issues of termination	Clarification and interpretation related to central conflicts and termination; clarification of unfinished issues and recommendations

As the subjects "dosed" themselves with more and more of the painful reality, they noted intrusive symptoms (Table 14.3) such as "flooding with memories in response to sudden reminders" (46%) and "unwanted thoughts about the surgery" (33%). At 1 year after the operation, more than a third of the subjects still noted experiences of denial (Table 14.1), with awareness of avoiding thoughts about the hysterectomy (38%) or of having a momentary sense of unreality that it had happened (35%).

In our psychiatric clinic, the presence of difficulty in completing the cognitive processing of a loss is generally linked to common painful meanings that must be warded off (Table 14.5). In the hysterectomy study, subjects who had a severe stress response syndrome were more likely to have experienced themselves postoperatively as a "changed woman" with deterioration in sexual function.

Whether or not the women had already borne children, the presence of a persisting wish for future children correlated with poor outcome; even women who had previously had tubal ligations experienced the hysterectomy as a more final loss. Within our limited sample, the presence of a stress response syndrome was not more common in the cervical dysplasia group or in those women who had had oophorectomies. What did seem to make the women particularly vulnerable to experiencing a stress response syndrome was poor adaptation to previous loss, a weak social support system, and lower socioeconomic level.

Clinical Typologies

Several clinical typologies can be described that distinguished the subgroups of women who exhibited different levels of stress response. Subjects with *no* stress response syndrome usually experienced the hysterectomy as providing considerable symptomatic relief or freedom from unwanted pregnancies. Their wish for children either had been satisfied or was not present. They had warm support from their families and generally valued activity and achievement. These subjects enjoyed independence and often saw the surgery as a way of taking control of a malfunctioning body. They tended to view themselves as both feminine and competent.

Women who experienced a *mild* stress response syndrome usually passed through a symptomatic period shortly after the surgery, with gradual resolution.

> Mrs. R., age 34, began exercising the day after surgery and was proud of her smooth recovery. Two months later she became depressed with guilt feelings for having cheated her husband out of a child. She said, "I felt like I'm nothing; I was completely empty. I was turning into a man." Every child or pregnant woman was a painful reminder. After several days of crying, the depression lifted and she resumed her characteristic coping style of being strong and in charge. She now notes increased energy and sexual pleasure but still broods over the fantasy of bearing a child.

Most women in this category gave a clinical impression of having considerable ego strength, and they responded to the loss as significant and needing to be worked through. A divergent subgroup of these women led a highly fragmented, turbulent life in which the hysterectomy only served as a temporary organizing focus for thought until a new stressful even superseded.

The women who experienced a *severe* stress response syndrome generally were emotionally isolated and lacked a cohesive system of social supports. They had been close to their own mothers and felt that they had not fulfilled a central life function, that of bearing children. Their future identity was linked to continued bearing of children, and they lacked acceptable alternative pathways to follow.

> Miss F., age 33, presented as an attractive young woman overwhelmed by depression. She had a hysterectomy on an emergency basis subsequent to an infection associated with an intrauterine device. Her initial response to the need for surgery was denial. She felt numb and asked the doctor, "Could you put it back in?" even though she intellectually knew this was impossible. When she tried to resume normal life she became overwhelmed by intrusive symptomatology. Miss F. experienced insomnia, nightmares, suicidal ideation, and unbidden visual images of dead flowers. She found herself especially sensitive to such triggers as the sight of a baby or discussion of a pregnancy experience. There was little resolution of the intrusive symptoms and considerable constriction in her life. She always felt tired and as if her body was dead. She noted a loss in sexual interest, with both decreased drive and difficulty in any close relationship with a man. Miss F. saw herself as a victim who was unable to trust men, symbolized by the doctors who created her intrauterine device and performed her surgery. She had always hoped to have a child—even without marriage—and saw potential offspring as providing an intimate relationship that would last a lifetime.

> Mrs. N., age 38, was a carelessly dressed obese woman who had a strong need to continue to produce children. Her initial response to the possibility of hysterectomy for menorrhagia was shock, and she drove around for hours in a daze. When she returned home, she lay shaking in bed but was unable to cry. After her husband reassured her, she told herself to be strong and count her blessings. After hysterectomy, she withdrew from all contact with her children, previously her greatest pleasure. There was marked change in her feminine self-concept. She said, "I feel like I am not a whole woman. Maybe if I had been something special or had a career, it would be different. But I always just wanted a home and kids; that's natural. If men know how I am inside, they wouldn't want me anymore." She felt that the inability to bear more children symbolized breaking of a special tie with her deceased mother, who raised a family of 15.

Discussion

The conceptual model of stress response syndrome appears to have a useful application to the experience of loss by medical patients who were studied in this pilot field study of premenopausal women after hysterectomy. The symptomatic pattern previously observed in our psychiatric population did occur in a mild (43%) to severe (18%) form in the field study and could be best understood by the phasic model. The initial reaction to the news of the hysterectomy may be an "outcry" of anger or desperation. Here the physician can carefully inquire about the wish for future children, stability of feminine self-concept, and concerns over sexual function, which may identify those at special risk of poor outcome. Previous poor response to loss and limited coping skills in a candidate for hysterectomy suggest the need for special supports.

It is often difficult for the physician to spend time in extensive preoperative counseling. Use of a woman nurse practitioner to discuss openly all aspects of the surgery could be most helpful, and the inclusion of a spouse in evaluation of the potential impact on sexuality would be good preventive medicine. Special caution in advising elective surgery is recommended in the group of young women with a history of hysterical symptoms (Martin et al. 1977). The younger woman might find it particularly useful to speak to a peer who has had a hysterectomy; such programs for women contemplating mastectomy have provided meaningful support.

Postoperatively, the physician who understands the phases of denial and intrusion will be alert to the patient who seems to be determined to carry on life as usual without acknowledgement of the implications of the surgical trauma. Sensitive inquiry at this stage can help the woman to become aware of the emotional numbing and warding off of ideas that will impede her processing of the psychological meanings of the loss. The possible later appearance of intrusive ideas, waves of feeling, and nightmares can be described to the patient, who otherwise may experience them as "going crazy." Support of family members, as well as the physician, and episodic minor sedation during the intrusive period can be of particular help.

Despite appropriate intervention by the physician, the particular meanings of loss such as a hysterectomy may trigger a strong response based on earlier neurotic problems, so that effective processing will not occur. In our field study of hysterectomy, 29% of the subjects were still symptomatic at 1 year but were hesitant to seek medical or psychological help because they felt they should be able to cope with this "normal" crisis. If the patient appears at any point to be overwhelmed by the intensity of the symptomatology, or if the symptoms persist more than 6 months after intervention by the general physician, then psychiatric referral for brief therapy is appropriate in the management of stress response syndrome.

PSYCHOTHERAPY OF STRESS RESPONSE SYNDROMES

The psychiatrist who sees a patient with an excessively intense or prolonged stress syndrome can organize treatment around three goals (Malan, 1976; Sifneos, 1972):

1. The patient needs to retain a sense of competence and self-worth. This necessitates accepting whatever unalterable limitations are placed on his or her life plans by the loss or injury. This should be done without loss of hope or a sense of meaning in life.
2. The person should continue realistic and adaptive actions, including maintenance of available relationships and development of new, adaptively useful ones.
3. In working through the reactions to such a serious life event, the situation should be used for additional growth and maturation.

The Pattern of Treatment

After a serious life event, individuals usually reconsider the meanings and plans for response to that event in a manner that is systematic, step-by-step, and dosed. When emotional responses become excessive or threaten flooding, the person initiates control operations. The recollection of the unfinished processing of sets of meanings will tend to counteract these controls. When the person cannot handle both the repetition compulsion (S. Freud, 1920/1955) and the defensive counters (A. Freud, 1936/1966), he or she seeks help. The therapist establishes a working alliance to assist the patient in working through his or her natural responses to the event and to the overall situation. In addition, efforts may be directed at modification of preexisting conflicts, developmental difficulties, and defensive styles that made the person unusually vulnerable to traumatization by this particular experience.

Therapy depends in part on establishing a safe relationship. Once this is done, work within the therapy alters the status of the patient's controls. With a safe relationship and gradual modification of controls, the patient can then proceed to reappraise the serious life event, and the meanings associated with it, and make the necessary revisions of his or her inner models of the self and the world. As this reappraisal and revision takes place, the person is in a position to make new decisions and to engage in adaptive actions. He or she can practice the altered models until they gradually become automatic. Overlapping with these processes is the necessity for working-through reactions to the approaching loss of the therapist and the therapy.

As individuals are able to accommodate to new levels of awareness, this process repeats itself. When they can relate in a still more mutual and intimate manner, they can examine themselves more deeply, and controls can be modified further. Additional work of this sort may modify aspects of character structure.

Within the time limits of a brief psychotherapy, the therapist works to establish conditions that will be helpful to the processing of the painful event. There is an early testing by the patient of both the safety of the relationship and the therapist's ability to help him cope with symptoms. Most commonly, patients will seek help for intrusive symptoms. These symptoms can seem less overwhelming when the therapist provides support, suggests some immediate structuring of time and events, prescribes medication if anxiety or insomnia is too disruptive, and gives "permission" for the patient to dose his feelings rather than to attempt to work them through as quickly as possible. Such interventions are often called for even during the period of acute medical hospitalization after trauma. Patients who are more handicapped by their symptoms of avoidance can be helped by encouragement from the therapist to recollect the stress even with associations and abreaction while working toward changing the attitudes that made the controls necessary.

Frequently, symptoms subside rapidly with the establishment of a good working alliance. The relationship of the stress event to the patient's various self-concepts can then become a focus. Introduction of the plans for termination of therapy several sessions before the final one leads to a reexperience of loss, often with a return of symptoms. But this time loss can be faced gradually, actively rather than passively, and in a communicative helping relationship. Specific interpretations of the link of the termination experience to the stress event are made, and the final hours center on this theme. At termination, the patient will usually still have symptoms, in part because of the time needed to process a major loss and anxiety about the loss of the relationship with the therapist. Follow-up evaluations suggest to us that the therapy serves as a catalyst for both symptomatic and structural change over the ensuing year or more. This very global and generalized overview for a model 12-hour therapy, as it has been applied in our center, is shown in Table 14.5.

In the course of these brief therapies, patients sometimes become aware of a particular style they have for not thinking about events, and they are able to alter that situation deliberately. It may be possible for them, by continued work on their own after therapy, to live out changes that may gradually alter habitual controls.

When a person experiences the impact of a serious life event such as a loss or injury, his most advanced and adaptive role relationships can be threatened. He may regress to earlier role relationships, or the meaning of the event itself may tend to create some new role relationship with unattractive, dangerous, or undesirable characteristics. The person may then enter a series of painful, strongly affective states based on altered self-images and the changed role relationship. As a consequence of therapeutic facilitation of normal processes, the disturbing role relationships or self-images can once again be subordinated to more adaptive, mature self-images and role relationships. Intensive work using a brief therapy model may both alter the symptomatic response to a stressful life event and facilitate further progress along developmental lines.

An understanding of reactions to serious life events will help the liaison psychiatrist to appraise the symptoms in the light of the phasic patterns of the stress response syndrome. Alertness of the medical care staff to recognition of the common signs and symptoms will lead to appropriate timing and focus for interventions. When warranted by the intensity or severity of the reactions, brief psychotherapy can allow the patient to work through the event and may trigger processes extending past the therapy period that will lead to alterations in the general repertoire of character defenses.

REFERENCES

Breuer, J., & Freud, S. (1955). Studies on hysteria. In J. Strachey (Ed. and Trans.), *The standard edition of the complete psychological works of Sigmund Freud* (Vol. 2). London: Hogarth Press. (Original work published 1895)

Caplan, G. (1961). *An approach to community mental health.* New York: Grune and Stratton.

Coehlo, G. V., Hamburg, D. A., & Adams, J. E. (1974). *Coping and adaptation.* New York: Basic Books.

Freud, A. (1966). The ego and the mechanisms of defense. In C. Baines (Ed. and Trans.), *The writings of Anna Freud* (Vol. 2). New York: International Universities Press. (Original work published 1936)

Freud, S. (1955). Beyond the pleasure principle. In J. Strachey (Ed. and Trans.), *The standard edition of the complete psychological works of Sigmund Freud* (Vol. 18, pp. 7–64). London: Hogarth Press. (Original work published 1920)

Horowitz, M. J. (1975). Intrusive and repetitive thoughts after experimental stress: A summary. *Archives of General Psychiatry, 32,* 1457–1463.

Horowitz, M. J. (1976). *Stress response syndromes.* New York: Aronson.

Horowitz, M. J. (1979). Psychological response to serious life events. In V. Hamilton & D. M. Warburton (Eds.), *Human stress and cognition: An information processing approach.* New York: Wiley.

Horowitz, M. J., & Kaltreider, N. (1979). Brief psychotherapy of stress response syndromes. In T. B. Karasu & L. Bellak (Eds.), *Specialized techniques in individual psychotherapy.* New York: Brunner/Mazel.

Horowitz, M. J., & Wilner, N. (1976). Stress films, emotion and cognitive response. *Archives of General Psychiatry, 30,* 1339–1344.

Janis, I. (1958). *Psychological stress.* New York: John Wiley.

Kaltreider, N., Wallace, A., & Horowitz, M. J. (1979). A field study of the stress response syndrome. Young women after hysterectomy. *Journal of the American Medical Association, 242,* 1499–1503.

Lazarus, R. (1966). *Psychological stress and the coping process.* New York: McGraw-Hill.

Malan, D. (1976). *Frontier of brief psychotherapy.* New York: Plenum.

Martin, R. L., et al. (1977). Psychiatric illness and non-cancer hysterectomy. *Disorders of the Nervous System, 38,* 974–980.

Parad, H., Resnik, H., & Parad, L. (1976). *Emergency mental health services and disaster management.* New York: Prentice Hall.

Parkes, C. M. (1972). *Bereavement.* New York: International Universities Press.

Sifneos, P. E. (1972). *Short term psychotherapy and emotional crisis.* Cambridge, MA: Harvard University Press.

15

Post-Traumatic Therapy

FRANK M. OCHBERG

Most victims of violence never seek professional therapy to deal with the emotional impact of traumatic events. If they did, they would be sorely disappointed. There are not enough therapists in the world to treat the millions of men, women, and children who have been assaulted, abused, and violated as a result of war, tyranny, crime, disaster, and family violence. When people do seek help, suffering with post-traumatic symptoms, they may find therapists who are ill-equipped to provide assistance. The credentialed clinicians in psychiatry, psychology, nursing, social work, and allied professions are only recently learning to catalogue, evaluate, and refine a therapeutic armamentarium to serve traumatized clients. There are, however, a cadre of clinicians who have shared insights and approaches, face-to-face and through written works, defining principles and techniques that address the worldwide problem of post-traumatic readjustment. A recent sampling of clinical insights (Ochberg, 1988) attempts to define the commonalities in assumptions and approaches to therapy. The common ground is the foundation of Post-Traumatic Therapy (PTT). The individual distinctions separating clinicians who share this common ground are the inevitable differences of creative minds.

THE FOUNDATION OF POST-TRAUMATIC THERAPY

Several principles are fundamental to PTT, and discussing these at the outset of therapy is usually advisable. Because traumatized and victimized

---

FRANK M. OCHBERG • Department of Psychiatry, Michigan State University, East Lansing, Michigan 48824. Correspondence regarding this article should be addressed to Frank M. Ochberg, 4211 Okemos Road, #6, Okemos, MI 48864. Reprinted from *Psychotherapy, 28*(1), 5–15.

Psychotraumatology, edited by George S. Everly, Jr. and Jeffrey M. Lating. Plenum Press, New York, 1995.

individuals are, by definition, reacting to abnormal events, they may confuse the abnormality of the trauma with abnormality of themselves. The first principle of PTT is therefore the normalization principle: *There is a general pattern of post-traumatic adjustment and the thoughts and feelings that make up this pattern are normal, although they may be painful and perplexing.* Reassurance ("This is normal") means that a healthy healing process is under way. Further explanation of the healing pattern allows the patient to participate actively in the recovery process, understanding the reasons for symptoms, the time course of reequilibration, and the signs of abnormal interference. The emotional healing process often includes reexperiencing, avoidance, sensitivity, and self-blame. These symptoms are easily described, explained, and set in a context of adaptation and eventual mastery. By sharing such information the second principle of PTT, the collaborative and empowering principle, is recognized: *The therapeutic relationship must be collaborative, leading to empowerment of one who has been diminished in dignity and security.* This principle is particularly important in work with victims of violent crime. The exposure to human cruelty, the feeling of dehumanization, and the experience of powerlessness creates a diminished sense of self. This diminution is normal when it is proportional to the victimization. Survivors of natural disasters experience powerlessness, too, although they are not subjected to cruelty and subjugation. They benefit greatly from a therapeutic alliance that is experienced as collegial and empowering. A third principle is the individuality principle: *Every individual has a unique pathway to recovery after traumatic stress.* Cannon (1939) and Selye (1956) may have identified common physiological and psychological reactions in states of extreme stress, but Weybrew (1967) and others note the complexity of the human stress response and the fact that one's pattern is as singular as a fingerprint. This principle suggests that a unique pathway of post-traumatic adjustment is to be anticipated and valued, not feared or disparaged. Therapist and client will walk the path together, aware of a general direction and predictable pitfalls, but ready to discover new truths at every turn.

These three principles can be expressed in various ways and supplemented with other important tenets. For example, an appreciation of coping skills rather than personality limitations allows therapy to proceed without undue emphasis on negative characteristics and the devastating implication that victimization is deserved. PTT begins with the assumption that a normal individual encountered an abnormal event. To ameliorate the painful consequences, one must mobilize coping mechanisms. How different this is from the hypothesis that PTSD and victimization symptoms are products of personality flaws and neurotic defenses that must be identified and treated according to traditional paradigms. Furthermore, an interdisciplinary approach, recognizing the contributions of biology, psychology, and social dynamics, stimulates clinician and client to see beyond any singular explanation for post-traumatic suffering and to search for remedies in many different fields. The contributions of pharmacology, education, nutrition, social work, law, and history are recognized and valued. Interventions may include introduction to a self-help network, exposure to inspirational literature, explanation of the victims' rights movement, establishment of an exercise regimen, or prescription of anxiolytics. PTT is interdisciplinary. The practitioner should therefore be aware of community resources that are of potential benefit and be willing to assess the merit of these adjuncts to his or her direct clinical intervention. Often, this requires personal meetings with colleagues from disparate fields.

TECHNIQUES OF POST-TRAUMATIC THERAPY

Many techniques have been used effectively to help survivors readjust after traumatic events. It may be useful to group the various methods into four categories. The first is *educational* and includes sharing books and articles, teaching the basic concepts of physiology to allow an appreciation of the stress response, discussing civil and criminal law with new participants in the process, and introducing the fundamentals of holistic health. The educational process is a two-way street. The client may have resources that he or she finds helpful and wants to share with the clinician.

The second grouping of techniques falls within the category of *holistic health.* Although the term has its critics as well as its supporters, it is offered in the spirit of Merwin and Smith-Kurtz (1988), who note how physical activity, nutrition, spirituality, and humor contribute to the healing of the whole person. The clinician who promotes these aspects of healing serves as a teacher and a coach, offering concepts that might be new to the client and shaping abilities that may be latent.

The third category includes methods that enhance *social support* and *social integration.* Family and group therapy could be included here. Exposure to self-help and support groups in the community is another example. But most important is the sensitive assessment of social skills, the enhancement of these skills, the reduction of irrational fears, and the expert timing of encouragement to risk new relationships. Traditional analytic tools and traditional social work skills are employed to promote healing in supportive human groups.

Finally, there are clinical techniques that are best categorized as *therapy.* These include working through grief, extinguishing the fear response that accompanies traumatic imagery, judicious use of medication for target symptoms, the telling of the trauma story, role play, hypnotherapy, and many individualized methods that are consistent with the principles of PTT.

These four clusters of techniques are not comprehensive. There are innovations that defy categorization, such as the Native American sweat lodge technique, discussed by Wilson (1988), and testimony of political repression, used as a therapeutic instrument (Cienfuegos & Monelli, 1983). But it is not necessary here to prepare an exhaustive catalogue of techniques. The intent is to explain those approaches I employ in residential (Ochberg & Fojtik, 1984) and outpatient settings with victimized, traumatized clients.

EDUCATION

Reading the DSM Together

> I will never forget the first time I brought out my green, hardbound copy of DSM-III (American Psychiatric Association, 1980), moved my chair next to Mrs. M, and showed her the chapter on PTSD. She was a thin, soft-spoken woman in her 30s who was assaulted and raped in South Lansing. She was referred by a colleague and had just finished telling me her symptoms 8 or 9 weeks after the traumatic event. She was frightened, guarded, perplexed, and sad. She had no basis for trusting me. But after she saw the words in the book as I read them aloud, she brightened, sat up tall, and said, "You mean, that's me, in that book! I never thought this could be real."
>
> Seldom have I found such a reversal of mood and such a sudden establishment of trust and rapport since Mrs. M, but I have never missed an opportunity to read the criteria list with a client when it seemed appropriate.

The responses vary from satisfaction that the symptoms are officially recognized to surprise that anybody else has a similar syndrome. Some patients take pride in making their own diagnosis, pointing out exactly which symptoms apply. Few show any interest in other sections of the book. Most seem to enjoy hearing explanations of the trouble in formulating the diagnostic category (how some of us argued for placing the description in the "V Code" section, with other "normal" reactions such as "uncomplicated bereavement," but others prevailed, and the practical consequence of placing this normal reaction to abnormal events in the chapter on anxiety is that insurance companies pay their fair share of the bill!)

Introducing Civil and Criminal Law

A therapist need not be a lawyer to know about the law. When our clients face the criminal justice system for the first time, they may be understandably concerned, confused, and overwhelmed.

> Mr. A was shot in the abdomen at close range by an intruder and almost killed. After heroic surgery, he awoke to the hubbub of an intensive care unit.

> Between hallucinations, he learned what occurred, received family visits, and began looking at mug shots. His introduction to the world of detectives, prosecutors, and judges was better than most. They appreciated his condition and worked slowly and sensitively after realizing the futility of expecting a positive identification. He appreciated their professional responsibilities and their regard for him. Would it were always so!

Victims of violent crime are often treated like pawns in an impersonal bureaucracy (Young, 1988). President Reagan realized this in commissioning the President's Task Force on Crime Victims (1982), and the U.S. Congress followed suit by passing the Victims of Crime Act of 1984.

Clients who are victims of violent crime may be offered several articles and brochures that explain their rights under state law and the role of the victim-witness in the American justice system. Michigan is blessed with a model victims' rights law (Ochberg, 1988, pp. 315–317; Van Regenmorter, 1989) and a crime victims' compensation board that provides financial aid. Clinicians who counsel victims could easily find resources and references in their own states.

A patient who is in the middle of a trial, cooperating fully with the prosecutor, may know nothing of the right to sue the assailant, to have a court injunction against harassment, to receive workers' compensation, and in some instances to receive representation from the *pro bono* committee of the county bar association. Finding the right lawyer is as difficult as finding the right clinician, so one should pay close attention to experiences with attorneys and maintain an up-to-date referral roster. Sharing information about legal resources is part of the education process.

Discussing Psychobiology

Few clients are interested in reading about autonomic nervous system activation, but some read voraciously. To understand the physiology of mammalian arousal during stress is to begin mobilizing the mind in pursuit of recovery. It is relatively easy to impart a basic understanding of the fight–flight mechanisms (Cannon, 1939) and the General Adaptation Syndrome (Selye, 1956). Merwin and Smith-Kurtz (1988) explain the concepts clearly, and Roth (1988) and van der Kolk (1988) discuss more complex implications in the same volume. Without turning therapy into a didactic exercise, and without burdening the client with unsolicited instruction, one can convey the fact that lethal threat has a powerful impact on body chemistry, that our adrenal glands are stimulated, that we are prepared to fight or to flee as if we were facing a wild beast, that all this circuitry is out of date and usually destructive when we face threats in modern society, that PTSD is the predictable outcome in general after extraordinary stress, and that everyone's individual pattern is different.

Furthermore, vigorous use of the large muscles is the intended result of adrenal activation, and physical activity is an advisable measure to ameliorate the effects of PTSD. This point leads to the next educational objective.

Reviewing Concepts of Fitness and Holistic Health

In designing the milieu and program of the Dimondale Stress Reduction Center (Ochberg & Fojtik, 1984), we hoped for a blend of a health spa, a community college, and a hospital. We maintained this balance for several years, but eventually the hospital bureaucracy crowded out the other elements. I was disappointed, but not surprised. American medicine, particularly hospital-based medicine, places the patient in a passive role and ignores the power of health promotion. We once called health promotion "hygiene" in elementary school. Gym teachers, not doctors, got the points across.

Patients should be educated about the benefits of exercise and nutrition; the syllabus is in Merwin and Smith-Kurtz (1988). My approach includes nagging, begging, and heartfelt approval when interest is shown.

PROMOTING HOLISTIC HEALTH

Physical Activity

Writing about the development of a healthy fitness routine for PTT clients, Merwin and Smith-Kurtz (1988) observe that "techniques of physical training have changed in recent years as the maxim 'no pain, no gain' has been discarded. Exercising past the pain threshold risks injury to muscles, joints, or tendons. The watchwords today are 'balance,' 'moderation,' and 'listen to your body.'" They go on to describe the three elements of a balanced program—strength, cardiovascular efficiency, and flexibility—and they note the generally accepted activities that provide these elements. Few clients nowadays are unfamiliar with these principles, but many lack the motivation to begin or to resume an interrupted routine. Some fear social interaction. Some have injuries that limit activity. Some are generally lacking in initiative, evidencing criterion C(4) of PTSD (APA, 1987), "markedly diminished interest in significant activities." Relatively early in therapy, I evaluate the client's potential for supervised physical activity. A recent medical examination should be performed to determine limitations or restrictions. If there are limitations, activity may be allowable, but only after consultation with the examining physician.

When there is resistance to exercise, the resistance itself must be confronted. The therapist should not assume to know an individual's underlying motive for avoiding healthy activity. A gentle, collaborative search for the obstacles and the construction of a path around them constitute an important chapter of PTT.

Therapists are advised to become familiar with supervised, structured fitness programs in their communities. A referral to a specific YMCA, health club, or aerobics instructor can assure that the milieu is appropriate, the regimen is reasonable, and the opportunity for reinforcement is available.

Nutrition

We never learned much about nutrition in medical school (outside of infant formulae in pediatrics). But it makes sense to evaluate a client's eating habits and look for the common mistakes that contribute to anxiety, irritability, and depression. This is part of good clinical work in general but is particularly important for post-traumatic patients who are vulnerable to mood swings and who may have neglected their nutrition.

Caffeine Intoxication. DSM III-R (APA, 1987) requires 5 out of 12 signs, plus the presence of recent excessive caffeine ingestion and the absence of other causes, to make the diagnosis of caffeine intoxication (or "caffeinism"). The 12 signs overlap with the hallmarks of panic, generalized anxiety, and aspects of PTSD: restlessness, nervousness, excitement, insomnia, flushed face, diuresis, gastrointestinal disturbance, muscle twitching, rambling flow of thought and speech, tachycardia or cardiac arrhythmia, periods of inexhaustibility, and psychomotor agitation. Clients who experience numbing may consciously or unconsciously increase their coffee consumption. A demoralized indifference to preparing and consuming adequate meals may result in excessive drinking of tea or coffee. And caffeine is found in soft drinks, candy, and certain desserts as well as coffee and tea. The incidence of true caffeine intoxication is relatively rare, but good clinical practice requires that we rule out the diagnosis when anxiety symptoms are present. Furthermore, a discussion of caffeine effects leads to the broader issues of diet, appetite, and meal rituals.

The Meaning of Healthy Eating. Food gathering, preparation, and consumption has ritual significance in most cultures. Food sharing is a critical aspect of nurturing and of family cohesion. When a traumatic event interferes with one's desire to eat, one's ability to face the ordeal of shopping, and one's participation in shared meals, more than nutrition is at stake. There is disruption of biochemistry, interpersonal relations, self-esteem, and connection to culture. PTT requires attention to all of these issues, agreement on desired objectives in the short-term and long-term future, and a collaborative search for remedies.

Mrs. A developed agoraphobia in addition to PTSD after being held hostage and surviving a sexual assault. Her therapy was prolonged, involving residential and outpatient treatment. She read every book she could find about coping with stress and understood the significance of reestablishing her role in her family and community. But a major obstacle was her fear of meeting people who knew about her assault and who felt compelled to make well-intentioned remarks about her recovery. We discussed this situation at length. As she learned to respond to the sympathetic comments of friends and acquaintances without feeling invaded, she overcame her "fear of the marketplace." The later phases of PTT were supportive and nondirective. She resumed her functions in the family, and meals became a source of pleasure rather than pain.

Referral to Nutrition Experts. It is relatively easy to identify competent colleagues. However, most are experienced in working with eating disordered patients, but not with victims of violence. Those therapists who do not have colleagues close by to assist with nutritional counseling are advised to review the basic facts and the supplementary reference list provided in Chapter 4 of Ochberg (1988).

Humor

Following the advice of a colleague who wrote the section on humor in the chapter just mentioned (Smith-Kurtz, 1988), I asked Mrs. R, an adult survivor of incest, to tell me about her ability to laugh. "Do you think my life is funny?" she fumed, casting a look at me that could wither an oak tree. My timing was awful. But usually I can succeed in initiating a discussion about humor, its salutary effect, and ways that we can improve our ability to laugh at ourselves. Smith-Kurtz cites the remarkable example of Norman Cousins (1979), a genius in marshaling humor as a coping mechanism for critical illness. Furthermore, she provides techniques and references to enhance the therapist's sense of humor.

The goal in adding humor to PTT is not for the therapist to be witty, but for the client to have the capacity to laugh. A clinician can facilitate the recovery and the improvement of a client's sense of humor by setting an example, by searching for instances when the client used humor well, and by providing a good audience when spontaneous humor arises.

A week after Mrs. R cut me down to size, I told her how clumsy a therapist can feel, trying to uncover humor and failing completely. She laughed. Now we can talk freely about her tendency toward sanctimonious ness and her neglect of humor as a healing art. She is interested in elevating her capacity for laughter, and that is a step in the right direction.

Spirituality

Long before psychology and psychiatry were invented, before medicine was a science, there were healers who treated the sick and the wounded. They sometimes used remedies with a chemical basis for efficacy unknown at the time (e.g., belladonna for diarrhea). But invariably there was a sacred, ritual dimension to the treatment. The medicine man invoked spiritual assistance. Sacrifices were required to the gods. Prayers were said, individually and collectively. There is abundant evidence that healing was facilitated. The power of prayer in surviving captivity and torture is well known (Fly, 1973; Jackson, 1973), although the mechanism of action is subject to debate.

Clinicians must evaluate every client's spiritual potential, or their ability to benefit from their own beliefs. For adherents to the major religions, this spiritual dimension may be conceptualized as feeling God's love. For others, spirituality may be described as a transcendent feeling of harmony and communion with humanity, nature, or the unknown reaches of space.

Merwin (1988) explains that "spirituality is a state of being fully alive and open to the moment." It includes a sense of belonging and of having a place in the universe. A deep appreciation of the natural world, an openness for surprise, a gratefulness for the gratuity of everything, joy and wonderment are all a part of spirituality. Although spiritual growth is a type of healing from which most of us could benefit, a victim's sense of spirit may be acutely dimmed for a period after the victimization. "Over time, however, as the victim heals in all areas, the potential for spiritual growth may become greater than ever before and greater than for many people who have not faced the reality of their individual death."

I usually avoid these issues early in therapy. Many patients have complained about clergy who focused on their own method of spiritual healing after a trauma, ignoring the feelings of the victimized individual. On the other hand, many clients have been helped by sensitive pastoral counselors and continue seeing them while seeing a therapist. The issue in therapy is not creating, *de novo,* a spiritual capacity, but identifying and overcoming the obstacles to feeling the embrace of one's faith.

An excellent example of personal triumph over childhood sexual assault, as well as the effects of racism and sexism, can be found in the autobiographical prose and poetry of Maya Angelou (1978). Her faith in her own indomitable spirit inspires others. I have referred her works to clients and students when the spiritual dimension of overcoming adversity was relevant. Here is a powerful poem of hers that can reach the right client at the right time:

And Still I Rise

You may write me down in history
With your bitter, twisted lies,
You may trod me in the very dirt
But still, like dust, I'll rise.
Does my sassiness upset you?
Why are you beset with gloom?
'Cause I walk like I've got oil wells
Pumping in my living room.
Just like moons and like suns,
With the certainty of tides,
Just like hopes springing high,
Still I'll rise.
Did you want to see me broken?
Bowed head and lowered eyes?
Shoulders falling down like teardrops,
Weakened by my soulful cries
Does my haughtiness offend you?
Don't you take it awful hard
'Cause I laugh like I've got gold mines
Diggin' in my own backyard.
You may shoot me with your words,
You may cut me with your eyes,
You may kill me with your hatefulness,
But still, like air, I'll rise . . .
Out of the huts of history's shame I rise.
Up from a past that's rooted in pain I rise . . .
Leaving behind night of terror and fear
I rise.
Into a daybreak that's wondrously clear
I rise.
Bringing the gifts that my ancestors gave
I am the dream and the hope of the slave.
I rise.
I rise.
I rise.

Quoted with permission from Random House.

Holistic health recognizes that the healing process is more than chemical reequilibration. Attention to exercise, nutrition, humor, and spirituality are important elements of the holistic approach. Beyond these elements is the human group, whether it is a family, a support network, or a community. The individual who is victimized cannot recover in isolation. Therefore the clinician must attend to the demands of social integration.

SOCIAL INTEGRATION

A supportive family is the ideal social group for healthy post-traumatic healing. Figley (1988) describes how such families promote recovery by "(1) detecting traumatic stress; (2) confronting the trauma; (3) urging recapitulation of the catastrophe; and (4) facilitating resolution of the trauma-inducing conflicts." After reviewing the first 50 admissions to the Dimondale victims' assistance program, a residential treatment facility with an average stay of 2 weeks, I was surprised to find that fewer than 10% of the patients had supportive families. It appeared that victimized individuals with loving effective families would rather recover at home than be separated from their primary source of nourishment. However, even the ideal family can be sorely strained after one or more members are seriously traumatized. There is an important role for the post-traumatic therapist in assessing family strengths and weaknesses, as well as assisting in the design and implementation of strategies for optimum recovery. Referral to support groups and self-help networks may complement or supplement the healing function of the family.

Post-Traumatic Family Therapy

Figley's (1988) formula for post-traumatic family therapy includes an assessment phase and four distinct treatment phases. Before summarizing these, it should be emphasized that family therapy is not necessarily the best approach, particularly when violation occurs within the family. For example, Herman (1988), cautions, "Following the crisis of disclosure, the incestuous family is generally so divided and fragmented that family treatment is not the modality of choice. Experienced practitioners who have begun programs with a family therapy orientation have almost uniformly abandoned this method except in late stages of treatment (Giarretto et al., 1978)." Stark and Flitcraft (1988) minimize family therapy and emphasize the shelter movement and individual, empowering therapy for battered women: "Assuming that violence has stopped, principal treatment objectives are to overcome the sense of physical and psychological violation and restore a sense of autonomy and separateness."

Family Assessment. Eleven criteria distinguish functional from dysfunctional families, according to McCubbin and Figley (1983): The traumatic stressor is clear, rather than denied; the problem is family centered rather than assigned completely to the victim; the approach is solution oriented rather than blame oriented; there is tolerance; there is commitment to and affection among family members; communication is open; cohesion is high; family roles are flexible rather than rigid; resources outside of the family are utilized; violence is absent; and drug use is infrequent. Standardized protocols can supplement clinical judgment, but ultimately the clinician and client together must decide whether family therapy is feasible.

Treatment Phase I: Building Commitment to Therapeutic Objectives. When the clinician and the client agree that family therapy is indicated, the first phase of treatment requires that as many family members as possible disclose their individual ordeals, and that the therapist demonstrate recognition of their suffering. Figley (1988) suggests that the therapist's sense of respect for each family member's reaction, coupled with optimism and expertise, promotes trust and commitment to therapy. Highlighting differences in individual responses leads to the next phase.

Treatment Phase II: Framing the Problem. Now each family member is encouraged to tell his or her view of the traumatic event, and to understand how each member was affected. The therapist reinforces discussion that shifts the focus away from the victimized individual toward the impact on the family as a whole. This is the time to recognize, explore, and overcome feelings of "victim blame." When positive consequences of the ordeal are mentioned (e.g., a greater appreciation of life after a close brush with death), they are duly noted.

Treatment Phase III: Reframing the Problem. After individual experiences, assumptions, and reactions are expressed and understood, the critical work of melding these view points into a coherent whole begins. "The therapist must help the family reframe the various family member experiences and insights to make them compatible in the process of constructing their healing theory," notes Figley (1988), illustrating this principle with an example from his work with Vietnam veterans. A combat veteran felt rejected by his wife, who avoided talking with him. She felt like a failure as a spouse because she couldn't help him overcome PTSD symptoms. In this treatment phase, "he began to reframe his perception of her behavior from a sign of rejection to a sign of love." Eventually, the whole family rallied, seeing obstacles as challenges to be overcome.

Treatment Phase IV: Developing a Healing Theory. The goal of posttraumatic family therapy is consensus regarding what happened in the past and optimism regarding future capacity to cope. An appraisal that is shared by all family members, that accounts for the reactions of each, and that contributes to a sense of family cohesion is a healing theory. Figley

(1988) suggests a fifth phase that builds upon this consummation, emphasizing accomplishment and preparedness. However the therapist chooses to clarify the closure of successful therapy, the family will know that they have fulfilled their potential as a healing, nurturing human group.

Alternatives to Family Therapy

Self-Help Groups. Lieberman and his colleagues (1979) described and evaluated self-help groups, noting how effective they are, particularly in those countries and cultures that do not rely upon the extended family for support. Self-help and mutual support groups tend to be specific, rather than generic. It is unusual to find a group for all victims of violent crime, but common to have groups for parents of murdered children, adult survivors of incest, and victims of domestic assault. Groups that endure tend to have extraordinary leaders, compatible members, and an optimum blend of ritual and flexibility. Often professionals are in the background, available for consultation and referrals but not intruding upon the autonomy of the group.

Therapists who work with victims of violence should become familiar with community groups that offer opportunities to share experiences, promote normalization, combat victim blame, and provide a nonthreatening social experience. Some groups will complement individual therapy. Some provide unique opportunities to help others, restoring a sense of purpose and potency. But some groups do more harm than good, encouraging premature ventilation, allowing self-styled "experts" to dominate, and confusing and demoralizing the new participant.

Dyadic Support. I have found several ex-patients who were willing to meet with current clients to share experiences. This usually worked best one-on-one at the ex-patient's home or a restaurant. Because I knew both individuals, I could arrange the meeting, giving a bit of background information to each. I would choose the pairs carefully, thinking about compatible personalities, common traumatic events, and timing with respect to each.

> For example, Mrs. L, a 35-year-old mother of two children and a survivor of rape by a man eventually convicted of serial rape and murder, told me after therapy that she would be pleased to help other women with similar terrifying experiences. Mrs. L was of considerable help to Mrs. A, the woman mentioned earlier who was held hostage and assaulted. Both were mothers, career women, and articulate and assertive. Mrs. A did not want sympathy from strangers, had difficulty returning to work, and feared entering a supermarket, but she rallied as therapy and self-help efforts progressed.
>
> Later Mrs. L assisted other clients. But when she went through a sep-

> aration and divorce from an abusive husband, she was not available to help. I therefore recommend that any attempt to promote contact between ex-clients and current clients be made with caution, knowing the current status of each and protecting confidentiality by withholding names and personal information until each has been consulted, each agrees, and the timing seems appropriate. A carefully screened dyadic "support group" can be extremely beneficial, however, and is well worth the effort on the part of the therapist. Most of my clients tell me they would appreciate an opportunity to assist others, and I believe them.

Support Services for Victims. Social integration refers to the use of sensitive, supportive companions in the course of recovery from traumatic events, and also to the goal of reentering society without fear. Victims of violent crime who participate in the criminal justice system have little choice about the timing of some very stressful social experiences. They are questioned, cross-examined, brought to crowded courtrooms, and sometimes forced to share a waiting room with the perpetrator. For them, social integration can be sudden and traumatic. Fortunately, efforts are under way in most states to provide specialized services for victims facing these stressful ordeals. Young (1988) points out the need for advocacy and assistance at every stage of the process, including the pre-court appearance, the trial, and the sentencing hearing.

There are victim-witness specialists who are trained to support an individual throughout the criminal justice gauntlet, but caseloads are overcrowded, budgets are tight, and too often the victim-witness is ignored. I have not hesitated to meet with prosecutors and to attend court hearings when my clients felt it would help. PTT objectives are advanced, particularly the objective of sensitive facilitation of social contact. Moreover, court personnel take more interest in the client. Some colleagues argue that this type of intervention fosters dependency and interferes with the therapeutic relationship. But PTT recognizes the reality of revictimization by busy bureaucrats and officious officials. Partnership between clinician and client in the pursuit of justice is both ethical and professional.

PSYCHOTHERAPY

Good therapists establish rapport easily, facilitate discussion of painful material gently, and help their clients or patients make informed choices about critical decisions, such as use of medication. PTT requires and employs these basic skills. There are several additional psychotherapy tools—specialized tools—that deserve mention. These are the timing of the telling of the trauma story, symptom suppression, the search for meaning, and the handling of coexisting problems.

Telling the Trauma Story

PTT is never complete if the client has not told the details of traumatization. This does not mean that a person who has seen several therapists must tell every detail to every clinician. Nor does it mean that one unemotional synopsis will suffice. Persons who suffer PTSD and victimization symptoms are still captured by their trauma histories. They are unable to recollect without fear of overpowering emotion. And they recollect what they do not want to recollect, when they are unprepared to remember. As a therapist, the purpose of hearing the details of the trauma story is to revisit the scene of terror and horror and, in so doing, remove the grip of terror and horror. The client should feel your presence at that moment. The purpose is more than catharsis; it is partnership in survival. It is painful.

There is no sense in exploring these corridors before a bond of mutual trust is established. One usually knows some details from a referral source before beginning the first session with a client, and these details may be mentioned in a matter-of-fact manner, but it should be clear from the beginning that there will be a time for sharing the details and that it will come later.

Highly charged events are filed in the brain's special filing system according to emotional tone, not chronologically and certainly not alphabetically. The objective with respect to traumatic memory is to file a memory of the two of us (client and clinician) revisiting the trauma right next to the original file. The co-location of this experience of controlled, shared recollection with the original, terrifying event allows mastery and respect to permeate the experience of lonely dehumanization.

Obviously, a mechanical retelling of events will not produce a memory file that ends up in that special drawer reserved for extreme emotion. And an uncontrolled, unanticipated abreaction lacks the healing quality of guided, collegial reexploration. There is an optimal emotional intensity, strong enough to assure association with the original trauma but not so strong as to obliterate the recognition of mastery and respect.

I have employed hypnosis and guided imagery to facilitate recall of trauma scenes, but always with continual reassurance that we are proceeding together, that safety is assured. With female sexual assault survivors I have always used a female cotherapist during hypnotic revisiting of trauma scenes. Occasionally the properly timed telling of the trauma story is the dramatic crux of therapy.

Mrs. M, a 60-year-old woman married to a man with advanced senile dementia, was driving with her lover on a snowy night. There was a crash, and he died in her arms. She could not share her horror with her daughters, and she had PTSD symptoms for over a year. A colleague, Alice Williams, worked with her on an outpatient basis and symptoms remained. But after 3 days in a residential unit, we revisited the terrible snowy night together, with Mrs. M in a light hypnotic trance. She cried and screamed as she narrated the events, then blurted out, "Alice, why didn't I do this before?" then cried some more. But now they were clearly tears of relief. The lonely terror was welded to the reenactment experience with a respected therapist. Symptoms abated completely. Telephone follow-up 2 years later confirmed enduring relief.

More frequently, the telling of the trauma story is not curative. One reenactment with a trusted clinician is not enough; aspects of the trauma are still hidden, implications of victimization are profound, and symptoms remain entrenched. PTT continues, with all applicable tools applied.

Symptom Suppression

Roth (1988) asks the pertinent question, "Is the treatment of a psychological disorder by biological means a short-sighted suppression of symptoms that robs the patient of the motivation and resources to solve his or her true underlying psychological problems?" He then provides an "integrated psychobiological viewpoint" of post-traumatic stress, justifying the temporary suppression of symptoms that interfere with adaptation. Whether medication, biofeedback, or behavior modification are offered to suppress symptoms, the client should have the opportunity to make an informed choice among effective options. Common post-traumatic symptoms that can be suppressed at any stage of PTT include insomnia, panic, and generalized anxiety. Medication can help with each of these, but there are pitfalls and contraindications. Roth (1988) and van der Kolk (1988) discuss these issues well.

Judicious use of sedatives (e.g., Triazolam, 0.125 mg every other night) often restores a normal sleep pattern without creating dependency. The dosage may be increased, but the client avoids using medication nights and discontinues the drug within a month. Some sleep disorders are very difficult to treat, however, with or without drugs.

Similarly, moderate use of tricyclics for panic and benzodiazepines for anxiety have allowed many patients to accelerate recovery, reenter social groups, and restore self-esteem. Both patient and therapist must know that symptoms are being suppressed to facilitate PTT, not to replace it.

The Individualized Search for Meaning

Catastrophic stress by definition shakes one's equilibrium, breaks one's attachments, and removes a sense of security. Confrontation with deliberate human cruelty inevitably strains one's sense of justice, shatters assumptions of civility, and evokes alien (sometimes bestial) instincts. Those clinicians who describe therapy with Holocaust victims and refugee survivors of violence and torture (Danieli, 1988; Mollica, 1988) recognize these profound effects, often transmitted to a second generation, cast in the shadow of cruelty.

Viktor Frankl, the famous Viennese psychiatrist, pondered the profound questions about life's meaning as he endured the Nazi concentration camp, and afterward as he provided therapy to fellow survivors. "Woe to him who saw no more sense in his life, no aim, no purpose, and therefore no point in carrying on," states Frankl, recalling the death camp (1959).

> What was really needed was a fundamental change in our attitude toward life. We had to learn ourselves and, furthermore, we had to teach the despairing men, that *it did not really matter what we expected from life, but rather what life expected from us.* We needed to stop asking about the meaning of life, and instead to think of ourselves as those who were being questioned by life—daily and hourly. . . . Life ultimately means taking the responsibility to find the right answer to its problems and to fulfill the tasks which it constantly sets for each individual. (p. 146)

It is a rare privilege to work with a client who reaches the philosophical stage of PTT, consciously formulating a new attitude toward life. But when patients are overwhelmed with symptoms, discussion of life's meaning has little relevance. As normalization restores a sense of dignity, as empowerment restores a will to endure, and as individuality restores a sense of self, however, the client does take "responsibility to find the right answer" for himself. His behavior demonstrates his fulfillment of Frankl's ideal, even if he lacks the ability or inclination to formulate a philosophy of life.

The therapist, however, should have the aptitude to guide a search for meaning, to recognize existential despair, to confront self-pity, to reinforce recognition of one's responsibility for one's own life. A final phase of PTT includes articulation of the meaning of life in terms that are specific to the individual, not general or abstract.

Coexisting Problems

PTSD may mimic personality and anxiety disorders. It may precipitate physical and psychiatric conditions. It may exacerbate preexisting disorders. It may be confounded by coexisting problems, including normal stages of life adjustment (Mowbray, 1988; Wilson, 1988). To illustrate this point, Wilson (1988) cites the remarkable findings of Green, Lindy, and Grace (1984) "that only 13% of a treatment seeking population of Vietnam veterans manifest a single diagnosis of PTSD." Therefore it is important for post-traumatic therapists to recognize coexisting problems and to clarify these in therapy.

Certain coexisting disorders, particularly borderline personality, may be impossible for the post-traumatic therapist to manage according to the principles of PTT. For example, collegiality may be misinterpreted as intimate friendship, and a willingness to intervene with criminal justice officials may lead to insatiable requests for help with personal affairs. Unfortunately, abused children may evidence combinations of borderline personality, multiple personality, and PTSD. This presents enormous challenges to the therapist. A treatment strategy must be individualized and may involve several therapists, concurrently or in sequence.

It is not unusual for a traumatized patient to request help with psychological issues that antedate the trauma. Several clients have embarked upon long-term therapy for dysthymia, avoidant personality disorder, or dependent personality disorder after achieving mastery of PTSD and victimization symptoms. In these cases the contract and the objectives must be clarified to avoid self-blame when working with victimization issues, and to promote self-reliance when treating the preexisting condition. There is no way to completely untangle PTSD and a personality disorder, treating one first and then the other. But the therapist can maintain the fundamental principles of PTT and use tools in the general armamentarium of techniques, as long as there is no contraindication as a result of coexisting problems.

CONCLUSION

The clinician and the client have no difficulty realizing when posttraumatic therapy approaches its conclusion. Symptoms subside, although they may be present to some degree. There is an understanding of the causes and significance of autonomic echoes. There is a sense of mastery and control. But most significantly, there is a shift from *victim* status to *survivor* status. To clarify this change of self-perception I wrote the "Survivor psalm" for use with clients to gauge progress and to mark termination:

- I have been victimized.
- I was in a fight that was not a fair fight.
- I did not ask for the fight. I lost.
- There is no shame in losing such fights, only in winning.
- I have reached the stage of survivor and am no longer a slave of victim status.
- I look back with sadness rather than hate.
- I look forward with hope rather than despair.
- I may never forget, but I need not constantly remember.
- I was a victim.
- I am a survivor.

With every client who travels that painful path from victim to survivor, there is a surge of hope for all of us who are engaged in the larger struggle for survival.

It is no accident that many of the same principles that guided the community mental health movement in the 1960s are rediscovered in the victims' rights movement of the 1980s. There is a vast, underserved population. There is a need to mobilize help from separate disciplines. There is a crescendo of attention that cuts across ideology. There is a scientific basis for humanitarian aid. There are atavistic approaches that do more harm than good, and that beg for reform. Treating rape victims on the same psychiatric unit as chronic schizophrenics is the modern equivalent of institutionalizing the mentally ill. Removing sexually abused children from their mothers rather than removing the abusive father is reminiscent of persecuting psychotic individuals as demons. And denying that thousands of Vietnam veterans and millions of refugees can benefit from clinical attention is tragically similar to the national myopia that culminated in President Kennedy's (1963) call for "action for mental health."

Participation in any aspect of the healing arts and sciences is a source of gratification and humility. The rewards are great; the problems are never ending.

REFERENCES

American Psychiatric Association. (1980). *Diagnostic and statistical manual of mental disorders* (3rd ed.). Washington, DC: Author.

American Psychiatric Association. (1987). *Diagnostic and statistical manual of mental disorders* (rev. 3rd ed.). Washington, DC: Author.

Angelou, M. (1978). *And still I rise.* New York: Random House.

Cannon, W. B. (1939). *Wisdom of the body.* New York: Norton.

Cienfuegos, A. J., & Monelli, C. (1983). The testimony of political repression as a therapeutic instrument. *American Journal of Orthopsychiatry, 53,* 43–51.

Cousins, N. (1979). *Anatomy of an illness.* New York: Norton.

Danieli, Y. (1988). Treating survivors and children of survivors of the Nazi Holocaust. In F. M. Ochberg (Ed.), *Post-traumatic therapy and victims of violence* (pp. 278–294). New York: Brunner/Mazel.

Figley, C. R. (1988). Post-traumatic family therapy. In F. M. Ochberg (Ed.), *Post-traumatic therapy and victims of violence* (pp. 83–109). New York: Brunner/Mazel.

Fly, C. L. (1973). *No hope but God.* New York: Hawthorne.

Frankl, V. E. (1959). *Man's search for meaning.* New York: Pocket Books.

Giarretto, H., Giarretto, A., & Sgroi, S. (1978). Coordinated community treatment of incest. In A. W. Burgess, A. N. Groth, L. L. Holmstrom, and S. M. Sgroi (Eds.), *Sexual assault of children and adolescents.* Lexington, MA: Heath.

Green, B., Lindy, J., & Grace, M. D. (1984). *Prediction of delayed stress after Vietnam.* Unpublished manuscript, University of Cincinnati.

Herman, J. L. (1988). Father–daughter incest. In F. M. Ochberg (Ed.), *Post-traumatic therapy and victims of violence* (p. 186). New York: Brunner/Mazel.

Jackson, G. (1973). *Surviving the long night.* New York: Vanguard.

Kennedy, J. F. (1963, February). In *Messages from the President of the United States relative to mental health and illness.* 88th Congress, Document House of Representatives No. 58.

Lieberman, M. A., Borman, L. D., & Associates. (1979). *Self-help groups for coping with crisis: Origins, members, processes, and impact.* San Francisco: Jossey-Bass.

McCubbin, H., & Figley, C. R.. (1983). Bridging normative and catastrophic family stress. In H. McCubbin and C. R. Figley (Eds.), *Stress and the family: Vol. I. Coping with normative transitions* (pp. 218–228). New York: Brunner/Mazel.

Merwin, M., & Smith-Kurtz, B. (1988). Healing of the whole person. In F. M. Ochberg (Ed.), *Post-traumatic therapy and victims of violence* (pp. 57–82). New York: Brunner/Mazel.

Mollica, R. F. (1988). The trauma story: The psychiatric care of refugee survivors of violence and torture. In F. M. Ochberg (Ed.), *Post-traumatic therapy and victims of violence* (pp. 295–314). New York: Brunner/Mazel.

Mowbray, C. T. (1988). Post-traumatic therapy for children who are victims of violence. In F. M. Ochberg (Ed.), *Post-traumatic therapy and victims of violence* (pp. 196–212). New York: Brunner/Mazel.

Ochberg, F. M. (1986). The victim of violent crime. In L. A. Radelet (Ed.), *Police and the community* (4th ed, pp. 285–300). New York: Macmillan.

Ochberg, F. M. (1988). *Post-traumatic therapy and victims of violence.* New York: Brunner/Mazel.

Ochberg, F. M. (1989). Cruelty, culture and coping. *Journal of Traumatic Stress, 2*(4).

Ochberg, F. M., & Fotjik, K. M. (1984). A comprehensive mental health clinical service program for victims: Clinical issues and therapeutic strategies. *American Journal of Social Psychiatry, 4*(3), 12–23.

President's task force on crime victims, final report. (1982). Washington, DC: U.S. Department of Justice.

Roth, W. T. (1988). The role of medication in post-traumatic therapy. In F. M. Ochberg (Ed.), *Post-traumatic therapy and victims of violence* (pp. 39–56). New York: Brunner/Mazel.

Selye, H. (1956). *The stress of life.* New York: McGraw-Hill.

Stark, E., & Flitcraft, A. (1988). Personal power and institutional victimization: treating the dual trauma of woman battering. In F. M. Ochberg (Ed.), *Post-traumatic therapy and victims of violence* (p. 127). New York: Brunner/Mazel.

van der Kolk, B. A. (1988). The biological response to psychic trauma. In F. M. Ochberg (Ed.), *Post-traumatic therapy and victims of violence* (pp. 25–38). New York: Brunner/Mazel.

Van Regenmorter, W. (1989). *Crime victim's rights act and other victim information.* Room 115, State Capitol, Lansing, MI 48913.

Weybrew, B. (1967). Patterns of response to stress. In M. H. Appley & R. Trumbull (Eds.), *Psychological stress.* New York: Appleton-Century-Crofts.

Wilson, J. P. (1988). Treating the Vietnam veteran. In F. M. Ochberg (Ed.), *Post-traumatic therapy and victims of violence* (pp. 262–268). New York: Brunner/Mazel.

Young, M. A. (1988). Support services for victims. In F. M. Ochberg (Ed.), *Post-traumatic therapy and victims of violence* (pp. 330–351). New York: Brunner/Mazel.

IV

The Prevention of Post-Traumatic Stress

Following the discussions of both strategic and tactical approaches to the treatment of post-traumatic stress in Part III, Part IV provides an introduction to the prevention of post-traumatic stress. Occupational groups that are at high risk for the development of post-traumatic stress disorder contain constituencies who might prosper the most from formal preventative efforts. Included among such high-risk groups would be law enforcement officers, fire suppression personnel, emergency medical personnel, disaster workers, the military, and most public safety and rescue personnel, and even mental health providers, just to mention a few.

In Chapter 16, Mitchell and Everly introduce the critical-incident stress debriefing (CISD) technology, an intervention technology used in response to accidents, homicides, suicides, community disruptions, and disasters in much of the world. CISD may be the most widely used formal group intervention for the prevention of post-traumatic stress within high-risk groups.

In Chapter 17, Talbot et al. continue the theme of prevention by presenting an excellent treatise on the psychological effects of crisis intervention upon those doing the intervention. The potentially burdensome and deleterious effects of providing crisis intervention and psychological support upon those trained to offer such services is too often overlooked. These authors examine the debriefing process as a useful technology for reducing the risk of vicarious post-traumatic stress among providers of psychological support.

16

Critical Incident Stress Debriefing (CISD) and the Prevention of Work-Related Traumatic Stress among High Risk Occupational Groups

JEFFREY T. MITCHELL and GEORGE S. EVERLY, JR.

The impact of post-traumatic stress upon society is most floridly apparent through the process of warfare. Indeed, it is hard to imagine a more destructive and psychologically debilitating process than warfare. Had there not been a Vietnam conflict, post-traumatic stress disorder (PTSD) may never have found its way into the official psychiatric taxonomy of the third edition (DSM-III) of the *Diagnostic and Statistical Manual of Mental Disorders* (American Psychiatric Association [APA], 1980). Yet warfare is not the only set of conditions, by far, capable of engendering post-traumatic stress.

Upon the publication of the revision of DSM-III (DSM-III-R; APA, 1987), it was made abundantly clear that PTSD could be engendered by trauma outside the realm of combat, including floods, earthquakes, rape,

---

JEFFREY T. MITCHELL • Emergency Health Services, University of Maryland, Baltimore County, Baltimore, Maryland 21228; and International Critical Incident Stress Foundation, Ellicott City, Maryland 21042. **GEORGE S. EVERLY, JR.** • International Critical Incident Stress Foundation, Ellicott City, Maryland 21042; Union Memorial Hospital, Baltimore, Maryland 21218; and Department of Psychology, Loyola College, Baltimore, Maryland 21210.

Psychotraumatology, edited by George S. Everly, Jr. and Jeffrey M. Lating. Plenum Press, New York, 1995.

large fires, airplane crashes, car accidents, and physical violence. Though almost anyone could be a potential primary victim of one or more of the aforementioned trauma, some individuals are at higher risk for experiencing PTSD by virtue of their career choice. Careers in the emergency services professions are prime examples of occupations that put their constituents at high risk for post-traumatic stress. For example, it is generally accepted that law enforcement, fire suppression, emergency medical services, and disaster response (just to name a few) are examples of professions that are at higher risk for engendering post-traumatic stress (see Mitchell & Everly, 1993).

Although we have learned much about the effective treatment of PTSD and related syndromes (see Part III of this volume), most would agree that prevention is clearly preferable to treatment (Butcher, 1980; Duffy, 1979; Kentsmith, 1980; Yandrick, 1990). This chapter will focus, therefore, upon the prevention of work-related post-traumatic stress through a structured group process that can be employed subsequent to exposure to a traumatic event. This process is referred to as critical-incident stress debriefing (CISD).

BACKGROUND

Critical-incident stress debriefing (CISD) and its parallel process, traumatic stress defusing, are group intervention techniques initially developed by one of the authors for implementation subsequent to a potentially traumatizing event so as to facilitate the prevention of post-traumatic stress among high-risk occupational groups, specifically fire suppression, law enforcement, emergency medicine, disaster response, emergency dispatch, and public safety personnel (Mitchell, 1983, 1988a,b, 1991). These processes have subsequently been adopted by the military, the clergy, and pupil personnel services as well as within high-risk business and industrial settings, (e.g., the banking industry, mining, oil discovery and refining operations, lifeguard services, and other recreational industries). The employee assistance program (EAP) industry has begun to heavily utilize the defusing and CISD processes as well. CISD and defusing employ both crisis intervention and educational theory and technologies.

At the time of this writing, there exist more than 300 formal trauma-response teams across the globe that utilize the CISD and defusing models in the prevention of post-traumatic stress. CISD and defusing protocols have been employed for more than 10 years in settings that range from small-scale traumatic incidents to large-scale disasters. CISD protocols have been employed in numerous major trauma venues, including the following:

Barneveld, Wisconsin, tornado (1984)
Mexico City earthquake (1985)
Cerritos, California, air disaster (1986)
El Salvador, earthquake (1986)
Palm Bay, Florida, mass shooting (1987)

Bridgeport, Connecticut, building collapse (1987)
San Francisco, California, earthquake (1989)
New York City, fire bombing with 87 dead (1990)
Charleston, South Carolina, Hurricane Hugo (1990)
Los Angeles, California, civil riots (1992)
Miami, Florida, Hurricane Andrew (1992)
Hawaii, Hurricane Iniki (1992)
Kuwait, Desert Storm, combat (1992)
Somalia, civil unrest (1993)
Yugoslavia, civil war (1993)
Midwestern U.S., floods (1993 and 1994)
Rwanda, civil war (1994)

In these and other settings, the primary emphasis has been the use of defusings and CISD with emergency response personnel, law enforcement, rescue workers, the military, and other public safety personnel for the mitigation or prevention of work-related post-traumatic stress.

The seeds of critical-incident stress teams were actually planted during combat situations in World Wars I and II. Brown (1918), Salmon (1919), and Appel et al. (1946) found that soldiers in the great wars were more prone to return to combat when given immediate psychological support after combat then when managed later in hospitals that were well behind the combat lines. More recently, the Israeli Defense Forces began to utilize group and individual psychological support after firefights in the Middle East. They concluded that the incidence of psychiatric disturbance was trimmed by as much as 60% following the inception of their support services (Breznitz, 1980).

The earliest formal CISD teams were begun in fire and emergency medical services units (Mitchell, 1983). There now exist more than 300 CISD teams across the globe designed to mitigate the adverse impact of crisis and trauma upon high-risk occupational groups. This makes the CISD process the most widely used structured intervention in the world for the prevention of post-traumatic stress. The success of the CISD intervention has spawned other similar group crisis intervention technologies, as well.

THE CISD TEAM

The CISD intervention is employed by a critical-incident stress debriefing team and is directed to the individuals who have become victims of the trauma (in this case, the workers in the high-risk environments). Critical-incident stress teams are in actuality a partnership between mental health professionals and emergency (or other high-risk) workers who are interested in preventing and mitigating the negative impact of acute stress on crisis, emergency, and other high-risk personnel.

Mental health professionals who serve on the teams have at least a master's degree in psychology, social work, psychiatric nursing, or mental health counseling. They are specially trained in crisis intervention, stress, posttraumatic stress disorder, and the critical-incident stress debriefing process.

Peer support personnel are drawn from the high-risk occupation groups, including military, police, fire, emergency medical services, dispatch, disaster response, and nursing personnel (especially those in emergency or critical care centers). Both the mental health professionals and peer support personnel form a pool of critical-incident team members from which a response team is developed. An incident that is predominantly police oriented is worked by police peers with the support of mental health professionals who are familiar with police activities and procedures. Likewise an incident that is predominantly fire oriented will have fire peers who provide the peer support services, and so forth. If an incident involves various response agencies, then a mixed cadre of peers is developed to provide support services.

CISD DEFINED

The CISD and defusing processes may be defined as group meetings or discussions about a traumatic event or series of such events. The CISD and defusing processes are solidly based in crisis intervention theory and educational intervention theory. They are designed to mitigate the psychological impact of a traumatic event, prevent the subsequent development of a posttraumatic syndrome, accelerate homeostatic mechanisms toward full recovery, and serve as an early identification mechanism for individuals who will require professional mental health follow-up subsequent to a traumatic event.

Table 16.1 Stages of CISD

	Phase	Objectives
Stage 1	Introduction	To introduce intervention team members, explain process, set expectations
Stage 2	Fact	To describe traumatic event from each participant's perspective on a cognitive level
Stage 3	Thought	To allow participants to describe cognitive reactions and to transition to emotional reactions
Stage 4	Reaction	To identify the most traumatic aspect of the event for the participants
Stage 5	Symptom	To identify personal symptoms of distress and transition back to cognitive level/domain
Stage 6	Teaching	To educate as to normal reactions and adaptive coping mechanisms (i.e., stress management); provide cognitive anchor
Stage 7	Reentry	To clarify ambiguities and prepare for termination; assess for follow-up

Note: See Mitchell and Everly (1993) for step-by-step guidelines. Used with permission.

The formal CISD process is a seven-stage intervention. These stages are delineated in Table 16.1 (Mitchell & Everly, 1993). The debriefing process has both psychological and educational elements, but it should not be considered psychotherapy. Instead, it is a structured group meeting or discussion in which personnel who have been directly affected by a traumatic event are given the opportunity to discuss their thoughts and emotions about that event in a controlled, structured, and rational manner. They also get the opportunity to see that they are not alone in their reactions.

As noted above, the debriefing is structured with seven major phases. It has been carefully structured to move in a nonthreatening manner from the usual cognitively oriented processing of human experience that is common to high-risk professional personnel through a somewhat more emotionally oriented processing of these same experiences. The debriefing ends up by returning the personnel to the cognitive processing of their experiences where they started.

1. Introduction Phase

The introduction to the CISD is crucial; it sets the stage for all of the other phases of the debriefing. If the introduction is not handled well, it is likely that the remainder of the debriefing will be difficult.

There are several objectives to be achieved during the introduction. The CISD team must do the following:

- Explain the purpose of the meeting
- Point out the team members
- Explain the process (overview)
- Motivate the participants
- Reduce resistance
- Explain the guidelines of the CISD
- Answer primary concerns, limit anxiety, and discuss confidentiality issues (the assurance of confidentiality is usually a critical point)

2. Fact Phase

The overall strategy for a CISD team during a debriefing is to start at the point that is easiest to discuss (usually cognitively based issues) and then move gradually into more emotionally intense discussions. After handling the intense emotional materials, the group is gradually brought back to the more cognitive issues until the discussion finally concludes.

Usually the easiest thing for a distressed worker to talk about is a description of the facts of an incident. Facts are a collection of items outside of oneself; they are impersonal. Discussions of facts are not as initially distressing as attempting to talk about how one feels, which is a very personal matter. This is especially so for emergency personnel and other high-risk occupational groups, who tend to be highly defended cognitively and to avoid most discussions of emotions.

To get participants talking about a situation in the fact phase, the team leader simply needs to state something like this: "The CISD team wasn't present during the incident. We only know some bits and pieces of the incident. It would be very helpful if we could get some understanding of what happened by having you tell us about the incident. So, we would like you to tell us *who you are, what your role was during the incident, and, briefly, what happened from your perspective.* It doesn't matter if what you experienced is different from what everyone else experienced. You all had an important part to play in the situation, and it would help everyone to have a big picture built by putting all your pieces of the incident together. If you choose not to speak, that is OK; just shake your head, and we will pass right over you. For the sake of organization, we are going to start over here on my left [or right] and go around the room. Again, what we need to know is (1) who are you, (2) what was your job or involvement during the incident, and (3) what happened from your point of view?"

The participants in the group will begin to tell their stories. The exact order of the telling does not really matter; the last to arrive at the scene might be the first to speak. All of the pieces will come together as everyone gets their chance to talk. The sorting out of the story comes naturally to an alert CISD team that has done its homework before the debriefing and learned something about the trauma.

3. Thought Phase

The thought phase begins when the team leader asks the participants to express their *first thoughts* or *most prominent thought* concerning the traumatic event. It is a transition phase between the factual realities and that which is close and personal. The facts are outside of a person; the thoughts are internal and part of him or her. It is impossible to respond to the questions about thoughts without some leakage of emotion into the discussion. CISD teams should expect this leakage as a natural by-product of the CISD process. Without it, it would be much harder for the team to get the participants to speak about their reactions to the incident. The CISD team should welcome such comments in the thought phase as a sign that the process is working and on schedule.

4. Reaction Phase

The reaction phase is typically the most emotionally powerful of all phases. If the introduction, fact, and thought phases have been focused and managed carefully, the reaction phase will flow relatively easily from the thought phase. The CISD team will find that its interactions in the group will quiet substantially during the reaction phase. In fact, most of the talking is done by the participants, not by the CISD team.

The question that triggers most of the discussion in the reaction phase is as follows:

- "What was the worse thing about this situation for you personally?"

There are numerous variations on the question that will bring about a discussion of the emotions associated with the event. They include the following:

- "What part of this event bothers you most?"
- "If you could erase one part of the situation, what part would you choose to erase?"
- "What aspect of the situation causes you the most pain?"

The discussion at this point is freewheeling. The process no longer involves going around the room, questioning each participant in the debriefing. Whoever wants to speak may speak; those who choose to be silent are silent. There is no order in discussion. *Going around the room is only done in the fact phase and in the thought phase.* The whole group is given the opportunity to speak if and when they choose in the reaction phase.

5. Symptom Phase

The symptom phase is another transition phase. The objective in this phase is to begin a movement of the group back from the emotionally laden content of the reaction phase toward more cognitively oriented material. Stopping the debriefing at this point in the debriefing process would leave people in a charged emotional state which could possibly be harmful to them. The debriefing is always continued to the end to complete the process and to restore people to the cognitive level so that they can resume their normal responsibilities in their lives.

The symptom phase is initiated when the team asks the participants to describe any cognitive, physical, emotional, or behavioral experiences they may have encountered while they were working at the scene of the incident. The debriefing team may need to give several examples of stress-related symptoms, such as trembling hands, inability to make a decision, excessive silence, or feelings of anger. Then the group spends several minutes talking about the various ways in which they experienced symptoms of distress while working at the scene, as well as symptoms that followed subsequently.

6. Teaching Phase

The teaching phase comes naturally after the symptoms phase. *It is easy to begin the teaching phase by pointing out several of the symptoms just described in the symptoms phase and letting the group know that those symptoms are normal, typical, or to be expected after the type of critical incident they experienced.*

All of the team members are very active in teaching the group. Team members describe the typical symptoms of distress that are usually encountered. Other team members forewarn the group about symptoms that might not have shown up yet but may develop in the future. The team spends a good deal of time teaching the group a variety of stress survival strategies (i.e., stress management). Instructions are given on diet, exercise, rest, talking to one's family, working with the supervisors to the initiate necessary procedural changes, and a wide range of other topics.

The teaching phase is very cognitive in approach. It is designed to bring the participants further away from the emotional content they had worked through in the reaction phase.

7. Reentry Phase

The last phase of the formal debriefing, the reentry phase, is the final opportunity to clarify issues, answer questions, make summary statements, and accelerate homeostasis. This phase puts closure on the discussions that have just occurred in the debriefing. Like most things that are human, debriefings have a beginning, a middle, and an ending. No part stands alone as vital without the others; only when an experience has an ending can the beginning and middle make any sense.

The reentry that ends the debriefing has several segments and several tasks that need to be performed. The participants in the debriefing will need to do the following:

1. Introduce any new material they wish to discuss
2. Review old material already discussed
3. Ask any questions
4. Discuss anything they wish would help them to bring closure to the debriefing

The debriefing team will need to do the following:

1. Answer any questions posed
2. Reassure and inform as needed
3. State any feelings or agendas that are suspected to be there, but have not been brought up by the participants
4. Provide appropriate handouts
5. Make summary comments
6. Provide referral sources as appropriate for psychological assessment, therapy, etc.

The summary comments made by CISD team are usually words of respect, encouragement, appreciation, support, gratefulness, and direction. Every CISD team member should make a summary comment in the last few minutes of the debriefing. The participants are welcome to comment if they wish, but they are not called upon to do so.

Table 16.2 Stages of Post-Trauma Defusings

	Phase	Objectives
Stage 1	Introduction	To introduce intervention team members, explain process, set expectations
Stage 2	Exploration	To discuss the traumatic experience via participants' disclosure of facts, cognitive and emotional reactions, and finally symptoms of distress related to the traumatic event
Stage 3	Information	To normalize cognitively and educate with regard to stress, stress management, and trauma

Note: See Mitchell and Everly (1993) for step-by-step guidelines. Used with permission.

This, then, is a brief overview of the seven-stage process. The CISD will routinely take from 2 to 3 hours, depending on the size of the group.

POST-TRAUMA DEFUSING DEFINED

The defusing process is typically a three-stage intervention. It may be considered a shortened version of the CISD. Defusings are designed to be (a) implemented immediately or shortly after a traumatic event, (b) shorter in length than a formal CISD (about 1 hour, compared to a 2–3 hour CISD), (c) more flexible than a CISD (with greater latitude in the three-stage format), and (d) used either to eliminate the need for a formal CISD or to enhance a subsequent CISD. The stages of a defusing are delineated in Table 16.2 (Mitchell & Everly, 1993).

MASS-DISASTER CISD

Recently, the basic formal CISD model has been slightly modified for mass disaster/community response applications. This variation of the CISD model was derived directly from our experiences working with large scale disasters such as Hurricane Hugo, Hurricane Andrew, the California earthquake, as well as disasters in the Middle East and Africa. Somewhat consistent with Herman's (1992) notions surrounding "complex PTSD," it may be argued that prolonged exposure to trauma, to trauma-related events or venues, or to repeated trauma can create special challenges to extant assumptions and traditional intervention tactics. Table 16.3 introduces the mass-disaster CISD model for use with prolonged trauma and/or repeated trauma as one might encounter in community or civil unrest, military action, natural catastrophes, and the like. The reader will note changes to stages 3, 4, and 5 that are better suited to mitigate a more complex PTSD as engendered by situations noted above.

Table 16.3 The Mass Disaster/Community Response Variation of the CISD

	Phase	Objectives
Stage 1	Introduction	To introduce intervention team members, explain process, set expectations
Stage 2	Fact	To have each participant describe the nature of their participation from a cognitive perspective
Stage 3	Thought Reaction	To solicit cognitive response to "What aspect held the most negative impact?" or "What aspect was the worst for you?"; then transition from cognitive to emotional processing
Stage 4	Emotional Reaction	Given the response to Stage 3, to solicit emotional reactions or consequences
Stage 5	Reframing	To transition from emotional domain back to cognitive: "What lessons could be learned from this experience?" and "What is something positive that you will take away from this experience?"
Stage 6	Teaching	To educate as to normal reactions and teach basic stress management, if applicable
Stage 7	Reentry	To summarize experience with emphasis on positive or learning aspects; assess for follow-up

Note: From Mitchell and Everly (1993). Used with permission.

MECHANISMS OF ACTION

CISD and defusing interventions appear to derive their effectiveness from several aspects of their phenomenology. It will be of value to any practitioner to understand the dynamic process harnessed in any intervention so as to be more capable of attending to truly unique or challenging circumstances. The CISD represents a complex amalgam of psychosocial dynamics; these are outlined below.

1. Early Intervention

CISD is most typically utilized as an early intervention strategy, often within hours or days of the traumatic event. Friedman, Framer, and Shearer (1988) found that early detection of—and early intervention with—post-trauma reactions led to lower costs and more favorable prognoses associated with the victims of trauma. Indeed, it is universally recognized that prevention and early intervention efforts are preferable to having to pursue traditional treatment of full-blown post-traumatic sequelae (Butcher, 1980; Duffy, 1978; Kentsmith, 1980; Yandrick, 1990).

2. Opportunity for Catharsis

Catharsis refers to the ventilation of emotions. CISD provides a safe, supportive, structured environment wherein individuals can ventilate emotions. In a review of studies specifically investigating the relationship between the disclosure of traumatic events and stress arousal, Pennebaker and Susman (1988) concluded that disclosure of traumatic events leads to reduced stress arousal and improved immune functioning.

3. Opportunity to Verbalize Trauma

CISD gives individuals the opportunity not only to release emotions but also to reconstruct and express specific traumas, fears, and regrets verbally. van der Hart, Brown, and van der Kolk (1989) recount the views of master traumatologist Pierre Janet, who noted at the turn of the century that the successful treatment of post-traumatic reactions was largely based upon the patient's ability not just to express feelings (catharsis) but also to reconstruct and integrate the trauma using the verbally expressive medium. The work of Pennebaker (Pennebaker, 1985; Pennebaker & Beall, 1986) appears to confirm the critical role that verbal reconstruction and expression of the traumatic event plays in the successful resolution of post-trauma syndromes for many individuals.

The collective value of catharsis and the verbalizing of the trauma appear to reside in their collective ability to lead to (a) reduced stress, (b) reduced strain on the homeostatic mechanisms of the body, (c) a reduced tendency to ruminate/obsess, and (d) an increased likelihood of "making sense" out of the trauma (reintegration of the Weltanschauung).

4. Structure

CISD provides a finite *behavioral structure*—that is, a group debriefing represents a finite beginning and a finite end superimposed upon a traumatic event representing chaos, suffering, and a myriad of unanswered questions. CISD is the antithesis of the cacophony of the traumatic milieu. Borkovec et al. (1983) found that providing a structured environment within which to worry actually reduced the overall tendency for worry to contaminate, or interfere with, other activities. Perhaps more subtly, CISD also provides an important *psychological structure*. The CISD process begins in the cognitive domain in order to match the existing defense mechanisms or to provide a stabilizing influence. The CISD then progresses into the affective domain to allow for emotional catharsis, then transitions back to the cognitive domain for normalization and stabilization.

5. Group Support

CISD, in its classic application, employs a group education model. The value of using a group format to address distressing issues is well documented. Yalom (1985) notes that the group format provides numerous healing factors intrinsic to the group format itself. Among them are the exchange of useful constructive information, catharsis, the dissolution of the myth of a unique weakness among individuals, the modeling of constructive coping behavior, the opportunity to derive a sense of group caring and support, the opportunity to help oneself by helping others, and, perhaps most importantly with regard to trauma, the generation of feelings of hope. As Jones (1985) commented on the value of using group discussion formats following trauma: "There is real value, especially for young men, in understanding that others feel the same strong emotions under such circumstances, that each is not alone in the strength of his shock, grief, and anger" (p. 307).

6. Peer Support

Although mental health professionals oversee the CISD process, it is a peer-driven process. Carkhuff and Truax (1965) long ago demonstrated the value of lay support models. Indeed, peer support interventions offer unique advantages over traditional mental health services, especially when the peer group views itself as being highly unique, selective, or otherwise different compared to the general population.

7. Allows for Follow-Up

The CISD process represents an entry portal where potential victims can engage in group discussion, information exchange, and support. It also represents a mechanism wherein individuals who do indeed require formal psychological care can be identified and helped so as to maximize the likelihood of rapid and total recovery.

SUMMARY

Critical-incident stress debriefing (CISD) and its parallel intervention, post-traumatic stress defusing, are interventions designed by one of the authors (Mitchell, 1983, 1988a,b, 1991) specifically for the prevention of post-traumatic stress and PTSD among high-risk occupational groups such as fire fighters, emergency medical personnel, law enforcement personnel, public safety workers, dispatch personnel, and disaster workers. The recently modified CISD appears especially suited for mass disasters and community response applications.

Greater emphasis is being placed upon prevention in all aspects of health care. The CISD process is one potentially useful mechanism for reducing the risk of incapacitating post-traumatic stress as it may be engendered in a myriad of occupational settings.

REFERENCES

American Psychiatric Association. (1980). *Diagnostic and statistical manual of mental disorders* (3rd ed.). Washington, DC: Author.

American Psychiatric Association. (1987). *Diagnostic and statistical manual of mental disorders* (rev. 3rd ed.). Washington, DC: Author.

Appel, J. W., Beebe, G. W., & Hilgardner, D. W. (1946). Comparative incidence of neuropsychiatric causalities in World War I and World War II. *American Journal of Psychiatry, 102,* 196–199.

Borkovec, T. D., Wilkenson, L., Folensbee, R., & Lerman, C. (1983). Stimulus control applications to the treatment of worry. *Behavioral Research and Therapy, 21,* 247–251.

Breznitz, S. (1980). Stress in Israel. In H. Selye (Ed.), *Selye's guide to stress research* (pp. 71–89). New York: Van Nostrand Reinhold.

Brown, M. W., & Williams, J. (1918). *Neuropsychiatry and the war: A bibliography with abstracts.* New York: National Committee for Mental Hygiene.

Butcher, J. (1980). The role of crisis intervention in an airport disaster plan. *Aviation, Space and Environmental Medicine, 51,* 1260–1262.

Carkhuff, R., & Truax, C. (1965). Lay mental health counseling. *Journal of Consulting Psychology, 29,* 426–431.

Duffy, J. (1978). Emergency mental health services during and after a major aircraft accident. *Aviation, Space and Environmental Medicine, 49,* 1004–1008.

Everly, G. (1989). *A clinical guide to the treatment of the human stress response.* New York: Plenum.

Friedman, R., Framer, M., & Shearer, D. (1988, September–October). Early response to post-traumatic stress. *EAP Digest,* pp. 45–49.

Helzer, J., Robins, L., & McEvoy, L. (1987). Post-traumatic stress disorder in the general population. *New England Journal of Medicine, 317,* 1630–1634.

Herman, J. L. (1992). Complex PTSD. *Journal of Traumatic Stress, 5,* 377–392.

Jones, D. R. (1985). Secondary disaster victims. *American Journal of Psychiatry, 142,* 303–307.

Kentsmith, D. (1980). Minimizing the psychological effects of a wartime disaster on an individual. *Aviation, Space, and Environmental Medicine, 51,* 409–413.

Lang, P. (1971). The application of psychophysiological methods to the study of psychotherapy and behavior modification. In A. Bergin & S. Garfield (Eds.), *Handbook of psychotherapy and behavior change.* New York: Wiley.

McCarthy, M. (1989, April 7). Stressed employees look for relief in workers' compensation claims. *Wall Street Journal,* p. 34.

Miller, A., et al. (1988, April 25). Stress on the job. *Newsweek,* pp. 40–41.

Mitchell, J. T., & Everly, G. S. (1993). *Critical incident stress debriefing: An operations manual for the prevention of trauma among emergency service and disaster workers.* Baltimore, MD: Chevron.

Mitchell, J. T. (1983). When disaster strikes: The critical incident stress debriefing process. *Journal of Emergency Medical Services, 8,* 36–39.

Mitchell, J. T. (1988a). History, status, and future of CISD. *Journal of Emergency Medical Services, 13,* 49–52.

Mitchell, J. T. (1988b). Development and functions of a critical incident stress debriefing team. *Journal of Emergency Medical Services, 13,* 43–46.

Mitchell, J. T. (1991). Law enforcement applications of critical incident stress debriefing teams. In J. T. Reese (Ed.), *Critical incidents in policing* (pp. 289–302). Washington, DC: U.S. Department of Justice.

Pennebaker, J., & Susman, J. (1988). Disclosure of traumas and psychosomatic processes. *Social Science and Medicine, 26,* 327–332.

Pennebaker, J. W. (1985). Traumatic experience and psychosomatic disease. *Canadian Psychologist, 26,* 82–95.

Pennebaker, J. W., & Beall, S. (1986). Confronting a traumatic event. *Journal of Abnormal Psychology, 95,* 274–281.

Salmon, T. W. (1919). War neuroses and their lesson. *New York Medical Journal, 109,* 993–994.

Rogers, O. (1992). An examination of critical incident stress debriefing for emergency service providers. Unpublished doctoral dissertation, University of Maryland.

van der Hart, O., Brown, P., & van der Kolk, B. (1989). Pierre Janet's treatment of post-traumatic stress. *Journal of Traumatic Stress, 2,* 379–396.

Yalom, I. (1985). *Theory and practice of group psychotherapy* (3rd ed.). New York: Basic Books.

Yandrick, R. (1990, January). Critical incidents. *EAPA Exchange,* pp. 18–23.

17

Debriefing the Debriefers

An Intervention Strategy to Assist Psychologists after a Crisis

ALISON TALBOT, MONICA MANTON, and PETER J. DUNN

In this chapter we describe the factors in crisis intervention that make the work particularly difficult or stressful. We discuss debriefing methods previously developed by others to deal with the effects of crisis work and propose a debriefing strategy especially for psychologist, social workers, psychiatric nurses, and psychiatrists. (For simplification, the word *psychologist* will be used to refer to all of these professionals.) The ideas and procedures put forward have evolved through our work with victims of violence, specifically armed hold-ups. We argue that psychologists, as distinct from other emergency responders (e.g., ambulance workers and the police), require *psychological* understanding and integration to be able to function and intervene effectively. We identify and discuss the elements involved in a debriefing and detail the task of the debriefer.

DISTINCTIVE FEATURES OF CRISIS INTERVENTION

For psychologists, crisis work has distinctive features that make it stressful. These features are related to the work itself, the role of the psycholo-

---

ALISON TALBOT, MONICA MANTON, and PETER J. DUNN • Staff Counseling Service, State Bank Victoria, Melbourne, Victoria 3000, Australia. Reprinted from the *Journal of Traumatic Stress*, Vol. 5, No. 1, 1993.

Psychotraumatology, edited by George S. Everly, Jr. and Jeffrey M. Lating. Plenum Press, New York, 1995.

gists, the countertransference, and the impact of the organization within which the crisis takes place.

First, there is the urgency and immediacy of the response. The crisis response is usually of an outreach nature, which means psychologists have no control of many aspects of the situation—when it happens, what the environment will be like, who will be there, and what functions will be required in each instance. Often there is no notice (of sudden events), no time for preparation, a limited amount of time for individual interventions, a lack of space, and unfamiliar surroundings. In a crisis psychologists need to be able to work speedily and effectively to stabilize the situation. The sheer volume of the work, both in terms of the number of people requiring attention in any one crisis and in terms of numerous successive crises, can have a debilitating effect (Rogers, 1987). In addition, the intensity of the emotions present is high, the victims are often regressed, and a large amount of energy is required on the part of the psychologist to contain them.

The role of the psychologist changes from being requested to provide intervention to offering intervention, and this can be seen as intrusive by victims. In addition, psychologists accustomed to structured therapeutic interactions may find themselves feeling powerless when confronted with trauma victims whose needs are for the most basic empathy and containment as opposed to more complex interventions. Often there is nothing to do but listen, and this is an extremely difficult task. As Kinzie (1989), in his work with traumatized refugees, says, "There are times for no intervention and no words can deal with the experience." The psychologist can only "enter the felt world of the patient" to gain the power to evoke and change feelings (Havens, 1972). The changing role also means that the psychologist has no knowledge of the premorbid or precrisis functioning of the victims.

Countertransference issues are of particular significance in crisis intervention because they tend to be about frightening aspects of one's life that are often unconscious and difficult to deal with, such as violence, abandonment, death, helplessness, degradation, and maiming (Kinzie, 1989; McCann et al., 1988). Countertransference refers here to the emotional response of the therapist that relates to an unresolved aspect of his or her past, causing misinterpretation or misresponding to the client in terms of the therapist's own difficulties (Arlow, 1979).

The crisis often occurs within an organizational context that makes particular demands on interveners. The organization's expectations of psychologists are often high and poorly defined, and these expectations may be in conflict with those of the victims, as well as with those of the psychologists themselves.

THE EFFECTS OF THE WORK ON CRISIS INTERVENERS

The very nature of crisis intervention can make stresses for psychologists and can have a range of effects. In the literature dealing with crisis intervention, there are numerous references to the effects of this work. Mitchell (1983), in his work with emergency service personnel, reminds us that rescuers are vulnerable human beings who have all the normal physical and psychological responses to the horror of human suffering. He comments that emotional aftershocks can appear at the scene or days, weeks, or even months later and can seriously affect the person's performance within the emergency organization as well as relationships with his or her family. He cites restlessness, irritability, excessive fatigue, sleep disturbances, anxiety, startle reactions to pressure, moodiness, muscle tremors, difficulties concentrating, nightmares, vomiting, and diarrhea as physiological responses or reactions to critical incidents. These reactions, though normal, are potentially dangerous to the emergency service worker's health, can sap energy, leave him or her vulnerable to illness, and be especially destructive when he or she denies their presence or misinterprets the stress responses as something wrong with him or her.

Berah et al. (1984) studied the effects of working with disaster on mental health professionals and found evidence that both their emotional and physical health were affected. A large majority felt shocked, confused, saddened, and very tired. About half became ill and/or had accidents, and all noticed changes in their eating, smoking, or drinking habits, recognized feelings of helplessness, and felt the need for team support. Even those with extensive training and experience in psychological trauma found they were considerably stressed. In the absence of clear role definitions on the one hand and of a therapeutic contract on the other, intense and intimate engagements with distressed victims often taxed all the empathy, emotional resources, and therapeutic skill of helpers. Berah et al. (1984) believe that if the team members had not often worked in pairs, ventilated to each other, and had regular debriefing sessions, the effects of stress might have been greater.

Raphael (1981), in a discussion of the helpers' perspective in the aftermath of the Granville disaster, describes the sense of helplessness and frustration felt by many of the workers. Many of them experienced dreams, nightmares, psychosomatic symptoms, irritability, anxiety, and depression after the event. Dealing with violence, death, and injury can trigger the awareness of one's own mortality, personal vulnerability, and survivor guilt (Raphael, 1981), so that not only the victims but also the helpers experience the intensity of personal disaster (Black, 1987; Raphael, 1977; Raphael, Singh, & Bradbury, 1980; Raphael, Singh, Bradbury, & Lambert, 1983–1984). Both must integrate the shock, denial, distress, helplessness, images, and encounter with death (Raphael, 1981). It is not just the encounter with death and existential issues that has ramifications for helpers but also the anguish and suffering of others. The human empathic response—together with the heightened arousal, engagement, and often intense relationships—means that the helper will become acutely aware of grief, pain, and distress. This distress may be awakened in the helper in addition to his or her own grief and anguish about what has happened (Raphael, 1986).

In their work with victims of armed holdups, we and our colleagues have experienced feelings, thoughts, and behaviors all of which have been variously cited in the literature as indicators of "burnout" (Beemsterboer, 1984; Kahill, 1988; Maslach, 1982; Miller et al., 1988; Raquepaw & Miller, 1989; Rogers, 1987; Savicki & Cooley, 1982). Whether that particular term is used or not, the experiences, as reported, clearly point to undue pressures or stress and indicate the need for some sort of intervention to minimize its effects.

After intervening following a holdup or a series of holdups, we and our colleagues have often found ourselves feeling isolated, angry, tense, powerless, hopeless, and anxious. We have also been emotionally exhausted, which manifested itself in feeling confused, tearful, overwhelmed, useless, and burdened with responsibility. As has often been reported in the burnout literature (Beemsterboer, 1984; Edwelwich & Brodsky, 1980; Kinzie, 1989; Miller et al., 1988; Raquepaw & Miller, 1989; Savicki & Cooley, 1982), we found that our clients' problems seemed either insurmountable or insignificant, and we were unable to be detached or tended to overidentify with them. We had a tendency to intellectualize, to be rigid in our thinking and resistant to change. We were often unaware of the way in which our work was affecting us (using denial as a protective strategy), and we found ourselves unable to differentiate between various armed holdups.

Behaviorally we experienced ourselves as exhausted, increased our alcohol intake, had numerous somatic complaints such as headaches and gastrointestinal disturbances, had sleep disturbances and nightmares, experienced an increased sensitivity to violence in general, and were emotionally demanding of family and friends. In addition, we found we were unable to concentrate and were tense, expecting the telephone to ring announcing another holdup. Finally, we were suspicious and fearful on entering banks as customers.

In summary, crisis workers, whether emergency service personnel (such as fire fighters, ambulance workers, or police) or mental health professionals (such as psychologists, social workers, psychiatrists, or psychiatric nurses), are affected by the circumstances in which they work. Trauma or disasters are not situations to which one can become accustomed rather there is a need to develop ways of dealing with such experiences.

TECHNIQUES FOR DEALING WITH EFFECTS OF CRISIS INTERVENTION WORK

Psychologists may have their own variety of post-traumatic stress reaction, and, as victims do, they require techniques to help them deal with the experience. Mitchell (1988) has developed a debriefing procedure for emergency service personnel, and Raphael (1986) details a psychological debriefing process for mental health workers.

Mitchell (1988) has made use of what he calls critical-incident stress debriefing, which is a group meeting of emergency personnel that aims to defuse the potential for post-traumatic stress disorder and other stress symptoms. The structured discussions emphasize normal responses to abnormal events and are scheduled 24 to 72 hours after the incident. The overall goal is to protect and support emergency response personnel and to minimize the development of abnormal stress response syndromes, which may cause lost time, a drop in effectiveness of work, and problems within the family. There is an initial defusing that needs an atmosphere that is positive, supportive, and based on care and concern for the team members. Free expression of feelings, with acceptance, support, and understanding from each other and their leaders, is encouraged. Mitchell states that the formal debriefing should be led by a skilled professional because the emotional content released during the session may overwhelm an untrained facilitator. The facilitator should be skilled in human communications and have a background in group dynamics or group interactions.

The aim of the psychological debriefing for mental health workers that Raphael (1986) describes is to help workers to deal with the stresses of this work so that problems do not subsequently arise. In a psychological debriefing the leaders of the working team may informally or formally provide an opportunity to review the disaster experience so that those involved may talk through their feelings, fears, frustrations, and successes. This provides catharsis and allows individuals to test their perceptions of the experience against those of others enabling them to review the experience actively and gain mastery. The debriefing explores the workers' initiation into the disaster role and their own experience in the disaster. It allows any frustrating and negative experiences, with associated feelings, to be ventilated, and positive aspects to be reviewed to balance the picture and help with integration. Personal relationships with coworkers and with family members are also explored, allowing for ventilation of feelings. There is gentle exploration by the debriefer of the workers' identification with the experience of the victim. This is particularly important for psychologists and enables them to recognize and shed some of the burden of empathy. Finally, workers are helped to integrate the disaster experience and make a transition back to everyday life. As Raphael (1986) concludes:

> This discussion promotes the processes of integration and mastery of the disaster, by actively defining, both concretely and at a feeling level, the experience and its consequences. The experience is given a cognitive structure, and the emotional release of reviewing it helps the worker to a sense of achievement and distancing. He will not forget the experience but neither is he likely to retain an ongoing stressful burden from it. (p. 286)

Mitchell's debriefings focus on the cathartic elements, whereas Raphael's debriefing extends this to a review of the experience of the work, the relationships of the workers, and integration of the experience.

As in all casework, psychologists need to know not only what happened, when, how, and where, but also *why*. That, is, debriefing is not just incorporating the experience but utilizing the knowledge gained from it. This allows an understanding from a theoretical perspective and enhances skills and psychological understanding for future work. A psychologist needs to be aware of psychological factors and to intervene with the knowledge of these. In order to continue to function *professionally*, he or she needs to have a psychological understanding of the trauma and his or her role in it personally and professionally—that is, the debriefing needs to attend to his or her personal and professional self. The debriefing that we undertake includes making psychological sense of what has occurred to the victims and the psychologists both professionally and personally.

DEBRIEFING THE DEBRIEFERS

The development of debriefing following crisis intervention work has been an evolutionary process. The most effective and clear-cut approach proved to be one where the debriefer did not belong to the team of crisis interveners, was not currently involved in firsthand crisis intervention work, but nevertheless had a familiarity with crisis work.

In the particular work that we undertake (Manton & Talbot, 1990), crises are attended to by teams of two or more psychologists. They debrief for the reasons discussed above and also to prepare for follow-up work the next day. The debriefings are held away from the crisis scene on the day of the crisis, the day of the first follow-up, and, if necessary, after other follow-up visits. The manner in which we work has particular relevance for the debriefing procedure. First, the victim group is always accustomed to working together within an organizational context. There are consequently pertinent issues related to the group's functioning and that of the organization that can affect the crisis work. Second, the psychologists as a team provide a second group whose functioning can affect the victims and vice versa, and this may need to be addressed.

The debriefing procedure incorporates the crisis event, the response to that event by the psychologists, and the processes occurring in the debriefing itself. Its aim is to tie in and make sense of the crisis and the counseling—what happened, when, where, to whom, and how, so that a clear total picture is formed. The debriefer is consequently dealing with a number of different levels of the crisis: the event itself, the victims' responses to the event, the psychologists' responses to the event, and the psychologists' responses to the victims. In addition, he or she needs to take account of the victims and each psychologist's professional and personal response to the events. Furthermore, each of these can be viewed in terms of the individual within the context of the group and the group as a whole. There are nine aspects to be attended to (Table 17.1), although not all may be relevant to every crisis.

What follows is a way of conceptualizing the process, rather than a prescriptive sequential procedure. A case study is used to illustrate this process.

> Three psychologists (Sarah, Ursula, and Isabelle) are employed by a bank to attend to the victims of an armed holdup. The debriefer, Don, is a consultant psychologist to the bank. In the branch itself there are 30 staff, including three senior staff accountants and a manager. A regional manager attends the branch immediately after the holdup to take over responsibility for the overall management of the crisis.
>
> Two psychologists, Sarah and Ursula, arrive first at the branch, which is some 30 minutes from the city. On arrival, they enter the branch (showing their identification to the police), stop inside the public area, and survey the bank chamber and the people in there. It is close to lunchtime. They observe that approximately 30 people are here; the staff are tidying up their units and desks with the help of four relief staff. The workers, mainly males, are noisily talking, drinking coffee and beer, and smoking cigarettes one after another. Some of the younger females are sitting in small groups of two or three. Two are sitting on their own, rocking, their faces downcast. One male accountant is banging drawers and moving around, his face tight and red.
>
> The more senior of the psychologists, Ursula, talks with the regional manager, who informs her that it was not a serious holdup. The armed bandit apparently waited in a queue for the teller nearest the front door, then passed over a note that read, "Put money in the bag and do not set off the alarm." The female teller took some money from her drawer; one of the other tellers noticed her looking pale and observed her actions. After the man left and hurried toward the door, the female turned and said, "It's a hold-up," and started to scream. The alarm was set off, and the staff secured the branch. Customers were spoken to by the manager of the branch. The police arrived a few minutes after the alarm, and the regional manager followed some 20 minutes later.
>
> The regional manager reports that no one was hurt, and the branch will reopen; only one female teller was involved and she was crying so much that the manager and regional manager thought she should go to the doctor and then home. This is contrary to bank instructions for action in armed holdups, as it is preferable to keep the group intact. The manager had organized his staff to continue working and to finish the tasks they were doing. He did not want them to "just sit and talk." The third psychologist, Isabelle, arrives, and the three consult about the way they will work. Reluctantly, the regional manager provides rooms for the two, Sarah and Ursula, while Isabelle works in the tea-room annex. The psychologists see the staff members one at a time before the staff leave the branch. As they do the regional manager moves around impatiently and seems to be in a hurry for the counseling to finish so that he can reopen the branch.
>
> After seeing a few of the staff, the psychologists meet to share information and also to find out how the others are progressing. Before she reenters her room, Sarah is approached by the manager and is told that the note also said, "and if you don't I will kill you." He has not told anyone else, and Sarah, realizing the other psychologists have resumed work, goes back to her room, too.
>
> At the completion of their task 3 hours later, the psychologists meet with

Table 17.1 The Elements of the Debriefing Process

	Individuals	Individuals in the Group	The Group as a Whole
	(a)	(b)	(c)
Victims	What happened to each person? Who is of concern? Is there individual pathology? What is the likely progress of the trauma response over time?	Individuals within the group that affect the psychological interventions or healing process of the group or other individuals in the group, e.g. Individual: –isolated during or after crisis –scapegoated –monopolist –psychotic –narcissistic –silent –helper/rejector –self righteous –moralist Role of: –mother/father –adolescent/child Important person: –not present/divisive/constructive	Group dynamics that affect individuals in the group or the group as a whole, and the psychological interventions or processes, e.g. Group –cohesive/fractured –affected/not affected –leaderless –subgroups –hierarchies –flight/fight Level of: –communication –self disclosure –conflict –risk taking

Psychologist professionally: How they worked in the trauma	(d) What did he/she do? What was productive? What would he/she do differently and how?	(e) Individual dynamics? roles within the group –leader/follower –supporter of others –isolate –observer –worker/drone Parallels with victim group	(f) Group dynamics of the psychologist –leaderless –split –cohesive –communicative Parallels with victim group; if it is different, why
Psychologist personally: How the trauma affected them	(g) How did he/she experience the event –feelings, thoughts, behaviors? Does this parallel the victims? Countertransference issues	(h) Counter transference or personal issues between members of the group, eg. Group member: –powerless –confrontational –silent –level of feeling –not expressing feeling –Parallels with victims?	(i) Historical issues for the group Pre-crisis functioning Does this parallel the victims' group? If it is different, why?

the regional manager and discuss the planned action for the next morning—they will be there before opening time to assist the staff as they arrive for work. The three psychologists gather at their cars and discuss the scheduled debriefing. Isabelle wonders if it is really necessary, as she says she is all right. Reluctantly she agrees to go, as the other two feel they require some debriefing.

Sarah and Ursula arrive first at the debriefing; both look pale and are talking earnestly in soft tones. Isabelle arrives a little later and sits slightly separate from the others in the room. She spends the initial part of the session tapping the chair with her hands and expresses a desire to complete the proceedings soon so that she can go home. She looks red, and her face is flushed. Still tapping her hand on the chair, she repeats that she doesn't need debriefing. She is fine, she sees the victims as fine, and the holdup was not as bad as some of the others she had been to—she has been to a lot lately. Ursula then tells the debriefer, Don, "I have just discovered that the note threatened the teller's life, and I am shocked." Ursula says that Sarah told her about the note in the car on the way to debriefing. Sarah adds that she didn't quite know what to do with that information. Isabelle responds, quite angrily, "How come I didn't know that?" A heated exchange follows. During the ensuing debriefing, Isabelle with encouragement and support from Don, is able to express her feelings both of isolation from and anger toward the other members of her team and is able to be included in the process of the group.

THE ELEMENTS OF THE DEBRIEFING PROCESS

Victims

The responses of *individual victims* (a) need to be looked at and understood and some prognosis made. In this instance, the main protagonist (the one whom the bandit confronts), having been seemingly banished for emoting, is likely to feel isolated. She needs to be contacted and urged to return the following day. In that way she can be integrated into the working group, her experience shared with the rest of the staff, and her recovery enhanced.

Within the *group context* (b) there may be individuals who affect the psychologists' work and the healing process of the group or of other individual victims. In the case example, the manager's indifference to other members of the branch left them feeling uncared for. His discounting of their experience encouraged denial by the victims (which can be inhibitive of healing), and this in turn affected their behavior. They went about their tasks as though nothing was wrong when many of them may have not wanted to. If the manager can express his guilt, fears, and anxieties and be available as a caring authority figure, the individuals in the group can seek comfort from this. In other holdups the absence of the manager during the event has left the victims feeling particularly vulnerable and exposed and, in some instances, has been conducive to further regression, exacerbating the crisis situation. Psychologists need to take into account these sorts of issues and tailor their interventions accordingly.

For *groups of victims* (c) there are dynamics that may affect individuals or the group as a whole and in turn the psychological interventions. A group that operates on high levels of communication and self-disclosure facilitates the healing process by normalizing experiences, reducing isolation, and facilitating a feeling of community and support for all victims. In a group that has subgroups, as in the case example, individuals or groups of individuals can become isolated and feel misunderstood. In this instance the ethos for the majority (group) is "we cope by loud conversation, convivial talk, and denial of our feelings." However, there is a smaller group of people who may be feeling a lot, are constrained from expressing those feelings, and are generally rendered powerless. Often during a crisis there is no time to think about or even know about all that is happening. Debriefing allows for a clarification of the victims' responses, giving a clear picture of the whole event. Just as one of the important elements of crisis intervention for each victim is to understand what happened, the psychologists need an avenue to do the same. What may seem an isolated and unimportant incident at the time of the crisis may be crucial in the overall picture of understanding the trauma and its effects.

Psychologist as Professional

The debriefer deals with and helps the psychologist to become aware of himself or herself as a professional and a person in the crisis situation. The way in which each psychologist operates as a *professional* (d) is important in the debriefing process. This is essentially a supervisory role for the debriefer in which each psychologist reaches an understanding of the interventions that he or she made, assesses those that were useful, explores possible alternatives, and decides on future actions.

Within a group of psychologists as with victims, *individual professionals within the group* (e) can affect the dynamics. For example, a leaderless group or one with an ineffectual leader can result in feelings of being lost and powerless. Alternatively if a psychologist isolates himself or herself from the group and begins working alone in a nonconsultative manner, then his or her functioning and perception of what happens can differ considerably from the rest of the group. Interventions can then be at cross purposes, causing friction and tension and possibly a splitting of the group. These dynamics become particularly important if they parallel what is happening in the victim group. *Parallel process* refers to the feelings, thoughts, and behaviors evident in a victim or group of victims that are replicated in a psychologist or group of psychologists (Talbot, 1990). In the case example, two psychologists are paired (they arrive and travel together) while one is separate, and the separation is exacerbated by the latter having to work in a smaller room. This has the potential to parallel the victim group, which, if the group is dysfunctional, is not useful for a working team. In addition, a psychologist who feels isolated may be unable to empathize with the experience of the victims who often feel isolated during and after an armed robbery.

Issues such as communication, cohesiveness, support, mutuality, and others related to *group functioning* (f) need to be addressed. The debriefer of the psychologists need to be aware of the dynamics of the professional group during the crisis. For example, a group that is not cohesive may leave individual psychologists working in isolation, which can make the professional work extremely difficult. Alternatively, a group that is cohesive, in the face of a victims' group that is not, avoids paralleling the process and is likely to be more effective in intervention and to provide a supportive environment from which to work. The debriefing provides a forum for psychologists as professionals to assess their work as a team and as individuals. There is an opportunity for them to share their experiences of the work, and to express concerns or satisfaction about the way it was done. In the case example, one of the psychologists was physically isolated and felt isolated from the other members of her team. Discussion of this between the team members facilitated her inclusion in the group, making it a more effective team.

Psychologist as a Person

For the *psychologists personally* (g), working in a crisis can be very traumatic. It is important to understand how the trauma has affected each of them, particularly where there has been violence and/or death. When psychologists experience anxiety related to their own personal life, the debriefer needs to be aware of the reality of this, the parallel process, and countertransference issues. For example, psychologists may find themselves feeling enormously sad and frightened (which is not unusual following a traumatic event), and the debriefer needs to normalize these experiences. Part of his or her responses may also be a parallel process in that the psychologist is experiencing what the victims have experienced. Past unresolved issues may also arise, however, particularly if violence or abuse has been experienced. It may not be appropriate to deal with the countertransference issues in the context of debriefing, but they need to be tabled and the psychologist may need a resource to resolve them. As in any therapeutic situation, if a psychologist has some understanding of what the countertransference is and what it is not, he or she is freer to continue working professionally. For example, during the debriefing Sarah was able to disclose that being the bearer of bad news is difficult for her: She found it painful to have to tell Ursula and Isabelle about the note. Her reluctance to impart this information affected them as people. It also affected their work; they were unable to respond to the enormity of the situation, because they didn't know about it.

The psychologists' personal issues may affect the *working of the group* (h). Isabelle, who arrived last and sat impatiently but said everything was all right, showed a discrepancy between her verbal and nonverbal behavior. This incongruence needs to be raised. She may be paralleling a member of the victim group, or this may be the way she functions normally in the group. Such issues need to be addressed with the person concerned and with the group by the debriefer. As a result of what happened during this hold-up, the team agreed that it was not useful for the psychologists to arrive separately. They decided they either needed to arrive together or, if they did arrive separately, to take time out from the work to meet as a team and establish contact to avoid any isolation.

Finally there are issues for the *professional group as a whole* (i). These include any historical issues of the precrisis functioning of the group.

The number of successive crises attended by psychologists may need to be addressed in this section. In the case example, one psychologist had arrived feeling overloaded with the amount of work she had been doing. The myth in this particular crisis, perpetuated by senior management, was that it was not a serious holdup because it had not been as dangerous as some of the other holdups. The psychologist wanted the victims to be all right because she felt she could not handle any more and conveniently accepted the myth. Here work felt unfruitful and unsatisfactory and was in addition untherapeutic for the victims.

This aspect of the debriefing allows for the airing of and dealing with personal issues, past and present, of individuals, between individuals, and of the group. This requires the debriefer to have skill, empathy, and a knowledge of group processes so that psychologists can express their feelings and thoughts in a supportive and safe environment.

THE TASK OF DEBRIEFING

To gain an understanding of these issues and to enhance the debriefing process the debriefer has quite a task. Table 17.2 elucidates this task by showing what the debriefer needs to do and examining the underlying thought processes. The debriefer's task involves observing and listening, responding and eliciting, and thinking about and making psychological sense of each individual, each individual within the group, and the group as a whole.

Like victims in crisis, psychologists may be only slightly affected or they may be traumatized, in shock, experiencing strong feelings and needing an opportunity to talk. The debriefer needs to be attuned to what is happening to psychologists individually and collectively, by attending and listening in order to establish rapport so that they can work together. He or she might do this by observing and listening to body language, feeling tone, interpreting

Table 17.2 The Task of the Debriefer

Debriefer	Individually	Collectively for individuals within the group and for the group as a whole
Observing and listening	Body language Words used (i.e., verbal messages and feeling tone)	Dynamics between individuals Who is communicating Who is isolated Who is silent Who is cohesive/split Who is vulnerable/coping Who is carrying emotion
Responding to and eliciting	Incorporating, the above, responding and eliciting feelings and cognitions Clarifying points, behaviors, and themes	Feelings and thoughts as they pertain to the group or individuals within the group
Monitoring own process	Looking at internal experience, for clues as to the individual's experience? Eg, if I feel X in response to this individual, what does it mean for him?	Looking at internal experience for clues as to the experience of the group. Eg, I am aware of fear—is this group frightened?
Thinking about	What happened at the crisis What is happening here What is similar What is different Why How	What happened at the crisis What is happening here What is similar What is different Why How
Makes psychological sense of the above by	Interventions: –Confronting –Putting into perspective –Tying in themes and personal issues –Making parallels –Using immediacy and congruence –Reframing –Forming alternatives for the future	As for individuals
Concludes	How is he/she now? Review	Summarizing Tying up Review

verbal messages, and looking at the dynamics between individuals in the professional group and of the group itself. In the case example, the debriefer would have noticed that two of the psychologists had white faces and appeared frightened or in shock. The third was red in the face, tapped her chair anxiously, was particularly garrulous, and seemed angry about the debriefing.

Part of the debriefer's task is to give individual psychologists and the group an opportunity to express and release emotions, provide containment, and be empathic. The debriefer needs to incorporate his or her observations and listening into this. He or she may need to elicit and respond to feelings individually and collectively. He or she may need to clarify points, elicit and respond to thoughts, and be starting to look for themes and hypotheses as to what is going on. The debriefer might note the pale faces—"Two of you look very pale and frightened. What happened? What did you do? What did you think? What did you feel?"—eliciting the story from the psychologists and empathizing with their experience.

The debriefer can use the way he or she is experiencing the individuals and the group to provide clues to what is occurring. In this instance, Don, the debriefer, feels distinctly uncomfortable; there is an argument occurring in front of him. He is aware of two people having information and of one person being uninformed, of two people feeling shocked and frightened and one person saying she feels all right. He asks himself what this means and how it is related to the whole picture. As the psychologists continue to talk, he hears them describe how the victims experienced themselves as unable to understand what was going on, and how some of the victims seemed very upset while others did not. He begins to see there is a similarity between what went on in the victim group and what is going on now with the psychologists; he wonders if this is a parallel.

To help the psychologists come to terms with the experience the debriefer needs to make sense of what is happening—what happened during the crisis, what is happening now, what is similar, and what is different to what has occurred overall. The debriefer would thus be making hypotheses about the event. For instance, the debriefer might note the isolation of one of the victims, the isolation of one of the psychologists, the denial by members of the group of victims, the denial by one of the psychologists, the shock and the enormous impact of the note on the victim and now on Ursula, and the feeling of enormous emotion in the room. When he sees the anger that Isabelle seems to be experiencing but not expressing, he might think of the red-faced accountant. He directs them to attend to what is occurring in the present moment, encouraging Isabelle to express her isolation and anger and all of them to express their shock and fear of the death threat. This mobilizes them and allows them expression of feelings about what has occurred. Catharsis and a chance to talk are insufficient; the debriefer needs also to impart understanding to the psychologists so that they comprehend personally and professionally what happened. This may include an understanding of countertransference and parallel process issues and how they affect professional and personal functioning. The debriefer forms a picture of what occurred and imparts this to them. For example, he might say, "You talked about how the main victim was very isolated, and I guess she is feeling much like you were feeling, Isabelle—isolated and possibly angry about it."

The debriefer has to make psychological sense of the psychologists' experiences in the crisis and in the debriefing. He or she does this by utilizing his or her knowledge of the victims as individuals and as a group, as well as of the psychologists as individuals and as a group and his or her understanding of psychological processes. In doing this he or she may need to be more confronting than psychologists are with victims or, for that matter, than debriefers might be with other emergency responders, such as police or firefighters. The aim ultimately is to tie in themes and personal issues, draw parallels, and put all of this into perspective. Countertransference issues may have also interfered, as discussed earlier.

The unconscious processes are denial by the manager, by the victim group, and subsequently by Isabelle. The effects of this denial are shown in the victim group by the red-faced accountant and the small group of victims who are isolated. This is paralleled in the psychologist group by Isabelle's isolation and unexpressed anger. The victim group has become split, and there is a potential for the psychologist group to be split, too. In the victim group the one who was sent home is carrying the trauma for the rest of the group, and this may inhibit her healing as well as that of the group. Similarly, one member of the psychologist group is carrying the emotion for all of the group (Isabelle the anger, and Sarah the secrets and the responsibility). The awareness of these processes in the debriefing paves the way for the psychologist group to be a cohesive team, and for them to be able to plan for appropriate interventions in the victim group to counteract any further splitting or disruption. The cognitive understanding gives them mastery of the situation, objectivity, and a theoretical base from which to make interventions. This is essential in order for them to continue to function as psychologists.

Finally, as in a therapeutic session, the debriefer needs to summarize, to contain and to make sense of what has occurred. It can be useful for individuals to verbalize what they have gained and learned from working in the crisis and from the debriefing. To continue personally and professionally psychologists need to have a sense of mastery of the experience as well as the assurance of feeling valued, worthwhile, and positive about themselves and their work. Without a debriefing they may not have an awareness of the complete experience and may be unable to comprehend it.

The debriefing, as described, is a model, and in any one debriefing not all elements may need to be addressed or be evident at one time. On some occasions it may be that there are particular issues relating to the work that need to be discussed, and at other times the personal experiences of the psychologists may be of more importance. In a crisis, victims respond differently and have a variety of needs—so, too, do psychologists in a debriefing. Whatever the components of any one debriefing, the crucial element is the psychological sense that is made of the entire crisis intervention episode. It means that a psychologist responds not only as a human being or a compassionate carer, but as someone who also clearly comprehends the meaning of the victims' experience, of his or her own experience, and of the way they interact to promote integration and healing.

CONCLUSION

Crisis intervention, because of its nature, has the potential to affect crisis workers. The post-traumatic stress reactions of psychologists who attend crises are similar to those of the victims themselves. Several studies describe the experiences, feelings, and behavior of psychologists as they carry out their crisis intervention work. Using a case study, we describe a process of debriefing that enables the psychologist who experiences such reactions—and most do—to still function professionally as well as personally. We consider the model proposed here to be essential for psychologists and have made it mandatory in our work. The model provides the ventilation and containment that Mitchell's (1988) critical-incident stress debriefing offers, as well as having the integrative function of Raphael's (1986) psychological debriefings. Most importantly, it assists the psychologists to a psychological understanding of the whole crisis, of the victims and their reactions, and of the ways in which they themselves are affected, both personally and professionally. With the use of this model, the psychologists are free to return to their work with a clarity that is otherwise not possible.

The proposed debriefing model has evolved in a specific work context and could be developed further to meet the particular requirements of the crisis itself or of other groups of mental health professionals. We believe that this model might be suitably adapted for use in a wide variety of crisis and trauma situations.

REFERENCES

Arlow, J. A. (1979). In R. J. Corsini (Ed.), *Current psychotherapies.* Itasca, IL: Peacock.

Bard, M., & Sangrey, D. (1980). Things fall apart: Victims in crisis. *Evaluation Change,* 28–35.

Beemsterboer, J., & Baum, B. H. (1984). "Burnout": Definitions and health care management. *Social Work Health Care, 10.*

Berah, E. F., Jones, H. J., & Valent, P. (1984). The experience of a mental health team involved in the early phase of a disaster. *Austr. New Zeal. J. Psychiatry, 18.*

Black, J. W. (1987). The libidinal cocoon: A nurturing retreat for the families of plane crash victims. *Hosp. Commun. Psychiatry, 38.*

Edelwich, J., & Brodsky, P. (1980). *Burnout: The staged of disillusionment in the helping professions*. New York: Human Sciences, Press.
Havens, L. L. (1972). The development of existential psychiatry. *J. Nerv. Ment. Dis.*, 154.
Kahill, S. (1988). Interventions for burnout in the helping professions: A review of the empirical evidence. *Canad. J. Counsel.*, 22.
Kinzie, J. D. (1989). Therapeutic approaches to traumatized Cambodian refugees. *J. Traum. Stress*, 2.
Manton, M., & Talbot, A. (1990). Crisis intervention after an armed hold-up: Guidelines for counsellors. *J. Traumatic Stress, 3*, 507–522.
Maslach, C. (1982). *Burnout: The cost of caring*. Englewood Cliffs, NJ: Prentice Hall.
McCann, I. L., Sakheim, D. K., & Abrahamson, D. J. (1988). Trauma and victimization: A model of psychological adaptation. *Counsel. Psychologist*, 16.
Miller, K. I., Stiff, J. B., & Ellis, B. H. (1988). Communication and empathy as precursors to burnout among human service workers. *Commun. Monog.*, 55.
Mitchell, J. T. (1983, March). When disaster strikes: The critical incident stress debriefing process. *Am. J. Emerg. Serv.*
Mitchell, J. T. (1988). *The psychological impact of the Air Florida 90 disaster on fire, rescue, paramedical and police officer personnel*. Paper presented at the International Conference on Stress and Trauma in Emergency Services, Melbourne, Australia.
Raphael, B. (1977). The Granville train disaster: Psychological needs and their management. *Med. J. Austr.*, 26.
Raphael, B. (1981). Personal disaster. *Austr. New Zeal J. Psychiatr.*, 15.
Raphael, B. (1986). *When disaster strikes*. London: Hutchinson.
Raphael, B., Singh, B., & Bradbury, L. (1980). Disaster: The helpers' perspective. *Med. J. Austr.*, 18.
Raphael, B., Singh, B., Bradbury, L., & Lambert, F. (1983–1984). Who helps the helpers? The effects of a disaster on the rescue workers. *Omega*, 14.
Raquepaw, J. M., & Miller, R. S. (1989). Psychotherapist burnout: A component analysis. *Prof. Psychol. Res. Pract.*, 20.
Rogers, E. R. (1987). Professional burnout: A review of a concept. *Clin. Superv.*, 5.
Savicki, V., & Cooley, E. J. (1982, March). Implications of burnout research and theory for counsellor educators. *Person. Guid.*
Talbot, A. (1990). The importance of parallel process in debriefing crisis counsellors. *J. Traum. Stress, 3*, 265–278.

V

Special Issues in Post-Traumatic Stress

This fifth and final section addresses special issues and concerns as they relate to dynamics that may be unique to certain populations of individuals affected by post-traumatic stress or issues surrounding unique types of traumatic stressor.

Chapter 18 is a valuable review of childhood traumatization by Terr. The chapter not only examines the nature of symptoms common to childhood traumatization but also sensitizes the reader to the role it may play in later life.

Chapter 19 reviews psychological trauma as engendered by sexual traumatization; the emphasis of this chapter is on coping and recovery. The chapter employs the concept of fundamental beliefs or worldviews, as discussed in our two-factor model (Chapter 3), as a vehicle for understanding sexual trauma and the coping process.

In Chapter 20, Figley addresses the family as a victim of post-traumatic stress and reviews the treatment process.

Chapter 21 represents a superb review of theoretical and practical issues related to the treatment of PTSD in Vietnam veterans.

Finally, Chapter 22 reviews a much neglected area of clinical import: issues pertaining to cross-cultural care for PTSD.

18

Childhood Traumas

An Outline and Overview

LENORE C. TERR

Mental conditions brought on by horrible external events in childhood present a wide range of findings. If one looks only at the clinical manifestations of trauma in a given day in the life of the traumatized child, one could diagnose conduct disorder, borderline personality, major affective disorder, attention-deficit hyperactivity, phobic disorder, dissociative disorder, obsessive-compulsive disorder, panic disorder, adjustment disorder, and even such conditions (as yet unofficial in the nomenclature) as precursors of multiple personality or acute dissociative disorder. If one projects this multiplicity of technically correct diagnoses onto a traumatized child's adulthood, one finds even more diagnostic leeway.

We must organize our thinking about childhood trauma, however, or we run the risk of never seeing the condition at all. Like the young photographer in Cortázar's short story (and Antonioni's film) "Blow Up," we may enlarge the diagnostic fine points of trauma into such prominence that we altogether lose the central point—that external forces created the internal changes in the first place. We must not let ourselves forget childhood trauma just because the problem is so vast.

Studies of adults in mental hospitals (Carmen & Rieker, 1984), adults suffering from multiple personalities (Bliss, 1986), adults who are borderline (Walsh, 1977), and adolescents who go on to commit murder (Lewis, Lovely, Yaeger, et al., 1989) show that these adults and adolescents very often were

---

LENORE C. TERR • 450 Sutter Street, San Francisco, California 94108. Reprinted from *American Journal of Psychiatry*, Vol. 148, 1991, pp. 10–20.

Psychotraumatology, edited by George S. Everly, Jr. and Jeffrey M. Lating. Plenum Press, New York, 1995.

abused or shocked in their own childhoods. Studies of adult rape victims demonstrate that they often were raped or incestuously abused as children and that they are quite prone to being raped again and again in their adult lives (Russell, 1986). Those who harm children have often been harmed themselves as children (Silver, Dublin, & Lourie, 1969). And some of those who indulge in self-mutilation or who make repeated suicide attempts give vivid past histories of long-standing childhood horrors (Herman & van der Kolk, 1987).

One could say that childhood trauma is so ubiquitous to the psychiatric disorders of adolescence and adulthood that we should forget it, that it cancels itself out. We know, however, that not every child is directly shocked or personally subjected to terror from the outside. Most children come from relatively kind, nonabusive families. Most youngsters are never enrolled in a pedophilic day-care center or happen upon a satanic cult. The chances of experiencing a frightening flood, hurricane, or earthquake are not that great. The chances of witnessing a murder or of being kidnapped are not overwhelmingly high. Numbers of children should be able to get through their childhoods without any direct exposure to a traumatic event or series of terrible events, and they apparently do so (Terr, 1983, 1990).

Even if we were to broaden the diagnosis of childhood trauma to allow any child mentally harmed enough by a single external event or a long-standing series of such events to qualify for a trauma-related diagnosis, as I will propose in this chapter, we could not possibly cover everything that we see in adults as a result of these early traumas—the borderline patients, the patients with multiple personality disorder, and the chronic victims or victimizers, for instance. We will still need our adult diagnostic schemes and our adult treatment plans. But perhaps if we looked in a more organized fashion at childhood psychic trauma and at what it does, we would recognize it as the important etiological determinant that it actually is. We could begin to see how childhood trauma works, and we could study it better.

Like childhood rheumatic fever, which causes a number of conditions in adulthood ranging from mitral stenosis to subacute bacterial endocarditis to massive heart failure, childhood psychic trauma leads to a number of mental changes that eventually account for some adult character problems, certain kinds of psychotic thinking, considerable violence, much dissociation, extremes of passivity, self-mutilative episodes, and a variety of anxiety disturbances. Even though heart failure and subacute bacterial endocarditis in adulthood look very different from one another and demand specific treatments, their original cause—the childhood rheumatic fever—gives an organizing pattern to the physician's entire approach. Every good internist thus knows how to obtain and assess a history of rheumatic fever, even though it was the pediatrician who originally diagnosed and treated the sick child.

In this chapter, I will define childhood trauma and point to four features that characterize almost all of the conditions resulting from extreme fright in childhood. These four features are seen in children suffering the results of events that were single, sudden, and unexpected (the classical Freudian traumas; Freud, 1920/1955; Pynoos, Frederick, Nader, et al., 1987) and in children responding to long-standing and anticipated blows—those resulting in the various child abuse syndromes (Green, 1983; McLeer, Deblinger, Atkins, et al., 1988) or survivor syndromes (Kestenberg, 1985; Kinzie, Sack, Angell, et al., 1986, 1989). These four features appear to last for years in the course of the condition. They are often seen in adults who were traumatized as children, even though the adults now carry other diagnoses. Only one or two of these four features may be evident in an individual traumatized as a child, but from the history it is often evident that the other features played an important part in the person's life.

I will divide all of the trauma-stress conditions of childhood into two rough categories and call them Type I and Type II childhood traumas. I will propose that children suffering from Type I traumas (the results of one sudden blow) differ in certain ways from children suffering from Type II traumas (the results of long-standing or repeated ordeals). I will conclude with a note on the crossover conditions: childhood traumas that appear to settle between the two major types that I propose.

This chapter is largely theoretical, although each point will be illustrated with a clinical example. It is based, in part, upon three studies: the Chowchilla kidnapping study (Terr, 1979, 1983, 1989), a retrospective study of 20 preschoolers suffering from a wide range of traumas that were documented by third parties (Terr, 1988), and a study of normal latency-aged children's and adolescents' responses to the Challenger space-shuttle explosion (Terr, 1990). The chapter is primarily based, however, upon my clinical notes taken from more than 150 individual children who came for evaluation or treatment after a variety of externally generated horrors. It is an attempt to provide a scheme of thinking about childhood psychic trauma. The chapter is not meant in any way as a last-minute addition to the DSM-IV process or as a proposal for a new and revisionary DSM-V. Instead, it is an outline and overview of a group of phenomena that may go their various ways into the adult diagnostic groups but that should still hold together in our thinking because of their association with the earliest traumas.

I will define childhood trauma as the mental result of one sudden, external blow or a series of blows that render the young person temporarily helpless and break past ordinary coping and defensive operations. As the reader will note, I have broadened the concept of trauma to include not only those conditions marked by intense surprise but also those marked by prolonged and sickening anticipation. All childhood traumas, according to my definition, originate from the outside; none is generated solely within the child's own mind. Childhood trauma may be accompanied by as yet unknown biological changes that are stimulated by the external events. The trauma begins with events outside the child, but once the events take place, a number of internal changes occur in the child. These changes last. As in the case of rheumatic fever, the changes stay active for years—often to the detriment of the young victim.

FOUR CHARACTERISTICS COMMON TO MOST CASES OF CHILDHOOD TRAUMA

There are several well-known characteristics that distinguish the traumas of childhood. Thought suppression, sleep problems, exaggerated startle responses, developmental regressions, fears of the mundane, deliberate avoidances, panic, irritability, and hypervigilance are prominent among these. I consider four characteristics, however, to be particularly important in traumatized children no matter when in the course of the illness one observes the child and no matter what age the child is at the time. They are (a) strongly visualized or otherwise repeatedly perceived memories, (b) repetitive behaviors, (c) trauma-specific fears, and (d) changed attitudes about people, aspects of life, and the future.

One note on traumatic dreams, the classic Freudian sign of trauma that I have not included in my list: The repetitive dream is a hallmark of trauma, but it is not always seen in childhood trauma, especially in children under age 5. Dreaming appears to be something that develops into a recognizable form by about age 3 or 4 (Mack, 1970). Before that, infants physically demonstrate that they are dreaming by making mouthing movements or little sounds in their sleep. Toddlers may scream during sleep without awakening, but this kind of dreaming is often too primitive and inexpressive to establish that traumatic dreams are actually taking place (Terr, 1987). In a study of 20 children with documented traumas that occurred before the age of 5, only 4 of them verbalized the contents of their dreams (Terr, 1988). In those children old enough to dream and to remember their dreams, traumatic dreaming may occur at intervals several years apart or in such deeply disguised forms that the process becomes extremely difficult to distinguish from other forms of dreaming.

Visualized or Otherwise Repeatedly Perceived Memories

The ability to resee or, occasionally but less frequently, to refeel a terrible event or a series of events is an important common characteristic of almost all externally generated disorders of childhood (Terr, 1985). Reseeing is so important that it sometimes occurs even when the original experience was not at all visual (Terr, 1985). Tactile, positional, or smell memories may also follow from long-standing terrors or single shocks, but the tendency to revisualize appears to be the strongest of all of these reperceptions in childhood trauma. Visualizations are most strongly stimulated by reminders of the traumatic event, but they occasionally come up entirely unbidden.

The vivid and unwelcome nature of returning traumatic visualizations marks them as special to these externally generated conditions. Children tend to see their traumas and old ordeals at leisure—during times when they are bored with classes, at night before falling asleep, and when they are at rest listening to the radio or watching television. As opposed to those traumatized as adults, traumatized children rarely find themselves abruptly interrupted by sudden, dysphoric visualizations.

Even those who were infants or toddlers at the time of their ordeals and thus were unable to lay down, store, or retrieve full verbal memories of their traumas tend to play out, to draw, or to resee highly visualized elements from their old experiences (Terr, 1988). In cases in which the facts of a sexual abuse are not known, for instance, children may indicate their internalized visions of the abuse by sketching what they see in their mind or acting it out almost like a movie picture. Such children may use their visual and positional senses, senses that may outlast the verbal memory itself, to draw pictures of themselves "at the most scary moments of [their] life." Of course, other post-traumatic features should be present, too, if the child actually was a trauma victim.

> Three and a half years after experiencing a series of traumatic events, a 5-year-old child was discovered (through pornographic photographs confiscated by U.S. Customs agents) to have been sexually misused in a day-care home between the ages of 15 and 18 months. The girl's parents did not dare speak to her about what they had learned from the investigators. They, in retrospect, realized that she had been sketching hundreds of nude adults beginning from the time when she had first begun to draw.
>
> While playing in my office, this child told me that a baby she had just drawn was "all naked" and "a bad girl." Unknowingly, she had just depicted herself. Despite the fact that the little girl's only verbal memory of the events was "I think there was grave danger at a lady—MaryBeth's—house," her volumes of drawings represented strongly visualized elements that she had retained and had needed to recreate from these very early, nonverbal experiences.

> A 40-year-old mental health professional began working at a facility for male juvenile delinquents. On his long rides home he began seeing himself as a toddler, attacked in a shack by a group of older children. The man drove to the town where he had lived until he was 4 years old, and he found the shack that he had "pictured." The shack stood catercornered to his old house.

Repetitive Behaviors

Play and behavioral reenactment are frequent manifestations of both the single blow and the long-standing terrors of childhood. Psychophysiological repetitions are less frequently observed in ordinary practice, but they gain particular importance in certain cultures (Kinzie, 1986). Post-traumatic play, defined by the players as "fun," is a grim, long-lasting, and particularly contagious form of childhood repetitive behavior (Terr, 1981). Although reenactments lack the element of fun, they also repeat aspects of the terrible events. Reenactment can occur as single behaviors, repeated behaviors, or bodily responses. Repetitive behaviors may even be seen in children who were exposed to traumatic events before the age of 12 months (Terr, 1988). In other words, children who have no verbal memory of their traumas may be seen to feel physical sensations or play or act in a manner that evokes what they experienced at the time of the event. The 5-year-old girl described in the previous case vignette, for instance, experienced "funny feelings" in her "tummy" every time she saw a finger pointed at her. The pornographic pictures confiscated by the customs authorities showed an erect penis jabbing the very spot on the child's belly that she had indicated when, more than 3 years later, she spoke of the "funny feelings."

The childhood survivors of single shocks and of long-standing terrors are usually entirely unaware that their behaviors and physical responses repeat something of the original set of thoughts or emergency responses. Thus the presence or absence of behavioral reenactment may at times be better determined from interviews with third parties.

Behavioral reenactments may recur so frequently as to become distinct personality traits. These may eventually gather into the personality disorders of adulthood, or they may recur physiologically so as to represent what seems to be physical disease. Long after most repeated nightmares have disappeared into deeply disguised form, reenactments continue to characterize the behaviors of traumatically stress children. Recent psychiatric investigation into the lives and works of important artists—Edgar Allen Poe, Edith Wharton, René Magritte, Alfred Hitchcock, Ingmar Bergman (Terr, 1987), Stephen King (Terr, 1989), and Virginia Woolf (Terr, 1990)—show that these artists reenacted childhood traumas behaviorally throughout their lifetimes and also played out their traumas in artistic works spanning their entire careers. If one could live a thousand years, one might completely work through a childhood trauma by playing out the terrifying scenario until it no longer terrified. The lifetime allotted to the ordinary person, however, does not appear to be enough.

> A 6-year-old girl walked into a circus tent and was suddenly attacked by a runaway lion. The animal tore open her scalp and bit into her face. The girl had to undergo several surgical procedures to repair what happened within a few seconds' time; she was left with an uneven hairline and a large bald spot. After the extraordinary experience, the little girl preferred "beauty parlor" to all other games of pretend. She combed her younger sister's hair repeatedly, often bringing the younger child to tears over the roughness of the combing. The little girl's dolls developed bald spots and uneven hairlines without anyone ever observing exactly how these anomalies came into being. The child, previously outgoing and friendly, stuck close to home and rarely ventured out into her neighborhood. At age 6, her main hopes for the future were to grow up and become a runway model or a "beauty parlor lady."

Trauma-Specific Fears

Some of the specific fears related to the shocks and long-standing extreme external stresses of childhood can be avoided by moving out of town or by changing houses or neighborhoods. Fears also can be conditioned away by repeatedly facing the feared object. Most extremely stressed or psychically traumatized children continue to harbor one or two trauma-related fears, however, well into adulthood. Fears of specific things that are related to experiences precipitated by traumatic events are fairly easy to spot, once one knows what the trauma might have been. This type of literal, specific fear is pathognomonic of the childhood traumas. Whereas neurotically or developmentally phobic children may fear all dogs, the dog-bitten youngster will fear the German shepherd, the Doberman, or whatever species actually created the traumatic state. Whereas neurotically anxious children fear growing up or getting married, traumatized youngsters fear (and re-create) oral sex, anal intercourse, or whatever particular sexual abuse they originally experienced.

Traumatized children tend also to fear mundane items—the dark, strangers, looming objects, being alone, being outside, food, animals, and vehicles, for instance. In fact, fears of the dark and of being alone are strongly connected with sudden shocks in the early years (Terr, 1990). But these mundane fears may also be connected with a number of other emotional disorders and developmental stages of childhood. The panic and extreme avoidances observed following terrifying events, in connection with this mundane group of fears, *do* make them important to childhood trauma. But the specific, literal kinds of fear noted in the preceding paragraph almost label the traumatic condition. When one sees this literal kind of fear lasting throughout the years despite the natural tendencies toward spontaneous desensitization, childhood trauma is the most likely cause.

> A girl was sexually misused by her father from age 5 to age 15, at which time she ran away from home, never to return. As a married adult of 38, she feared sex with her husband unless she initiated the act herself. She responded to the female-on-top or side-to-side positions, positions that had not originally been taken by her father. Any sexual positioning that was evocative of the incestuous set of sexual postures stimulated fear, pain, and revulsion.

Changed Attitudes About People, Life, and the Future

The sense of a severely limited future, along with changed attitudes about people and life, appears to be important in the trauma and extreme stress disorders originating in childhood. The limitation of future perspective is particularly striking in traumatized children because ordinary youngsters exhibit almost limitless ideas about the future. Truisms such as "I live one day at a time" or "I can't guess what will happen in my lifetime" come from the rethinkings that occur in the years after traumatic events. Ideas such as "You can't trust the police" or "You can't count on anything or anyone to protect you" also follow from single and long-standing, repeated traumas. Sexually traumatized girls may shrink away from men or accost them with overfriendly advances. Part of this behavior is reenactment, but part reflects attitudinal changes.

Limitations in scope and future perspective in childhood trauma victims seem to reflect the ongoing belief that more traumas are bound to follow. Traumatized children recognize profound vulnerability in all human beings, especially themselves. This shattering of what Lifton and Olson (1976) call "the shield of invincibility" and what Erikson (1950) terms "basic trust" and "autonomy" appears to characterize almost all event-engendered disorders of childhood. The feeling of futurelessness to the traumatized child is quite different from that of the depressed youngster. For the traumatized, the future is a landscape filled with crags, pits, and monsters; for the depressed, the future is a bleak, featureless, landscape stretched out to infinity.

> A 17-year-old boy, searching for a freeway shoulder on which to stop his disabled car, was hit from the rear by a speeder. The boy's automobile exploded. He flew out completely unscathed but watched helplessly as his best friend burned to death in the passenger seat.
>
> For months after the event the boy could not work and spent most of his days moping. He was plagued with bad dreams and fears of further disaster. He began psychotherapy, and when I said to him at the end of an early session, "See you next week," he asked, "How do you know it will be next week? Who knows? I may die on my way out of your office. I may be killed out there on the sidewalk. I don't count on seeing you next week. I live day to day—day to day."

> A 15-year-old girl came for psychiatric treatment because, since she was attacked at age 8, she had failed to volunteer or speak up in class. Since her acceptance in an academic high school, she could achieve no more than Bs because she was too quiet.
>
> The girl had experienced significant changes in her attitudes about life and people while she was lying in a hospital room for 3 months, following repairs to her vagina, anus, and peritoneum. A man had grabbed her from a Chinatown sidewalk on her way home from school, taken her into an abandoned garage, and attacked her vagina with a pair of chopsticks. The girl had decided after her ordeal that she was "chosen" by the deranged man because she had "showed too much." Never again, she had vowed to herself, would she ever "show." People could not be trusted, she believed; life had to be endured, not savored.

FEATURES CHARACTERISTIC OF TYPE I DISORDERS

The Type I traumatic conditions of childhood follow from unanticipated single events. These are classical childhood traumas, as defined by Anna Freud (1969). They are also the most typical post-traumatic stress disorders that one finds in childhood, usually meeting the criteria of repetition, avoidance, and hyperalertness that represent the major divisions in DSM-III-R. Those children who suffer the results of single blows appear to exhibit certain symptoms and signs that differentiate their conditions from those resulting from more complicated events. The findings special to single, intense terrors are (a) full, detailed, etched-in memories; (b) "omens" (retrospective reworkings, cognitive reappraisals, reasons, and turning points); and (c) misperceptions and mistimings. Type I traumas do not appear to breed the massive denials, psychic numbings, self-anesthesias, or personality problems that characterize the Type II disorders of childhood.

Full, Detailed Memories

With the exception of youngsters below the approximate age of 28 to 36 months, almost every previously untraumatized child who is fully conscious at the time that he or she experiences or witnesses one terrible event demonstrates the ability to retrieve detailed and full memories afterward (Terr, 1988). Verbal recollections of single shocks in an otherwise trauma-free childhood are delivered in an amazingly clear and detailed fashion. Children sometimes sound like robots as they strive to tell every detail as efficiently as possible. As a matter of fact, children are sometimes able to remember more from a single event than are the adults who observed the same event (Terr, 1981). A few details from a traumatic event of childhood may be factually wrong because the child initially misperceived or mistimed the sequence of what happened. But children with Type I disorders seem to remember the event and to give impressively clear, detailed accounts of their experiences.

This remarkable retrieval of full, precise, verbal memories of almost all single-blow traumas makes one conclude that these memories stay alive in a very special way, no matter how much conscious suppression the traumatized child is attempting. Memories of prolonged or variably repeated childhood abuses, in contrast, appear to be retained in spots rather than as clear, complete wholes (Terr, 1988). Amnesias, as a matter of fact, are often reported in children who seem to be heading for the multiple personality disorders of adulthood (Kluft, 1985). Children who have been repeatedly physically or sexually abused may waver in their accusations of abusers and in the completeness and the detail of their memories. But children who have been traumatized a single time do not often forget. As Malle says at the conclusion of his autobiographical film *Au Revoir Les Enfants* (1987), a tale of a single, terrible event from his boyhood in occupied France: "Over 40 years have passed, but I will remember every second of that January morning until the day I die."

> The first time that he visited the psychiatrist, a 5-year-old boy minutely described his stepfather's murder of his baby brother. The incident had occurred 2 weeks earlier. The boy knew just where under the television table in a motel room he had been hiding. He reported exactly where he had been

sitting and lying before taking cover. He described the types of blows that fell upon his younger sibling and meticulously repeated the attacker's phrases and threats. He said that he had been trying to forget all of this but could not. The boy's teacher had been reprimanding him for repeatedly hiding under the desks and tables at school, but neither teacher nor student recognized the significance of this "bad behavior."

Omens

During and after single-blow shocks, children tend frequently to ask themselves "Why?" and "Why me?" In this way they attempt to gain retrospective mastery over the randomness, the lack of control, and the inhumanity of the trauma that they endured. When children traumatized by a single event belatedly develop a reason why everything happened, a purpose to the entire affair, or a way that the disaster could have been averted, considerable mental energy goes into these reworkings of the past. I have termed these belated reshiftings, reasons, and warnings "omens" (Terr, 1979), whereas Pynoos et al. (1987) call them "cognitive reappraisals"; I believe, however, that we are describing the same phenomenon. This kind of rethinking and reworking occurs much more often after one sudden external shock than it does after a prolonged series of terrible experiences. Children who have found omens or reasons to explain why they suffer often feel intensely guilty. Although victims of Type II childhood trauma also experience profound guilt, the sense of guilt does not often consciously align itself to the "Why me?" question. The repetitions and long-standing nature of the Type II stressors make "How could I have avoided it?" a far less pressing question than "How will I avoid it the next time?"

The omen or cognitive reappraisal is a belated way in which the singly traumatized child tries to deal retroactively with what had been entirely unexpected—a sudden, surprising psychological blow. Because repeated horrors encourage a sense of anticipation and expectation, different means of coping come to be employed. These means of coping eventually create the defining characteristics of the Type II disorders, characteristics that are unmatched in the Type I disorders.

An 8-year-old boy's mother bought him a fancy skateboard, admonishing him to ride only on the sidewalk. The first Saturday morning the boy rode his skateboard on the sidewalk, he was run over by a car backing out of a neighbor's driveway. The boy commented years later, "I can't help thinking many, many times about what Mom said about riding skateboards on sidewalks."

A 16-year-old girl received a slice of pizza from her best friend as a birthday present. Biting into the pizza, she was poisoned by a corrosive toxin. The girl suffered from internal injuries for more than 6 weeks. Even though the real source of the poison was found by health officials at the pizza parlor, the injured girl thought again and again about the nature of her relationship with the friend who had purchased the pizza. In minutest detail she tried to figure out at what point her friend had decided to kill her.

Misperceptions

Misidentifications, visual hallucinations, and peculiar time distortions often occur to children who have experienced single, intense, unexpected shocks (Terr, 1985, 1990). In contrast to this, the long-standing, extreme external stresses that affect children are often engineered by perpetrators known to them—caretakers, teachers, or family members, for instance. Because of a child's familiarity with such perpetrators, the chances of early misperceptions become slim. Two important exceptions to this general rule are when a Type II victim thinks that he or she "sees" a once-familiar abuser years after losing track of the person and when a known, long-standing perpetrator was never perceived correctly by the child because of a disguise that he or she was wearing (as in satanism and cults).

Many of the Type I childhood traumas include visual misperceptions and hallucinations. These perceptual distortions may seem to indicate organic mental conditions or psychoses, but a few bizarre sightings do not "make" a brain disorder or a schizophrenic episode. Visual hallucinations and illusions are observed in children shortly after traumatic events and, at times, long after sudden, unanticipated shocks. Massive releases of neurotransmitters in the brain at the time of the terror may account for these problems with perception, but the types of substances and mechanisms are as yet unknown.

A 7-year-old girl rode in a station wagon alongside her sister and two cousins on a family outing to the mountains. A loose boulder from an adjacent hillside smashed into the roof of the girl's car, killing one cousin and the girl's older sister while sparing the girl and her other young cousin. For the ensuing year, the surviving girl "saw" her sister at her bedside almost every night. The dead sister visited the living child dressed in pink, green, and orange outfits. She appeared alive and uninjured, but said nothing. The young survivor felt upset by a sense of menace emanating from her sister's "ghost," yet at the same time she felt oddly comforted by the sight.

FEATURES CHARACTERISTIC OF TYPE II DISORDERS

Type II disorders follow from long-standing or repeated exposure to extreme external events. The first such event, of course, creates surprise, but the subsequent unfolding of horrors creates a sense of anticipation. Massive attempts to protect the psyche and to preserve the self are put into gear. The defenses and coping operations used in the Type II disorders of childhood—massive denial, repression, dissociation, self-anesthesia, self-hypnosis, identification with the aggressor, and aggression turned against the self—often lead to profound character changes in the youngster. Even though a repeatedly abused youngster may not settle into a recognizable form of adult character disorder until the late teens or early 20s, extreme personality problems may emerge even before the age of 5.

The emotions stirred up by Type II traumas are (a) an absence of feeling, (b) a sense of rage, or (c) unremitting sadness. These emotions exist side by side with the fear that is ubiquitous to the childhood traumas. Type II disorders, under the scrutiny of able mental health professionals, may come to be diagnosed in childhood as conduct disorders, attention-deficit disorders, depression, or dissociative disorders. Recognition of the expanded group of traumas that I am suggesting here may help to define a common etiology and range of findings for many of these childhood conditions. Of course, if a child originally was traumatized, one would expect to find vestiges of the repeated visualizations, repeated behaviors and physiological sensations, specific fears, and revised ideas about people, life, and the future that appear to characterize the childhood traumas.

Denial and Psychic Numbing

Denial and psychic numbing have long been considered classic findings of the post-traumatic stress disorders. Diagnostic problems often arise, however, because massive denial and emotional shutdown are so often evanescent or absent in children who have gone through single shocks (Terr, 1979). Although conscious suppression of thoughts will take place in any kind of trauma, and although brief, limited denial and numbing may last from moments to hours after a shocking event, massive denial and psychic numbing are primarily associated with the long-standing horrors of childhood (i.e., Type II traumas). Children who experience this type or stress may employ such extreme numbing and denial that they look extremely withdrawn or inhuman. When very young, they may assume the guise of "hospitalism" babies (Spitz, 1945) or of "hail fellow well met" superficiality (Terr, 1970), both of which are signs of failure in attachment and in personality organization.

Children who experience Type II traumas do not complain of going numb. The sense of "going dead" is one that depends upon years of subjectively knowing what it was to feel alive. Children who have been repeatedly brutalized or terrorized, though, do exhibit massive denial to the eyes of the trained observer. Such children avoid talking about themselves. They often go for years without saying a thing about their ordeals. They valiantly try to look normal at school, in the neighborhood, and on the playground. They may tell their stories once or twice and entirely deny them later. (This is quite different from some children who have experienced Type I traumas, who may tell their stories even at kindergarten show-and-tell.) Children who experience Type II traumas often forget even whole segments of childhood—from birth to age 9, for instance. Where one sees the difference between these "forgetful" children and ordinary youngsters is in the multiply traumatized child's relative indifference to pain, lack of empathy, failure to define or to acknowledge feelings, and absolute avoidance of psychological intimacy. Repeatedly brutalized, benumbed children employ massive denial—and when their denial-related behaviors cluster together, the resultant childhood personality disorder (one that cuts across adult narcissistic, antisocial, borderline, and avoidant categories) is massive.

Profound psychic numbing in children occurs as an accommodation to the most extreme, long-standing, or repeated traumatic situations. Childhood physical and sexual abuse represent two of these extremes. What still makes the underlying idea of trauma the correct etiology and pathogenesis here is the fact that the specific fears, the repeated play, the behavioral and physiologic reenactments, the tendencies toward visualizations, and the revised ideas about life, people, and the future seem to persist in so many of these children for years after the last abuse stops.

> Suzanna was 6 years old when her teenaged brother began sexually molesting her. (It turned out that he, in turn, had been sexually molested by a junior high school teacher before he began abusing Suzanna.) Suzanna once tried to tell her mother, "Nobody's supposed to touch you in your—" [she pointed at her genitals]. But after that she said nothing further to her parents, teachers, or friends until the school nurse discovered what was happening 2½ years after it began.
>
> On psychiatric examination when she was age 9, Suzanna spent much of the first hour pushing her index finger back and forth through a small hole she had made with the rest of her fingers. She repeatedly rubbed the loose couch pillows over one another. She said of her experiences with her brother, "He put his penis where I pooped. It hurt. I told him it hurt, but he said nuttin' back. I didn't like that at all. It didn't really frighten me. Not really, I just made up my mind to think about other things."
>
> When Suzanna was asked how she was able to do this mind trick—"to think about other things"—she replied, "I say 'I don't know' over and over to myself. When I say my prayers I keep saying the last word of the prayer. Sometimes I do it a hundred times. I say 'I don't know' a lot of times in my mind each day. . . . Sometimes now I find myself not feeling things. I don't feel sad or mad when I should be. I'm not afraid when I should be. I act silly and crazy a lot. The people at my school think I'm funny because of it."

Self-Hypnosis and Dissociation

Spontaneous self-hypnosis, depersonalization, and dissociation are important outcomes of Type II traumas. Children who have been the victims of extended periods of terror come to learn that the stressful events will be repeated. Some of these children—the ones, perhaps, who have an innate ease of hypnotizability—spontaneously fall upon the technique of self-hypnosis. This mechanism enables a child to escape mentally. Suzanna, the child described above, used the repetition of a single word (the last word of her prayers) to accomplish this escape from pain and worry. She also lulled herself into minitrances by saying "I don't know" in her mind. The children at school recognized her affect to be unusual, but only the child herself could recognize the self-hypnosis.

Traumatized children who use a great deal of self-hypnosis may in fact go on to develop adult multiple personality disorders (Spiegel, 1984). This is probably a rare condition. Spontaneous dissociation, however, accounts for a number of more commonly observed findings in abused children: bodily anesthesias, feelings of invisibility, and amnesias for certain periods of childhood life.

Multiple personality disorder, a syndrome in search of its own place in our diagnostic manuals, belongs here, at least in terms of etiology—the repeated, extreme, long-standing traumas of childhood. In children, periods of time that cannot be accounted for, problem behaviors, visual and auditory hallucinations, and headaches appear to indicate that the child is suffering from multiple personality precursors (Lewis, 1985). Most self-hypnotizing children who are Type II trauma victims, however, fall short of the multiple personality or precursors diagnoses. They instead develop anesthesias to bodily pain, sexual anesthesias, and extreme emotional distancings. Children who come to expect the repetition of terrors remove themselves in any way that they can; these emotional removals are not possible for the ordinary Type I trauma victim.

> Frederick was 7 years old when he was sent to live with his aunt because his mother found out—through a tape recording set up to catch her husband at infidelity—that Frederick's stepfather had been throwing him against walls while she worked the evening shift. Frederick did not tell anyone his yearlong story, despite two visits to the emergency room and one neighbor-instigated protective service investigation.
>
> While in his aunt's custody, Frederick glanced down at the playground pavement one day and saw blood. After several seconds of searching for a wounded companion, Frederick realized that it was *he* who was bleeding. The boy realized he could feel no pain.
>
> In a psychotherapy session I asked Frederick how he could make this sort of thing happen. "It jus' happens now," he said. "I used to pretend I was at a picnic with my head on Mommy's lap. The first time my stepdaddy hit me, it hurt a lot. But then I found out that I could make myself go on Mommy's lap [in his imagination], and Winston couldn't hurt me that way. I kept going on Mommy's lap—I didn't have to cry or scream or anything. I could *be* someplace else and not get hurt. I don't know how many times Winston punched me out. I wasn't always payin' attention. Like I told you, first I'd be at a picnic on Mom's lap. Later I didn't have to think of no picnic—jus' her lap. Now if something makes me bleed, I don't think of no lap at all. I jus' don't feel no pain."

> Jamie was repeated abused by his alcoholic father. He had also repeatedly observed his father beating his mother. At age 8, he saw his mother

shoot his father to death. When he was 9, Jamie was psychologically evaluated. At that time he told me, "I started some planets. I made my planets up as a game. But it's real now. It's no game anymore." Jamie described a safe planet he had invented long ago, his own planet. He also had invented a number of very unsafe planets where people "got killed." He said that he had come to achieve invisibility by repeatedly visiting his own safe planet and avoiding the unsafe ones. "Starting when I was 6," he said, "I began to feel invisible. When my Mom pointed a gun at my Dad . . . I was thinking like I didn't see it, like 'This didn't happen.' I blinked to see if I was dreaming. . . . I remember at first pretending I wasn't there—that didn't see it—that I was on my own planet. I had gone there a lot before. When Mom and Dad would fight, I would try not to hear, not to see. I'd try to go to sleep. Normally I couldn't. I'd try to get out of the room where they were. I'd try to visit my planet. But now my mind, yes, it just goes blank. Mostly it happens at home. A few minutes at a time."

Jamie repeatedly dreamed at night about his father's death, and he visualized the killing by day. But from the moment that his dad was shot, Jamie wondered if he himself could turn invisible. "I know I can," he said. "I do it here on earth. I do it all the time on my planet. You're just going to have to believe me. My friends believe it. . . . When my father was being shot I felt invisible. But if I turned invisible in front of everybody, they'd take away my powers."

Rage

Rage, including anger turned against the self, is a striking finding in those post-traumatic disorders that are brought on by repeated or long-standing abuses. One observes rage and its negative, extreme passivity, in those Type II disorders originating in places where trust originally resided. Dorothy Otnow Lewis and her group reported that among adolescent delinquents who go on to commit murder, chronic physical abuse is a key finding within a cluster of several other key findings (Lewis, Moy, Jackson, et al., 1985). The rage of the repeatedly abused child cannot safely be underestimated.

Reenactments of anger may come so frequently in the Type II trauma disorders that habitual patterns of aggressiveness are established. The rage may become so fearsome to the child as to create extremes of passivity as well. Wild fluctuations of both active anger and extreme passivity may so dominate the clinical picture that the young person is eventually given a diagnosis of borderline personality. Defenses against rage (such as passive into active and identification with the aggressor) also put their own peculiar stamps on the Type II child. Type II children have been known to attack their own bodies; self-mutilations or physically damaging suicide attempts occur. The festering anger of the repeatedly abused child is probably as damaging a part of the condition as is the chronic numbing. Both the numbing and rage, in fact, probably figure later in the antisocial, borderline, narcissistic, and multiple personality diagnoses that are so often part of the picture of the Type II traumatized child when he or she has grown up.

> A 5-year-old boy whose new stepmother had been tying him with ropes and leaving him locked up in closets behaved well at kindergarten. At home, however, he took scissors to his stepmother's best lingerie. He sprinkled India ink twice into the family wash. He consistently managed not to eat the food his stepmother prepared for him. The boy's stepmother said he was asking for the punishments she gave him—and so the abuses escalated.

> A 45-year-old woman had been a teenager in summer camp when the atomic bomb destroyed her home in Hiroshima. (Her immediate family was spared; all were out of town on August 6, 1945.) As an adult, the woman could not get along well with her American-born husband, alternately accusing him of laziness, ineptitude at work, and infidelity. From the time her daughter turned 13, the woman began believing the girl to be promiscuous, a liar, a drug addict, and a thief. The woman could not get along with her coworkers at an international law office. She was able, she said, to relate only to customers from Japan; they reminded her "of the people [she] used to know at home when [she] was a girl." I invited the woman to come to my office to talk about her experiences with the bomb. She made two appointments for this purpose but failed to appear for either. Obviously, too much time had lapsed to prove any cause-and-effect hypothesis here. It is interesting, however, that the woman's anger and suspiciousness rested only with American and American-influenced people. Native Japanese persons—the victims, not the perpetrators of the atomic bomb—were entirely spared her wrath.

CROSSOVER TYPE I–TYPE II TRAUMATIC CONDITIONS OF CHILDHOOD

When a single psychological shock takes a child's parent's life, leaves a child homeless, handicapped, or disfigured, or causes a child to undergo prolonged hospitalization and pain, the ongoing stresses tend to push the child toward the changes characteristic of the Type II childhood traumas. In these cases one often finds features of both the Type I and the Type II conditions. Those children with permanent handicaps, long-standing pain, or loss of significant objects are often forced into making significant character changes or using numbing tricks to minimize their pain. They may still retain, however, the characteristics typical of responses to single events—clear memory, perceptual distortions, and omens.

Perpetual Mourning and Depression

Psychic shock interferes with childhood bereavement, and vice versa (Eth & Pynoos, 1985). The combined psychological effects of shock and grief continue to drag on throughout childhood. As times goes by and the childhood mourning does not proceed through its ordinary stages (Osterweis, Solomon, & Green, 1984), the young trauma victim is reinjured—from the inside this time—through prolonged exposure to sadness and loss. The psychological condition of mixed mourning and trauma in youth may take the guise of major affective disorder and may have to be treated as such, at least at first. There is a high rate of depression in refugee children from brutal regimes (Kestenberg, 1985; Kinzie, Sack, Angell, et al., 1989). An explanation for this finding may be the unresolved trauma that potentiates and extends the unresolved grief, the grief that furthers the trauma, or both.

A 4-year-old boy watched his older sister's evisceration in a freak accident in a children's swimming pool. Before the disaster she had asked him to play, but he had refused. The little girl then sat down on an exposed drain pipe. The boy spent a couple of years after the accident using wooden blocks to build his own perfect pool. He blamed himself for not agreeing to play with his sister—an act, he felt, that caused his sister's injury. The boy retained a clear memory of all of the events and showed symptoms typical of Type I trauma.

Following his sister's death in transplantation surgery 2 years after the accident, the boy began to retreat from his friends, avoid participating in class, and stay silent much of the time. His teachers complained about his extreme passivity and said he was losing ground in subjects in which he had already proved himself. He lost some weight and stopped sleeping through the night. He lost his playfulness and began losing his friends. His 2 years of mourning had introduced Type II characteristics into a previously pure Type I disorder.

Childhood Disfigurement, Disability, and Pain

Children who are physically injured in psychically traumatic accidents tend perpetually to mourn old selves, personas that were previously intact and perfect. Even when perpetual grief is not the problem, post-traumatic physical handicaps frequently demand considerable personality reorganization so that the child can live with a new, limited self. In children, character rearrangements may become massive. To deal with the pain and procedures accompanying traumatic accidents, children may employ self-hypnosis. They may experience self-revulsion, unremitting guilt and shame, impotent rage at peers who shun and tease them, and sadness. Suicide attempts are not infrequent in this group. Robert Stoller (1989) suggested that some extremes of adult sadomasochistic behavior may originate in painful illnesses, injuries, and procedures during childhood: Rather than self-hypnotizing, these children may divert themselves from the pain by self-stimulating, and thus may perpetually associate their pain with sexuality. Childhood syndromes of injury and shock do not consistently qualify as post-traumatic stress disorders under DSM-III-R criteria (Stoddard, Norman, & Murphy, 1989). But these mixed syndromes of depression, numbing, rage, and fright often carry many of the four characteristics that I associate with childhood traumas. Adjustment to a sudden surprise, coupled with a prolonged ordeal, often lies at the origin of the problem.

> A kindergartner climbed onto a large department store display table, causing it to fall over onto her face as her grandmother paid the clerk for a purchase. The child's facial bones were smashed, and although they were beautifully reconstructed, she looked quite different than she had before the accident. Old friends did not recognize her, and other kindergartners told the child that she must be pretending to be Belinda—she could not actually *be* Belinda.
>
> The little girl, previously outgoing, mischievous, and vivacious, took on a quiet, remote, and perfectly well-behaved mode of behavior. Two years after the accident she said, "I was a devil before, but I was punished for it. Now I'm good." Despite the fact that she experienced bad dreams, liked to play alone under chairs, and tended to mutilate her dolls' faces, Belinda's character change dominated all other post-traumatic findings.

SUMMARY

There appears to be a group of problems brought on in childhood by the experience of extreme fright generated by outside events. Some of these childhood problems are created by one external shock, and others are created by a multiplicity of blows. Untreated, all but the mildest of the childhood traumas last for years; the child's responses, in fact, may create a number of different kinds of problems in adult life.

There are four characteristics, however, that seem to affect almost everyone subjected to extreme terrors in childhood. These findings seem to last and can be retrieved in histories. They include repeated visualizations or other returning perceptions, repeated behaviors and bodily responses, trauma-specific fears, and revised ideas about people, life, and the future. These four findings appear to remain clustered together in childhood trauma victims even when other diagnoses seem more appropriate. Like rheumatic fever, childhood trauma creates changes that may eventually lead to a number of different diagnoses. But also like rheumatic fever, childhood trauma must always be kept in mind as a possible underlying mechanism when these various conditions appear.

If one takes all of the disorders of childhood brought on by extreme external events and puts them into the general category of trauma, they can be roughly subdivided into two groupings: Type I, which is brought on by one sudden shock, and Type II, which is precipitated by a series of external blows. Crossover conditions are quite common and develop when one blow creates a long-standing series of childhood adversities.

REFERENCES

Bliss, E. (1986). *Multiple personality, allied disorders, and hypnosis.* New York: Oxford University Press.

Carmen, E., Rieker, P. P., & Mills, T. (1984). Victims of violence and psychiatric illness. *American Journal of Psychiatry, 141,* 378–383.

Erikson, E. (1950). *Childhood and society.* New York: Norton.

Eth, S., & Pynoos, R. (1985). Interaction of trauma and grief in childhood. In S. Eth & R. Pynoos (Eds.), *Post-traumatic stress disorder in children.* Washington, DC: American Psychiatric Press.

Freud, A. (1969). Comments on psychic trauma. In C. Baines (Ed. and Trans.), *The writings of Anna Freud: Research at the Hampstead child-therapy clinic and other papers* (Vol. 5, pp. 221–241). New York: International Universities Press.

Freud, S. (1955). Beyond the pleasure principle. In J. Strachey (Ed. and Trans.), *The standard edition of the complete psychological works of Sigmund Freud* (Vol. 18). London: Hogarth. (Original work published 1920)

Green, A. (1983). Dimensions of psychological trauma in abused children. *Journal of the American Academy of Child Psychiatry, 22,* 231–237.

Herman, J., & van der Kolk, B. A. (1987). Traumatic antecedents of borderline personality. In B. van der Kolk (Ed.), *Psychological trauma.* Washington, DC: American Psychiatric Press.

Kestenberg, J. (1985). Child survivors of the Holocaust—40 years later. *Journal of the American Academy of Child Psychiatry, 24,* 408–412.

Kinzie, J. D. (1986). Severe posttraumatic stress syndrome among Cambodian refugees. In J. Shore (Ed.), *Disaster stress studies.* Washington, DC: American Psychiatric Press.

Kinzie, J. D., Sack, W., Angell, R., et al. (1986). The psychiatric effects of massive trauma on Cambodian children. *Journal of the American Academy of Child and Adolescent Psychiatry, 25,* 370–383.

Kinzie, J. D., Sack, W., Angell, R., et al. (1989). A three-year follow-up of Cambodian young people traumatized as children. *Journal of the American Academy of Child and Adolescent Psychiatry, 28,* 501–504.

Kluft, R. (1985). Childhood multiple personality disorder. In R. Kluft (Ed.), *Childhood antecedents of multiple personality.* Washington, DC: American Psychiatric Press.

Lewis, D. O., Lovely, R., Yaeger, C., et al. (1989). Toward a theory of the genesis of violence. *Journal of the American Academy of Child Psychiatry, 28,* 431–436.

Lewis, D. O., Moy, E., Jackson, L. D., et al. (1985). Biopsychosocial characteristics of children who later murder: A prospective study. *American Journal of Psychiatry, 142,* 1161–1167.

Lifton, R., & Olson, E. (1976). The human meaning of total disaster. *Psychiatry, 39,* 1–18.

Mack, J. (1970). *Nightmares and the human conflict.* Boston: Little, Brown.

McLeer, S., Deblinger, E., Atkins, M., et al. (1988). Post-traumatic stress disorder in sexually abused children. *Journal of the American Academy of Child and Adolescent Psychiatry, 27,* 650–659.

Osterweis, M., Solomon, F., & Green, M. (1984). *Bereavement.* Washington, DC: National Academy Press.

Pynoos, R., Frederick, C., & Nader, K., et al. (1987). Life threat and post-traumatic stress in school age children. *Archives of General Psychiatry, 44,* 1057–1063.

Russell, D. (1986). *The secret trauma.* New York: Basic Books.

Silver, L. B., Dublin, C. C., & Lourie, R. S. (1969). Does violence breed violence? Contributions from a study of the child abuse syndrome. *American Journal of Psychiatry, 126,* 404–407.

Spiegel, D. (1984). Multiple personality as a post-traumatic stress disorder. *Psychiatry Clinics of North America, 7,* 101–110.

Spitz, R. (1945). Hospitalism. *Psychoanalytic Study of Children, 1,* 64–72.

Stoddard, F. J., Norman, D. K., & Murphy, J. M. (1989). A diagnostic outcome study of children and adolescents with severe burns. *Journal of Trauma, 29,* 471–477.

Stoller, R. (1989). Consensual sadomasochistic perversions. In H. Blum, E. M. Weinshel, & F. R. Rodman (Eds.), *The psychoanalytic core.* New York: International Universities Press.

Terr, L. (1979). Children of Chowchilla. *Psychoanalytic Study of Children, 34,* 547–623.

Terr, L. (1981). Forbidden games. *Journal of the American Academy of Child Psychiatry, 20,* 740–759.

Terr, L. (1983). Life attitudes, dreams, and psychic trauma in a group of "normal" children. *Journal of the American Academy of Child Psychiatry, 22,* 221–230.

Terr, L. (1985). Remembered images in psychic trauma. *Psychoanalytic Study of Children, 40,* 493–533.

Terr, L. (1987). Children's nightmares. In C. Guilleminault (Ed.), *Sleep and its disorders in children.* New York: Raven.

Terr, L. (1987). Childhood trauma and the creative product. *Psychoanalytic Study of Children, 42,* 545–572.

Terr, L. (1988). What happens to the memories of early childhood trauma? *Journal of the American Academy of Child and Adolescent Psychiatry, 27,* 96–104.

Terr, L. (1989). Terror writing by the formerly terrified. *Psychoanalytic Study of Children, 44,* 369–390.

Terr, L. (1990). Children's responses to the Challenger disaster. In *New research program and abstracts of the American Psychiatric Association* (143rd annual meeting). Washington, DC: American Psychiatric Association.

Terr, L. (1990). *Too scared to cry.* New York: Harper & Row.

Terr, L. (1990). Who's afraid in Virginia Woolf? *Psychoanalytic Study of Children, 45,* 531–544.

Terr, L. C. (1970). A family study of child abuse. *American Journal of Psychiatry, 127,* 665–671.

Terr, L. C. (1983). Chowchilla revisited: The effects of psychic trauma four years after a school-bus kidnapping. *American Journal of Psychiatry, 140,* 1543–1550.

Walsh, R. (1977). The family of the borderline patient. In F. Grinker & B. Werble (Eds.), *The borderline patient.* New York: Aronson.

19

The Process of Coping with Sexual Trauma

SUSAN ROTH and ELANA NEWMAN

The work that has been done at Duke over the past several years has led to a very simple conclusion: In coping with sexual trauma, the survivor must come to understand the emotional impact of the trauma so that she is no longer preoccupied or driven by negative feelings, and must grapple with the meaning of the trauma until an adaptive resolution is achieved. This process can lead to a variety of adaptive or maladaptive schemata, and a strong fear of overwhelming affects. Psychotherapeutic intervention is often required for successful completion of the process. In this chapter we present a conceptual system that characterizes this process, along with clinical examples and preliminary reliability findings in measuring the process. We selected case examples from the course of a group psychotherapy for female survivors of sexual trauma to illustrate potential use of the system in describing the process of coping changes over time. As a background, data on sexual trauma and the theoretical material that has guided our work will be briefly presented.

SEXUAL TRAUMA: RISK FOR PSYCHOLOGICAL DISORDER

Many studies that have utilized large random or probability samples provide estimates of the prevalence of sexual abuse in childhood, peer sexu-

SUSAN ROTH • Department of Psychology, Duke University, Durham, North Carolina 27706. **ELANA NEWMAN** • National Center for PTSD, Boston Medical Center, Boston, Massachusetts 02130. Reprinted from *Journal of Traumatic Stress*, Vol. 4. No. 2, 1991.
Psychotraumatology, edited by George S. Everly, Jr. and Jeffrey M. Lating. Plenum Press, New York, 1995.

al abuse among adolescents, rape among college students, and rape and sexual assault among adult women (see Koss, 1987, 1989, for reviews). Though the estimates vary, there is no question that they reflect the reality of a major social problem. As Koss (1987) notes, up to 40% of women experienced sexually abusive contacts as children. Completed or attempted rape was reported by 5% to 12% of adolescent girls, by 28% of college-age women, and by up to 44% of adult women. A significant proportion of these incidents are perpetrated by close friends or family members.

Not only are these instances of sexual trauma prevalent, they also present a serious mental health hazard (see Koss, 1987, for a review of these data). In addition to large community surveys (e.g., Burnam et al., 1988) that report a significantly increased risk of major mental disorders attributable to sexual assault, studies of hospitalized psychiatric patients, patients diagnosed with multiple personality or borderline personality disorder, psychotherapy outpatients, prostitutes, and prisoners overwhelmingly point to the mental health significance of sexual trauma (see, e.g., Jacobson, 1989; Koss, 1987). For example, Jacobson (1989) elicited a 48% prevalence of sexual trauma from an interview study of male and female outpatients, and Herman et al. (1989) found a 68% prevalence rate among subjects with borderline personality disorder.

THE PROCESS OF RECOVERY FROM SEXUAL TRAUMA

Sexual trauma confronts individuals with affects (e.g., rage, helplessness) and meanings (e.g., self-blame, challenged to the ability to trust) that are extremely difficult to manage and that may have long-term effects (Roth & Lebowitz, 1988). The emotional impact may be overwhelming, and the life implications of the meanings associated with the trauma may be disruptive and disturbing to face. Working through the trauma may require a major reexamination of one's beliefs and may result in an untenable view of the world or oneself. For example, sexual trauma victims may internalize the implicit and explicit communications of their attacker. In the vulnerable state that accompanies a sexual attack, the meaning of the rapist's actions (e.g., that the victim is an object, that she exists for his needs, that her own are irrelevant) may become an important part of how the victim comes to perceive herself, particularly when the rapist is an intimate. The range and depth of affective response is so great, at least in part, because of the range and depth of meaning that the assault may have. Epstein (1991), Horowitz (1986), Janoff-Bulman (1985), and McCann et al. (1988) all view cognitive schemata as playing a central role in the recovery process. Traumatic events challenge people's core beliefs about themselves, others, and the world and force people to search for an integrated meaning.

In the ideal case of coping (see Dye & Roth, 1991), an individual would gradually dose herself with manageable amounts of emotional material.

That is, she would be trying to come to both an emotional and cognitive understanding of the meaning of the trauma, and the impact it has had, a process that involves a reexperiencing of the affect associated with the trauma in the context of painful memories. Over the course of time, this process would lead to a reduction in symptoms and to successful integration of the trauma experience. For integration to occur, conceptions of the event(s) and conceptions of self and world must evolve until a match or fit is achieved (Horowitz, 1986).

Individuals faced with traumatic experiences, however, are often unable to undergo this ideal coping process, and they find themselves unable to integrate adaptively or recover from the trauma without psychotherapeutic treatment. Treatments can be viewed as effective to the extent that they facilitate a healthy integration process. Though integration may not be possible for some people because of their lack of psychological or social resources, or in some situations because of the severity of the trauma, we view the goal of integration as an appropriate one in most cases. The cost of avoiding thoughts or feelings associated with the trauma can be great in the long run. In the case of sexual trauma, the trauma often continues to unconsciously affect the individual in maladaptive ways, as when there is an increased vulnerability to repeated victimizations and/or to symptoms of severe post-traumatic distress. Even the more experimental research on coping strategies (see Roth & Cohen, 1986, for a review) is consistent with the conclusion that avoidance of stressful material is not the optimal adaptive end point.

AFFECT AND SCHEMA CHANGE

The system we will describe is designed to represent the coping or change process described above. This system defines affect and schema categories that describe the experience of sexual trauma, and these are drawn in part from the work by Roth and Lebowitz (1988) on sexual trauma themes. These categories can be described along a dimension that represents movement toward trauma resolution, which is the extent to which there has been both an emotional and cognitive understanding and resolution of the meaning of the trauma and the impact it has had.

The system is designed for representing a victim's accounts of her experiences in a situation where the discussion is focused on her trauma, whether it should occur within the confines of psychotherapy or not. The system documents the underlying coping process in terms of affect and schemata, and it does not address causes of or interventions that promote these changes. Though there are many similarities between the ultimate goals of our work and those of psychotherapy process researchers (Greenberg & Pinsof, 1986), we are not examining the psychotherapy process per se. We are examining the psychological process of coping that can occur in any number of contexts. The case examples we use in this chapter, however, are from a trauma-focused psychotherapy group.

Affects

The affects experienced by sexual trauma survivors include helplessness, rage, fear, loss, shame, guilt, and diffuse affect. Although guilt, shame, and self-blame (one of the schemata) are often hard to distinguish, guilt and

Table 19.1 Affect Categories

Helplessness. Helplessness describes not only the reality of and feeling inherent in being sexually traumatized, but also the longer-term effects of having experienced a profound loss of agency. Victims often describe feeling that someone else had absolute power over them; this feeling can generalize beyond the actual moments of the assault(s) to characterize other encounters with people, particularly men.

Rage. Rage can be manifested in different ways. Sometimes women will express anger directly at their attackers or about the event(s). Sometimes anger is focused at mothers for not protecting them, or at people who were not helpful in the aftermath of the trauma. Women also express anger indirectly, through describing the difficulties they have had with it. Problems with anger can include feeling ambivalent or guilty about one's anger, the fear that one's rage could prove to be emotionally overwhelming, and the fear that the expression of anger would further endanger the self.

Fear. Fear can result from fearing for one's life during the event(s) or as a consequence of reporting it, as well as from fear of the event being repeated. Fearfulness is usually seen in avoidant, phobic, and protective behavior that many women describe engaging in. It can be a central issue underlying the constricting effect that trauma has on many women's lifestyles. Fear of being reminded of the trauma (i.e., fear of affect) is not included here except when it relates to protecting oneself from further trauma.

Loss. Women often feel that their life has been altered by sexual trauma. This alteration can entail either a loss of a previous way of being and experiencing the world, or a loss of what they believed could have been theirs. Women sometimes conceptualize trauma as event(s) that stole something from them.

Shame. Women who have been sexually abused often describe deep feelings of embarassment, humiliation, and mortification for their exposure to sexual trauma. These feelings may be a result of the actual traumatic experiences in which the victim was humiliated, or a consequence of the stigmatization and secrecy surrounding the event(s). They may also refer to survivors' embarrassment about their reactions at the time of the abuse, or the present effects of the abuse including the power of their feelings.

Guilt. Guilt refers to survivors' feelings of culpability, the emotional self-reproach for having any role in the sexual trauma. Guilt may be experienced for enjoying the attention of the perpetrator, or experiencing some physiological pleasure in the contact. It may refer to victims' feelings surrounding disclosure or lack of disclosure, and may include feelings about the effects of the abuse or disclosure on other family members. Guilt may also arise from ambivalence about surviving the event(s).

Diffuse Affect. Trauma survivors often describe intense emotions that are nonspecific, such as pain, misery, discomfort, and hurt. Such expressions would be coded in this category.

Table 19.2 Affect Dimension

1. **No conscious awareness of affect, but evidence that it is there**
   A victim in a support group, for example, might tell another victim how angry that victim should be about what happened to her, although the first victim feels no anger about her own situation at all.
2. **Movement toward consciously acknowledging affect, but movement that is tentative in some way**
   A victim describes, for example, how she has to shut off the TV if the story has anything to do with a child losing something or someone important to her, because it reminds her of bad feelings she has.
3. **Acknowledgment of affect, but not directly associated with trauma**
   A rape victim, for example, discusses how fearful she is whenever she's driving alone, or is alone in her house at night.
4. **Awareness that affect is associated with trauma**
   An incest survivor discusses, for example, how ashamed she feels about what her father forced her to do to him.
5. **Attempt to deal with bad feelings**
   For example, an incest survivor decides to talk with her mother about what her father did to her in the hope that her mother will absolve her of some of her guilt.
6. **Resolution**
   For example, a rape victim realizes that her assailant no longer has any power over her and that she is in fact not as helpless to defend herself now that she has learned methods of self-defense.

shame were nevertheless added to the Roth and Lebowitz (1988) list of affects. Guilt and shame are more likely to come up in clinical contexts, particularly ones that extend over a longer period of time.

Affect dimensions are designed to be descriptive of the extent to which the victim has come to understand the emotional impact of the trauma and is no longer preoccupied with or driven by these feelings. Dimensions do *not* reflect the extent to which the person is feeling overwhelmed by emotion, as this could happen at any point in the recovery process. Tables 19.1 and 19.2 include the definition of the affect categories and the dimensions for affects.

We have chosen examples that illustrate the essence of the categories and dimensions and illuminate the potential use of the system in documenting the process of affect change over the course of weekly group psychotherapy. To achieve this goal, we will focus on the statements of one survivor, **N** (all initials have been changed), although we will also include a couple of examples from other survivors at the end to give a sense of all the dimensions. **N** is in her early 40s, and had been in a previous survivor group at Duke for 1 year before the start of the current group. Her statements over the first 5 months indicate movement toward resolution, primarily from dimension 4 to 6, although in the third month, there is a clear tentativeness in her acknowledgment of her feelings. In the statements that follow, for the sake of simplicity, we have indicated the most salient category when more than one category is discussed. The examples appear in chronological order.

> **N:** [having just remembered that her grandmother and cousin sexually abused her, in addition to the years of sexual abuse by her father that she had been conscious of for some time] I think that I have convinced myself that so many good things had happened, I just wasn't prepared for any of this [crying]. I think I thought I knew basically everything that was there to be confronted. I thought I knew most of the bad stuff in my life [sighs]. I would like to say I want to go home, but I can't go home because it's not safe. I'd like it all to stop. I can't stop. There are no options. The only option is to go forward. I know this part of the process, but . . . how do we label any of this? What it seems to me is new information to feel guilty about. [GUILT, DIMENSION 4; Session 3]

> **N:** There are just certain things I'm familiar with that seem like everyday stuff to say. You know, "Your shoe is burgundy." That doesn't hurt me. Saying that my father fucked me the day of my birthday doesn't hurt me, you know, it doesn't. But to say the other things I haven't said just seems so painful. I'm not sure if I'll be able to say them. I know I want to. Maybe I just have this false idea that it will make me feel more familiar . . . When you talk about me saying those things about my grandmother, that information came up very quickly. Those images, those feelings, and it sort of just knocked the breath right out of me. [DIFFUSE AFFECT, DIMENSION 4; Session 3]

In the two statements above, **N** is directly discussing the emotional impact of remembering new memories of sexual abuse by other family members. In the first example, she is describing feelings of guilt. She is also questioning the ways in which she has experienced the world as kind and good to her (benign world). In the latter example she is describing powerful uneasy feelings, which we consider diffuse affect. In both examples, she is clearly aware that her reactions are connected to the sexual abuse, thus dimension 4.

> **N:** What has happened is that I've got myself in a place where I feel very devastated. And where, almost on an hourly, minute by minute by minute by minute, that I have to do some kind of visualization. I have to do some kind of imagery. I have to pull up my totem pole, you know, to get through daily. And it is, it's left me verbally unable to articulate what's going on. I mean it's almost as if I'm disintegrating . . . It's left me out of control. [DIFFUSE AFFECT, DIMENSION 2; Session 11]

Although **N** is aware she is feeling intense negative feelings, she describes ways she needs to avoid actively her feelings so she is not continually suffering. Because there is no discussion of her feelings in relation to the trauma and she is clearly overwhelmed, we consider this statement to represent tentative movement toward acknowledging her feelings (dimension 2 under diffuse affect).

> **N:** I dislike the idea of coming so far to the point where I'm stripping myself and finding there's nothing about myself that I can claim as my own yet. Being 41 years old and having nothing that is mine—I did this with my life. So I think I'm experiencing more anger at that, the lack of having skills so that I would have some direction. **W** [group member] has talked about, "O.K., I'll be the brain." I didn't even, I couldn't even hold up that. There was nothing. I've never been able to say that before, but I really believe it now. It was all taken away from me. It was never there to begin with. And what chances I had of doing certain things that could've been called that, because I lacked the skills, my parents lacked the skills of parenting, it couldn't be developed. I grew up in fear. I grew up in shame. When I used to sing, and this, that, and the other, I went out with great trepidation, I was physically ill. I mean I discovered the other day that one of the reasons I don't eat breakfast is, I remember that's when my father would get me a lot of times. And I would go to school sick. I couldn't figure out why I'm always nauseous in the morning. Now I understand why going to work I had to stop at bathrooms, you know? It makes much more sense about the colitis all these years. It's like, Jesus Christ, did the man ever stop? You know? It was just, I went to see a nutritionist and she was telling me I had to eat in the morning. I was like, "What do you mean I have to eat in the morning?" That was a real big deal! And it was the first time I had remembered that. And finally I'm remembering a lot of things that I don't have any memory of. I think disclosing that information to **K** [individual therapist] last week, I think that it's been sitting up there like a dam. So I think, at the same time, here I remember all this other stuff that I didn't know was there, that if I knew I just wasn't acknowledging. So there's the whole mourning for my childhood. I mean I had no childhood. And now that I'm 41, I want to go through my childhood. And that's why I've been so despondent. That's why I've been so depressed. [LOSS, DIMENSION 4; Session 13]

In this unit, **N** is acknowledging the ways the sexual abuse prevented her from experiencing a safe and nurturing childhood which should have fostered, not hindered, her development (loss). She is angry at her parents for their thoughtless behavior, and this rage is also relevant. **N** is clearly associating her present feelings of loss and anger with the sexual abuse (dimension 4).

> **N:** S [the therapist] asked you [another group member, **C**] if you think your father intentionally meant to hurt you, and your voice got quieter. Maybe it didn't, but it seemed that way to me. And you said, "Not intentionally," but I wanted to slap somebody around. How you said it is how I feel sometimes. I felt timid and shy, not wanting to blame anybody, be generous and taking all the blame for something. And how could you possibly be responsible? In a way, just in a way, I wanted to shake you, and I wanted you to be angry for me. [talking now to the therapist] I've gotten angry in here and it was pretty intense. And I was aware of wanting to shake **C** so she'll get angry and I'll feel better. I'm angry at her father. I felt anger, but it's difficult to feel that toward my father. [RAGE, DIMENSION 4; Session 14]

N: The big thing I can remember is being fucked on Christmas Eve and then waking up the next day and having these goddamn Christmas presents under the tree. Now I'm angry. Then it was just another day. [RAGE, DIMENSION 4; Session 14]

Again, **N** is clearly connecting her current angry feelings with her experiences of sexual victimization.

N: Um, this is not such a big deal, but I do want to acknowledge your observation that I'm doing better. Um, I think that is true, um, and I'm not quite sure why, because I think that a lot of the issues that have come up have struck me as being pretty overwhelming. But I don't have the same kind of—they didn't have the same kind of effect on me as, say, as have the other memories or recollections or the actual feeling that I was going through the experiences with my father or mother or whatever that the first group had. I think that what you said, awareness, has really been the key issue. It's taken me so long to, um, be able to hold the awareness close to me. It still—something will happen and I will react quite passionately. I called you, if you remember. It was about the situation with **W** and **O** [group members], and my reactions to that, because I had a very difficult time that group and was in a lot of pain, and I couldn't quite figure out why it was, and I'm really grateful to you for realizing that and also doing something about it . . . Because when I called you and I though I was hysterical, I don't know if I sounded that way, but I was crying, I was upset, but as soon as I got off the phone, I was able to go about putting on my clothes and going to work and functioning and facing these people, and it wasn't until the weekend that I realized that I had actually dealt with it, and it was really a funny kind of feeling. I've often used the word of just throwing up my feelings and vomiting them out, but I realized that actually what happened was that I have absorbed some of the information and had been able to make some decisions about it and it wasn't as painful as it had been previously. And, um, I think that's part of what's happening now is the dealing with the feelings, the unexpected realization that I am actually feeling what's happening to me, and that I'm acknowledging them, those feelings. And it's just such a surprise that I survived through those feelings. Um, um, I would like some of the things that happened to go away, but I think that I'm probably taking a little more, that I'm capable now of taking more responsibility whereas before I think that I was so fragile in many ways and even though that fragility comes back, but it's not quite the same. I'm doing this very poorly because it's still so new to me, but, um, I just have this sense of being more responsible, taking more responsibility for my feelings . . . It doesn't mean that the pain has gone away, because they don't, um, but it's not as frightening. Um, I know that I can make it through the night where I used to not believe that was true. I haven't been howling in a corner. I haven't reduced myself to crawling around on all fours. Um, there are times when I feel very uneasy and what I've been doing is, I rather acknowledge that fear where I used to carry a baseball bat around the house or lock doors behind me. I was telling **K** [therapist] today, that it's really significant that I can take a shower without locking the door or blocking it or to sleep at nighttime on my stomach without having covers up around my neck. It's so many ways I've tried to protect myself that I see those things falling away. It's really, it's pretty neat, you know? It's like, do normal people feel—are normal people grateful [laugh]? If they're not, let me tell them about it. [DIFFUSE AFFECT, DIMENSION 5; Session 19]

In this example, **N** is describing how she is learning to accept her negative feelings and, if necessary, take action to gain support or information. Dimension 5 is indicated because this depicts efforts to deal with diffuse affects. This example is also dealing with fear, as **N** describes facing her fears (dimension 5).

N: [talking to another group member] I think it takes a long time to realize that you've made progress. I really think that what you're going through is part of a movement, and it's a motion in a forward movement, but I think even when you're going through what you're doing now, it's very difficult to realize that's what's happening, because it is so painful. It is so scary. Because, you know, it's somebody telling us that we should, we need to deal with these feelings. We need to feel the anger, we need to talk about what happened to us. And what happens is, that my expectation when I came in was, "So I'll get better." Well, I didn't get better at first, I got worse. And I really thought that I couldn't survive. There are many times when I came in here and I would just say, "I'm not sure I'll live long enough to get well." I never really talked about suicide, but I really didn't believe I could get through it. You know, the things that you're talking about, and the kinds of things that you're becoming aware of, um, are familiar to me. And it's funny for me sitting here listening to you talking about your mother, you know? I can relate to that, because my mother has never touched me in an affectionate way, and still does not touch me, and has never told me that she loves me. And I now accept the fact that she never will, and I now no longer reach for her and give her a kiss, you know? Because I no longer want to have her like this. And now, I mean, usually that was such a big deal to me. It still is to a certain extent, but it's not as painful. It just—I'm saddened by it now. And it's come to the point where the sadness I feel about things is not as overwhelming as the recognition of those things in the beginning, or even in the middle of the process. It's sort of, now that I can look at things, and I'm sorry it didn't happen, I'm sorry I didn't have a childhood. I'm sorry, like you, I can't remember things. I don't remember any special birthdays. I don't remember even, like I know I went to dances when I was a teenager, but I don't remember any of 'em. I just don't remember any of that kind of stuff. What I remember is protecting myself from my father, or doing exactly what he wanted, or keeping peace in the family. Those are the things that I remember. I don't remember all the other stuff. I'm sure some stuff went on, but I just don't remember. But for some reason now, I don't know why, it doesn't seem quite as devastating. Like I can hear it from you now. It's such a queer kind of feeling right now to hear you and know how I felt when I began to recognize those things. I just want to tell you that I really believe it's going to get better for you. [LOSS, DIMENSION 6; Session 19]

In this unit, **N** has acknowledged the magnitude of her losses, but no longer experiences the loss or is driven by it. We consider this a resolution and indicate dimension 6. In this unit, too, **N** seems to have resolved many of her negative feelings (diffuse affect).

Two additional examples from two different survivors illustrate dimensions 1 (no conscious awareness) and 3 (general acknowledgment). In the first example, the therapist needed to point out the way in which **B** has projected her own feelings of loss onto her niece. This is an example of the client not being aware of her own feelings (dimension 1). This example illustrates "people trustworthy," dimension 1, because **B** is addressing issues of betrayal.

> **B:** She [niece] is really the most important person in the world to me now, and she's like a picture, so innocent. She's not to the point yet of thinking anyone's bad except the dog when it barks or something. She's so innocent, so outgoing. She's lovable. I guess I see her as—I don't want her to lose that, all the trust she has. She's so trustworthy [she means trusting]. And she knows when you hold her she's not going to fall. I don't want her to lose it.
>
> Therapist: Like you lost it?
>
> **B:** I guess so. [LOSS, DIMENSION 1; Session 14]
>
> **C:** When I start to get really aggravated, it's because I really feel that I am sort of helpless, or feeling like I don't know how to do something, or just because—I'm helpless because I feel like he's controlling the argument or topic of conversation; helpless a far as the way I'm reacting. Does that make sense? I think that's what really gets me going! [HELPLESSNESS, DIMENSION 3; Session 14]

In this unit, the client labels her feelings of helplessness in regard to her husband's behavior, but is not addressing her sense of helplessness in regard to her trauma. The therapist believed, however, that the origin of the feeling was the traumatic event. This acknowledgment of affect distinct from the trauma is thus dimension 3. This unit also deals with rage, dimension 3.

Schemata

We have adopted Epstein's (1991) four fundamental beliefs as our four major schema categories. Epstein argues that there are four fundamental beliefs that are likely to be invalidated by a traumatic event: (1) the world is benign, a source of pleasure, a rewarding place; (2) the world is meaningful, predictable, controllable, and just; (3) the self is worthy (lovable, good, competent); and (4) people are trustworthy and worth relating to. The invalidation of these beliefs leads to a compensatory search for meaning. The construction of a modified belief system that can assimilate the traumatic experience is required, and this belief system can be either adaptive or maladaptive. The essence of an adaptive resolution is the modification or accommodation of a belief system in a manner that permits realistic coping with, and enjoyment of life, while recognizing its limitations. Maladaptive solutions tend to maintain a chronic state of negative affect, and provide an overly restrictive and biased way of relating to the world (Epstein, 1991). On the basis of the Roth and Lebowitz (1988) work and our clinical experience, we have added several subcategories under "self worthy," which are self-blame, reciprocity, alienation, and legitimacy.

Dimensions for schema material are designed to be descriptive of the extent to which the victim has grappled with the meaning of the trauma and achieved an adaptive resolution, and they parallel the dimensions for Affect. Tables 19.3 and 19.4 include the definitions of the schema categories and the dimensions for schemata.

To illustrate the various categories and show the system's potential utility in describing the process of schema change over time, we will focus again on statements by **N** from group psychotherapy sessions. In the following series, covering the first 5 months of the group, there is clear movement toward **N** resolving that she is a worthy person. As before, we have indicated the most salient category in each case. The examples appear in chronological order.

> **N:** I can't remember the actual event, but I was with **K** [individual therapist], and we were discussing something. And there was a realization, like a breakthrough, just one of my memory lapses. I can't remember exactly what it was, but it was extremely painful. And I was facing her and was looking at her, but what was happening inside was I had lowered my head, and when I raised my head up, what I saw was the horizon, and there was nothing there, and I was alone against the horizon. It was nothing to hold on. And at that moment, I felt as if I were, as, if I had a gun, I would kill myself because the pain was so unbearable. And it was the realization that if what we had just discovered was true, which it was, then I had lost everything that I had worked for, everything that I had done, leaving **R** [husband] [crying]. And **K** [individual therapist] was very perceptive about that, and she—I was able to tell her what was happening. She said something, I guess, and I was actually telling her as I was experiencing something, and she immediately asked me to think of something I—that I could hold on to. Was there something that I could hold onto? And this totem pole just came up. It was taller than the horizon, and I cannot see the top of it. And it goes down to the core of the earth and it's made of rock. And it's solid rock. So no matter what would happen, even if parts of it were to crack or break or shatter or whatever, it is so strong that it would never disintegrate. And so far there are only two masks completed. And one is terribly, terribly, terribly ugly, with holes and gaping holes and snarls and it's black. It's blacker than the black. It's uglier than anything you could imagine. And it took me a while to realize that is all the ugliness I feel about myself. It's someplace to deposit it. And then there's another mask that has some colors, green and yellow and blue, and there are some sort of smiles, but not really yet. But it's still, it makes me feel good to see it. It makes me feel hopeful. [SELF WORTHY, DIMENSION 5; Session 3]

Table 19.3 Schema Categories

Benign World. Survivors of sexual trauma may question notions of the goodness and benignity of the world. As a consequence of their experiences, they may see the world as malevolent, dangerous, and/or unrewarding. An adaptive resolution would allow for a recognition of danger and the like in the world, but within limits.

Meaningful World. Sexual trauma challenges a victim's ideas about order and meaning in the world, raising concerns about fairness or justice, predictability, and control. A victim may learn to experience the world as unpredictable, uncontrollable, and unjust. An adaptive resolution would allow for recognition of these things, but within limits.

People Trustworthy. Sexual trauma involves a severe violation at the hands of another person. It challenges one's ideas about interpersonal relationships, often leading to expectations of others being dangerous, unhelpful, unfair, capable of deception, betrayal, and exploitation, and generally untrustworthy. An adaptive resolution requires the recognition that some, but not all, people may have these qualities, or that any particular person is trustworthy within limits.

Self Worthy. Lowered self-esteem following sexual trauma may derive from several possible sources. A person's sense of her own competence may be diminished because trauma, by definition, involves a condition of profound helplessness. A person's sense of inadequacy is likely to be heightened by the presence of problematic post-trauma symptoms. In addition, a person is likely to irrationally blame herself for not meeting unreasonable demands which she places on herself about what she could have or should have done in the situation. She may also feel diminished by the loss she has experienced. Finally, she may have a sense of being flawed, or damaged as a result of experiencing the traumatic event(s). One's sense of her own vulnerability must be cut down to size, and not be a cause for her generalized sense of unworthiness.

Self-Blame. Self-blame is defined as a woman holding herself responsible in some way for abuse perpetrated against her, and/or her behavioral responses to it (i.e., arousal). Though self-blame might serve a number of self-protective functions, such as restoring a sense of control, avoiding the sense of helplessness or the experience of rage, it is not adaptive for victims to maintain the belief they were to blame in any way for the abuse and its aftermath.

Reciprocity. Sexual trauma victims may feel that as a consequence of the abuse, they are not worthy of equal relationships in which they can both give and receive support, and in more intimate relationships, feel unworthy of both giving and receiving love.

Alienation. Feelings of alienation are related to the extremity of the experience of trauma, which leads women to feel different and set apart from other people. They often perceive that others cannot understand or relate to their experiences. The feeling of alienation is also related to keeping the abuse a secret. A consequence of the feeling that one must keep an important part of one's experience a secret is that it leads to a discrepancy between one's inner and outer experience of self, thereby promoting alienation. People can feel detached, disconnected, and fractured from their own self-definition.

Legitimacy. Legitimacy refers to whether the victim believes that the trauma can account for her emotional experience. Victims often describe feeling deviant in their reactions, that their feelings are somehow not valid, and that they reflect a deficit in their functioning.

Table 19.4 Schema Dimensions

1. **No conscious awareness that there has been any disruption or invalidation of schema, but evidence for same**
   A victim might describe interpersonal encounters that suggest an extreme lack of trust of others, for example, without in any way acknowledging that this is an issue.
   Note: We are aware that in cases of early and chronic childhood abuse, it is difficult to talk about a disruption or invalidation of schemas such as the world is benign, meaningful, etc. It is perhaps more appropriate to talk about the early trauma as formative in the development of schemas we would consider maladaptive. In any case the event must come to have some other meaning that would allow for the development of more adaptive schemas.
2. **Movement toward consciously acknowledging that there is uncertainty about some beliefs, or that there is a maladaptive schema, but movement that is tentative in some way**
   A victim says, for example, that lately she's confused about how the world works and that she's been avoiding going to church because some uncertainty about her faith in God makes her too anxious to think about it.
3. **Acknowledgment that some basic beliefs feel threatened, or acknowledgment of a maladaptive schema, but not directly associated with trauma**
   A victim states, for example, that she feels poisonous some of the time, and very different from other people most of the time. This makes it hard for her to have any close relationships.
4. **Awareness that basic beliefs have been challenged by the trauma, or awareness that one has, as a result of the trauma, adopted a schema that is maladaptive**
   For example, a victim describes how she holds herself responsible for what happened with her father. She discusses how she should have done something to stop him, and how her lack of action makes her culpable. She recognizes how badly this makes her feel about herself.
5. **Attempt to resolve discrepancy trauma presents, or to change maladaptive schema**
   For example, an incest survivor realizes that, in spite of how unrewarding her life has been so far because of the incest, that maybe the world isn't all bad, and she resolves to concentrate her efforts on finding pleasurable and rewarding experiences.
6. **Resolution**
   An incest survivor discusses, for example, how she's learned to discriminate trustworthy from untrustworthy men.

In this segment, **N** is describing how visualizing a totem pole helps her resolve the discrepancy she perceives about her negative self-appraisals. Because **N** is actively grappling with a means of changing her self-concept, we see it as an attempt to change her maladaptive self-worth schema (dimension 5).

> **N:** He had said something around Christmas, and I can remember thinking to myself, what if I just said, 'I'm really having a hard time, daddy. I'm wondering if you remember what happened when I was a little girl?' And if he said, 'Yes,' I would say, 'Well, can you tell me why it happened?' [crying] It felt like if I could do that—but I am still so hung up on his anger, even though I see him differently. When I hear myself say those words, I see him

falling to pieces. And I hear my mother saying, 'Save his life. Don't do anything to upset him.' I'd like to just have a day in peace. I just feel so responsible if anything like that would happen. I don't think I could handle it. I don't . . . I keep coming back to the fact it must have to do something with me, because what I remember with my other two sisters, I think it's because my mother saw them as needy and she didn't see me as needy. At some point, I became her friend. She talked to me about daddy. She cried to me about daddy. And just as I was calming daddy, I was protecting my mother. [SELF-BLAME, DIMENSION 4; Session 14]

In this unit, **N** is examining her own role in her family in the context of the incest, and it describes dimension 4 under self-blame because she is associating her sense of responsibility directly to the sexual abuse.

N: I still have a lot of difficulty with interpersonal situations, and um, all those things are related to the inability to develop skills as a child to relate to people, and what was proper and what was normal, what's acceptable, um, the lack of negotiating as a child. Um, so I still don't know how to do that as an adult. And it's something that I would really like to be able to work on. Because that's where I feel like there's often times when my behavior is inappropriate.

C: [group member] What kinds of things are hard for you to negotiate?

N: Anything. If you want something, you get it. If I wanted something else, I don't.

C: Negotiating needs?

N: Right. And it doesn't matter what level those needs are. When I have victories, when there is a situation where I've been able to put my needs forward and I don't take away entirely from that other person . . . it's a victory . . . but . . . it's really hard to do. [RECIPROCITY, DIMENSION 5; Session 19]

N is asking for help to deal with her difficulties in asserting and accepting her interpersonal needs. She clearly sees this behavior in the context of her incestuous abuse and is trying to alter her behavior and views about it, thus we see it as reciprocity, dimension 5.

N: Going to Washington with these people, um, I went to Washington with three other women whom I do not know very well. I drove my car. Usually I'm very—I have to know people. You can't share a lot of things with people. I slept in a room with a woman that I barely know. Well, I know her, but I don't know her. It's sort of an acquaintance. I met another woman there. Then another woman that I've only met one other time. I mean, this was a really big deal to me. I went to Chinatown, walked all over Washington without any regard to where bathrooms were. I mean, this is a real significant thing to me. Had an attack of colitis on Saturday morning as we were going to the museum to see the O'Keefe exhibition, and they're already down to the corner from the building lined up 15 deep, and I'm saying to these women, "I can let you out because I have go find a bathroom." No, they were coming with me. And I didn't fight them. I didn't spend 14 hours saying, "Get out of the car, I'll do it on my own." And I didn't feel badly. I mean I felt sort of badly about that this was happening, and we were going to be late, and this and that and the other things, and we might not get tickets, you know, and they joked about it too. Well, if we didn't get tickets, I was saying, I would tear the building down brick by brick, because I was going to see her today. Because I was sure she was in there, not really, but you know, it was O.K. I put myself in a situation where I knew things would happen that would, quote, be out of my control. But that's what I meant about responsibility. I felt like I was being responsible to me. I was acknowledging that I have some rights. I'm worth taking care of. It's a really big deal, you know. Um, we drove all over Washington. I had wanted to see, I like the Lincoln memorial and the reflecting pool and the Vietnam memorial and I always go there. I'm always one of those that does this and that's something I really wanted to do along with the exhibit, and I was able to say that without sounding like, at least I didn't feel like I was being dominating. And I got to walk by the reflecting pool and it was pouring down rain and I did—felt as if I was really free. It was some sense that I allowed these women to sort of tolerate my frailties, and I was exposed, and I couldn't tear myself away from the exhibits, you know? I'd go back and forth and it didn't matter to me at all that these women were already gone. Two women didn't like it and two of us just [trails off]. And when I saw this other woman sort of hovering around this picture, it was just great. It was wonderful. And after we left and we got downstairs and they sort of were waiting, I said, "I hope I didn't keep you too long," and "No, this is an opportunity of a lifetime." And that's what I felt. So what if they had to wait? That's great, that was fine. It's OK with them. So that was pretty exciting. Walking in Georgetown at nighttime, you know, like 10:30 to 11:30 at night, going in these itty bitty, tiny weeny shops, trying to get into a bathroom, finally telling a person, "I want the key to the bathroom, there are six of us and we all have to pee." It was just really neat, and people didn't look to me like, "You crazy woman," you know, "You have to go to the bathroom, that's not our concern." I mean, these were just really—it was just really neat. And there were all these people, these kids walking arm and arm slurping on each other, and I found that wasn't as offensive as it's usually been. It's just a lot of different things, "Oh, that's OK, and this is all right too." It was like, bam, bam, bam, bam, bam. It was like finally a culmination of where the last, almost two years have been. So, I think, you know, in the last group, I think I told you one of the reasons I came was that I sort of had a brief encounter with what I call an illusion of peace . . . It's less an illusion, it's not complete, but there are times and longer periods of time of experiencing that. And it's, um, it was the right decision [working on the incest]. I mean, sometimes I've lamented over the decisions that I've made, and the upheaval that my life has been in the last four years, and the loss of my marriage, the loss of time spent with my son, because I've had to put so much time in this. But, it's all been worth it, so I'm doing better. [SELF WORTHY, DIMENSION 6; Session 19]

This unit illustrates **N**'s ability to accept herself and take her needs as worthy. We consider this experience to represent a resolution in her self-concept (dimension 6). Since she also expresses her ability to negotiate with others and recognize her reactions and needs as valid, this also illustrates reciprocity and legitimacy, dimension 6.

Two additional examples from two different survivors illustrate the "people trustworthy" category at an earlier point in the coping process. The first example portrays a woman who is aware she has difficulty trusting but has no insight about the relationship of trust to the abuse. This illustrates dimension 3 under trust (as well as helplessness and rage). The latter unit demonstrates the client's ability to understand her trust difficulties in the context of the sexual abuse (dimension 4).

> **O:** I think trust issues are becoming a big deal for me again. I find myself—you asked me a couple of weeks ago if I was angry at you, and I couldn't understand why. Um, why you were getting that, and it's just, really, I'm getting myself in this terrible . . . predicament. Why am I continuing to act in ways which are distasteful to me, um, a lot? . . . The fact that I thought about it and I realized that . . .
>
> Therapist: You were angry at me? [Therapist and **O** laugh.] Good. What were you angry at me about?
>
> **O:** I wasn't angry at you. It was—see—I, um, guess I [trails off]. It's the moving forward and trusting, and then the fear, "Oh my God". . . I've been moving so much and trusting you that I was really starting to resent the whole major nature of everything. I've been seeing that happen elsewhere.
>
> Therapist: Like where else?
>
> **O:** Well, nothing on the level of intensity I feel about you . . . I don't try and trust people, you know. But with my friends and **Q** (husband), and just in general with other people, I feel like I've been expressing anger and in turn being snappy.
>
> Therapist: What in relationships do you start to resent?
>
> **O:** Well, I'm not really sure.
>
> Therapist: Feeling dependent?
>
> **O:** Yeah, you're quick [laughs], and I guess the other part is helpless and out of control. Some minor issues [laughs]. [PEOPLE TRUSTWORTHY, DIMENSION 3; Session 12]
>
> **C:** I mean, I guess like I said, reading that article, it just really hurt because it was as if someone else was telling me what I had never been aware of for so long, is that I had really been taken advantage of and was treated so wrongly! And it was by someone who was supposed to be just the opposite, you know,

> and have my best interest [trails off]. In some ways it's shocking to me, maybe because I had my own perception of the way my family was for so long. This new finding, I don't know . . .
>
> Therapist: What do you remember about your father when you were a kid?
>
> **C:** Well, he wasn't around a lot. He worked 'till about eight o'clock. As a kid, I remember my father out in the yard a lot. You know, I would be helping him with cutting the bushes and a lot of time would be spent outside doing those kinds of things. Um, I would always go, like on Sunday morning, I would always—he would go drive and get the paper, and we'd go get ice cream or something. . . . You know, we would go get ice cream and the paper, what not [crying as she speaks]. And I remember we would go to the park, you know, and feed ducks or go on the swings. And those are really good memories. I'm not sure why I'm crying. I'm lost for words. I don't know, maybe because I have some really good memories of him. And I did, I was idolizing him, he was so good in those days [sobbing]. And then he just shit on me later and I was so deceived. [PEOPLE TRUSTWORTHY, DIMENSION 4; Session 16]

RELIABILITY IN MEASURING THE COPING PROCESS

As we believe our clinical examples illustrate, our conceptual system has potential for measuring the coping process in a systematic way. We have begun the work of gathering information that will allow other researchers and clinicians to benefit from our work. For the purpose of establishing an initial level of reliability for the use of the system in measuring the coping process, ratings were made from transcripts of five sessions from the trauma-focused psychotherapy group of female survivors. The group consisted of six female survivors who met with two psychotherapists for 2 hours weekly. The group met for 54 weeks, although three members terminated earlier, at weeks 25, 29, and 35, and several new members joined at week 36. The particular sessions for the reliability round (19, 23, 24, 25, 26) were not chosen in any systematic way, but were chosen according to transcript availability. One of the raters (EN) was one of the therapists in the group. The second rater relied only on information from the transcripts, although she was familiar with the members of the group from early observations in conjunction with her training in the system. The asymmetry between the two raters was a clear disadvantage, as material was often interpreted differently according to the amount of information available.

Relevant material for coding was material expressing feelings or thoughts in the present that were defined by one of the coding categories. All relevant material was broken up into units, which were defined simply as clinically meaningful, self-contained statements with no restrictions as to length. Each unit was then coded with as many categories as were thought relevant, and each category was given a dimension rating. The total number of units coded was 37, with the average length of a unit 1½ pages. Dimension reliabilities were based on categories chosen by both raters.

The percentage agreement for the categories as a whole was 54, and was somewhat higher for the affects (69) than the schemata (41). The corresponding kappa statistics (Cohen, 1960) are 0.49, 0.62, and 0.31, respectively, indicating moderate agreement for schemata, and excellent agreement for affects (Landis & Koch, 1977).

The percentage agreement for the dimensions as a whole was 47, and was higher for the schemata (60) than the affects (41). The corresponding kappa statistics are 0.30, 0.43, and 0.21, respectively, indicating moderate agreement for schemata, and poor agreement for dimension ratings for affects. Some of this disagreement has been addressed in the system that is described above. Subsequent to the reliability trial, definitions of both categories and dimensions were clarified to address problems of disagreement between the raters. We believe we have a very promising system in terms of reliability, although this is clearly a difficult coding system that requires considerable training for raters.

CONCLUSION

We hope we have illustrated the preliminary reliability and viability of our system, and the underlying assumptions we have used in constructing our system. We believe that we have opened up the way for future research efforts to characterize recovery from sexual trauma and have provided clinicians with a way to conceptualize psychotherapeutic change. We are currently planning a research effort to more systematically track change in affects and schemata over periods in the psychotherapy process. Though we will use periodic structured interviews as the primary indicator of change, we will continue to rely as well on the more spontaneous productions of our clients to weave the story of change as they present it. Through this work we hope to continue to improve our coding system so that it may ultimately be used by other researchers and clinicians to facilitate the process of recovery in survivors of sexual trauma.

ACKNOWLEDGMENTS. This research was reported at the Meeting of the Society for Traumatic Stress Studies, San Francisco, October, 1989. The authors are grateful to Bonnie Dansky for her help as the second coder for the reliability data. The coding manual is available upon request from the first author.

REFERENCES

Burnam, M. A., Stein, J. A., Golding, J. M., Sorenson, S. B., Forsythe, A. B., & Telles, C. A. (1988). Sexual assault and mental disorders in a community population. *J. Consult. Clin. Psychol., 56,* 843–851.

Cohen, J. A. (1960). A coefficient of agreement for nominal scales. *Ed. Psychological Meas., 20,* 37–46.

Dye, E., & Roth, S. (1991). Psychotherapy with Vietnam veterans and rape and incest survivors: An evaluation of the treatment literature and an examination of underlying assumptions about the coping process. *Psychotherapy, 28*(1), 103–120.

Epstein, S. (1991). The self-concept, the traumatic neurosis, and the structure of personality. In D. Ozer, J. M. Healy, Jr., & R. A. J. Stewart (Eds.), *Perspectives on personality* (Vol. 3). Greenwich, CT: JAI.

Greenberg, L. S., & Pinsof, W. M. (1986). *The psychotherapeutic process: A research handbook.* New York: Guilford.

Herman, J. L.,, Perry, C., & van der Kolk, B. A. (1989). Childhood trauma in borderline personality disorder. *Am. J. Psychiatry, 146,* 490–494.

Horowitz, M. (1986). *Stress response syndromes.* New York: Basic Books.

Jacobson, A. (1989). Physical and sexual assault histories among psychiatric outpatients. *Am. J. Psychiatry, 146,* 755–758.

Janoff-Bulman, R. (1985). The aftermath of victimization: Rebuilding shattered assumptions. In C. R. Figley (Ed.), *Trauma and its wake* (pp. 15–35). New York: Brunner/Mazel.

Koss, M. P. (1987). *The women's mental health research agenda: Violence against women.* Paper presented at the National Institute of Mental Health National Coalition for Women's Mental Health Meeting, Washington, DC.

Koss, M. P. (1989). *Rape incidence and prevalence: A review and assessment of the data.* Unpublished manuscript.

Landis, J. R., & Koch, C. C. (1977). The measurement of observer agreement for categorical data. *Biometrics, 33,* 159–174.

McCann, I. L., Sakheim, D. K., & Abrahamson, D. A. (1988). Trauma and victimization: A model of psychological adaptation. *Counsel. Psychologist, 16,* 531–594.

Roth, S., & Cohen, L. (1986). Approach, avoidance and coping with stress. *Am. Psychologist, 41,* 813–819.

Roth, S., & Lebowitz, L. (1988). The meaning of sexual trauma. *J. Traum. Stress, 1*(1), 79–107.

20

Systemic PTSD

Family Treatment Experiences and Implications

CHARLES R. FIGLEY

As human beings we retain membership in social systems, and our experiences are shaped and perceived within these social contexts. This is why we seek the comfort of those we care about when we are exposed to traumatic events. Boehnlein (1987) has noted that cultural belief systems, along with traditional family and social role expectations, greatly affect psychosocial adjustment in individuals recovering from severe trauma.

Thus any assessment or treatment of traumatic stress or stress disorders must consider not only the social context but the cultural context as well. Yet much of the traumatology literature, and the psychotherapy literature generally, is dominated by Western-oriented conceptions of mental health and focused almost exclusively on individual functioning. When viewed as a system, the family responses to stress—including traumatic stress—provide considerable insight into how individuals cope with stress and why.

The purpose of this chapter is to review the extant scholarly and practice literatures that focus on some aspect of *systemic* PTSD in order to demonstrate how families are exposed to traumatic material, attempt to cope and recover from it, and how various treatment programs help to facilitate the recovery process. The first part of the chapter reviews the scholarly literature on the impact of traumatic stress on families and other systems. The

---

CHARLES R. FIGLEY • Psychosocial Stress Research Program and the Marriage and Family Center, Florida State University, Tallahassee, Florida 32306-2024.

Psychotraumatology, edited by George S. Everly, Jr. and Jeffrey M. Lating. Plenum Press, New York, 1995.

next section notes how families naturally react and recover from these sources of stress, followed by a review of the practice literature. Here are described various ways in which families are helped to cope with PTSD. The final section is an extended description of a generic approach to treating a wide variety of families suffering from PTSD.

SYSTEMIC TRAUMATIC STRESS

Although considerable research and writing exist on the assessment and treatment of PTSD in victims of various types of catastrophes (e.g., Figley, 1983, 1985, 1986), relatively little attention has been given to social relationships. Among the first efforts to recognize the role of social relationships was the classic study of World War II veterans' families by Hill (1949). Most observers consider Hill to have originated the concept of family stress; he was the first to suggest that the system of the family is greatly affected by crisis events such as war and postwar reunion. This sociological orientation emerged into what was later to be called the ABCX model of family crisis (Hill, 1949; Hill & Hansen, 1965) and has evolved into the current Double ABCX model (McCubbin et al., 1980) and subsequent models (e.g., McCubbin & Patterson, 1983).

Montgomery (1982), in addition to providing a family psychological perspective of family crisis and stress, suggests that these families must "maintain a balance between integration (keeping the family together) and instrumentality (getting things done or dealing with the stress)" (p. 33). Moreover, he contends that families must balance consistency (being predictable in their actions) with flexibility (enabling the family to change existing patterns whenever they contribute to the family's stress). The family's capability of dealing with stress depends on the effectiveness of both its execution (task completion) and correction (decision-making) patterns. Montgomery also suggests that capability can be enhanced by family value congruency and value–behavior agreement on the part of family members.

Although the sociological and psychological explanations are helpful in understanding and appreciating families under extraordinary stress and crisis, neither provide a clear-cut direction in helping families recover, particularly from traumatic events and circumstances. There are only a few studies that document the difficulties faced by families struggling with various types of traumatic stress.

Lavee, McCubbin, and Olson (1987) focused on the effects of stressful life events and transitions on family relationships in a survey of 1,140 families. Among other things, they found that both marital adjustment and appraisal were positively related to well-being, thereby counteracting the effect of the pileup of stressful experiences. Interestingly, these factors play-different intervening roles between demands and well-being: Apparently, marital adjustment is a mediating factor, whereas appraisal of the situation plays a stress-buffering role.

Lewis (1986) has offered a theoretical model of the relationship between normative and severe stresses and a family's organizational structure. The model, in contrast to those that are oriented only at the individual level of functioning, provides direction in planning treatment intervention for families at several levels of functioning: competent, dominant-submissive, chronically conflicted, and severely disturbed.

Solomon (1988) has noted the effect of combat-related PTSD on the family. Acknowledging that the literature on the detrimental effects of combat-related PTSD indicates guilt feelings, emotional withdrawal, and elevated levels of aggression in the returning veteran, the study hypothesized that those with PTSD would have a greater negative effect than those without PTSD. In other words, the former group's experiences would make it difficult, perhaps even impossible, to resume fully the formal roles of father, husband, and breadwinner, and thus wives and children of veterans would begin to show psychiatric symptoms themselves.

Despite these hardships, the families are generally reluctant to seek professional help. Subsequent research by Solomon and her associates has supported such a perspective. For example, Verbosky and Ryan (1988) studied the female partners of Vietnam veterans, suggesting that they experienced the stress of war by "proximity." In their retrospective, descriptive study of 23 female partners of Vietnam veterans receiving treatment for PTSD, the authors focused on the effects of PTSD on the female partner of the veteran; the presence of any interrelationship between issues of PTSD and the identified women's issues; and the relationship, if any, between the veteran's symptoms and the woman's coping skills. Results showed a significant relationship between PTSD symptoms and the female partner's poor self-esteem, limited coping skills, and ineffective use of overcompensation to deal with problems. Verbosky and Ryan conclude, as do others (Figley, 1983; Figley & Sprenkle, 1978; Hogancamp & Figley, 1983; Stanton & Figley, 1978), that the perpetuation of the dysfunctional family system is therefore enhanced both by the presence of PTSD in one family member (e.g., the war veteran) and the existing (or resultant) characteristics of the partner.

Similarly, Maloney (1988) focused on PTSD in the Vietnam-veteran partner through open-ended, semistructured interviews with a convenience sample of 6 wives of Vietnam veterans with PTSD. The results indicated conflicted relationships between these women and their mothers, idealized relationships with the fathers, the importance of children, beliefs that their husbands have not grown past adolescence, conflicted feelings about the military, and a lifelong history of alcohol and physical abuse in their lives, as well as the deleterious effect of post-traumatic stress disorder on family life. Unfortunately, Maloney did not utilize a control group to contrast these respondents with those in a different context.

Solomon, Mikulincer, Freid, and Wosner (1987) looked at family characteristics and PTSD as a follow-up of Israeli combat stress reaction casualties. The study investigated the role of family status and family relationships in the course of combat-related PTSD; the data source was medical records and questionnaires and scale data on a sample of 382 Israeli soldiers who suffered a combat stress reaction episode during the 1982 Lebanon war. In contrast to theories and studies that suggest that intimate relationships help in the recovery from traumatic experiences, the results obtained by Solomon et al. did not show this. One year after the war, married soldiers had *higher* rates of PTSD than did unmarried soldiers. It is revealing to note that the authors also found higher rates of PTSD associated with low expressiveness, low cohesiveness, and high conflict in the families. This lends support to the notion of the deleterious impact of war-related PTSD on families and challenges the simplistic notions that the availability of a family of procreation automatically ameliorates the symptoms of PTSD. Without information about the functionality of the family *prior* to the war, however, we are unable to conclude that PTSD caused the dysfunction found among these families.

One of the most recently reported reports was a study of the most comprehensive investigations of the long-term psychosocial effects of war. A nationally recognized set of research teams (Kulka et al., 1990) investigated 2,867 Americans who were recruited from a national, random household survey. The teams carefully interviewed not only Vietnam theater veterans but also their families. The results were both startling but not entirely unexpected. First, the researchers found that family members tended to confirm the accounts of Vietnam-veteran family members. This lent support and credibility to the claims of long-term combat-related problems described by Vietnam veterans for years. Second, "There are more problems in the families of Vietnam veterans with PTSD than in the families of Vietnam veterans without PTSD" (Kulka et al., 1990, p. 237). Third, wives of vets with PTSD were significantly less happy and satisfied and have more general distress, including feelings as though they might have a nervous breakdown, than wives of vets without PTSD (Kulka et al., 1990, p. 237). Fourth, PTSD-inflicted veteran families had more marital problems and family violence than veteran families there were not PTSD-inflicted (p. 237). Fifth, veterans with PTSD were less effective as family members in fulfilling their roles as father and husband. Sixth, veterans with PTSD tended to have been married to or living with their spouse/

partner for significantly less time than veterans without PTSD (averages of 10 years vs. 16 years, respectively). Seventh, children with a veteran parent with PTSD had significantly more behavioral problems than did children of veteran parents without PTSD.

THE ROLE OF THE FAMILY IN THE TRAUMA INDUCTION/RECOVERY PROCESS

Thus there is ample empirical evidence that families are affected by traumatic events. Figley (1983, 1989a) has suggested that families are effective in helping their members either mitigate or ameliorate the unwanted consequences of traumatic events.

Before we review programs reported to be effective in treating traumatized families, it is important to note how families cope *without* professional intervention, for better or worse. It is certainly true that families are sources of traumatic stress themselves, as in the case of family abuse (Figley, 1983). But for the most part, when people are exposed to highly stressful situations—especially stressors originating outside the family—members of the family, friends, and others in one's social support network play a vital role in the recovery process (Figley, 1983, 1988a). As an intimate social support system, family members promote recovery in at least four separate and related ways: detecting traumatic stress, confronting the trauma, urging the recapitulation of the catastrophe, and facilitating resolution of the trauma-inducing conflicts.

Detecting Traumatic Stress

The concept of the family is derived from the Latin term *familia,* the root word of *familiar.* It means "household" and includes everyone who lives there (e.g., family members, housekeepers, boarders, live-in relatives, friends). Anyone bound by a household—be they tied by blood or law—becomes well aware of the habits, dispositions, and patterns of behavior of fellow inhabitants. Add to this the similarities of inherited and acquired traits of family members, and what emerges in most families is a remarkable feel for the normative behavior of fellow family members.

Thus, in a healthy family, when one family member is having a bad day, others know it immediately. When a family member has experienced a catastrophe, he or she is expected to behave differently. Even when a family member displays symptoms of post-traumatic stress disorder for which the cause may be unknown, other family members detect the changed pattern of behavior almost immediately.

Confronting the Trauma

Once the traumatic or post-traumatic stress reactions are noticed, family members are also in a position to help the victim. This may be done by simply linking the victim's behavior to the traumatic event. The method of confrontation is most often tailored to the individual needs and style of the victim in a way that only another family member could know. For some, the direct approach is used; for others, a more subtle method of confronting the victim has proven more effective over the years.

Urging Recapitulation of the Catastrophe

Once the traumatic experiences are confronted, supporters often urge the traumatized person to review the circumstances of the traumatic event and the various meanings attached to it. Typically, there are five questions that are often reviewed: what happened; why did it happen; why did I and others act as we did then and since then; and, if something like this happens again, will I be able to cope more effectively? In the process of recapitulation, the family member enables the victim to recall facets of the trauma that are critical in answering the other victim questions.

Facilitating Resolution of the Conflicts

Finally, the family can be extremely useful in helping the victim work through his or her traumatic memories and accompanying conflicts. Most importantly, families help victims by "reframing" or offering alternative ways of viewing the highly stressful event and the event-related consequences in a more positive or optimistic light: for example, the traumatic event was "God's test of our faith," or "it made us more aware of how other victims feel." In doing so they help the victim formulate a "healing theory" (Figley, 1979) in which all five of the victim questions can be answered to the satisfaction of the victim. Knowledge about the traumatized family member is especially useful here in reminding the member of past struggles and achievements or tendencies to over- or underestimate issues, or other characteristics that would facilitate resolution of the conflict.

Many families facilitate resolution through a variety of strategies. Most often these include (a) clarifying insights, (b) correcting distortions, (placing blame and credit more objectively), and (c) offering or supporting new and more "generous" or accurate perspectives on the traumatic event (Figley, 1989).

Clarifying Insights. In studies of successful families we (Figley and McCubbin, 1983) found that family members were effective in helping other members, including those most troubled by highly stressful events, to clarify insights, perspectives, frame-works, and discoveries about their ordeal. This skill involves family members listening carefully to another's views or insights in a nonjudgmental and caring manner, then succinctly paraphrasing these views in a way that demonstrates both understanding of the facts and acceptance of the feelings.

We (Figley & McCubbin, 1983; Figley, 1989a,b) have found that families nearly always possess the capacity for coping with nearly all of their traumatic stressors. By listening carefully to what they say and feel and feeding this information back to each other, family members are able to work through most of their traumatic experiences. Moreover, they are able to learn from their experiences so that they will feel more competent and confident about future challenges.

Correcting Distortions. Also, successful families tend to place blame and credit more objectively than less successful families. Based on their years of shared experience, they are able to gently guide a fellow family member to view various situations from a different perspective. This is a part of what could be called basic family-relations skill. Often parents, for example, show an extraordinary capacity to help their children sort out blame and credit for their actions. This may be attributable in part to some parents spending more time with the children, knowing them better, and, being skilled interpersonally.

Recovering from traumatic stress is the process of developing more effective memory management. With regard to this skill, families enable fellow members to manage memories more effectively by correcting distorted views or conclusions in a way that will lead to effective recovery.

Supporting Reframes. Similarly, effective families are able to offer or support new and more generous or accurate perspectives on the catastrophe, the traumatic and post-traumatic stress, and stress reactions. This involves, for example, positively connoting what is currently viewed as negative. These new perspectives are the final major building blocks for constructing a healing theory for the family, and thus they are critical for helping family members work through their traumatic experiences.

These naturally occurring actions within the family system are the basis for my approach in helping families: using methods found to be effective in other families and teaching them to families who are impaired in some way. But, at the same time, there is a cost of caring.

TREATING SYSTEMIC PTSD

A brief overview of the treatment literature yields approaches that can be grouped into five categories: evaluation, crisis intervention, psychoeducation/prevention, grief therapy, and family psychotherapy. This last category will receive the most attention, because it provides the most comprehensive approach to the assessment and treatment of systemic traumatic stress.

Evaluation

Some argue that effective assessment/evaluation is critical for treatment of traumatic stress or disorders. This has been claimed generally (Eldridge, 1991; Lyons, 1991), in terms of rape (Atkeson, Calhoun, Resick, & Ellis, 1982), with regard to combat-related problems (Keane, Caddell, & Taylor, 1988) in developing the Mississippi Scale and multidimensional assessment approaches to assessment of combat-related PTSD (Hyer, Woods, & Boudewyns, 1991; Lyons, Gerardi, Wolfe, & Keane, 1988; Malloy, Fairbank, & Keane, 1983; Schlenger et al., 1992; Wolfe, Keane, Lyons, & Gerardi, 1987) and by VA clinicians (McFall, Murburg, Smith, & Jensen, 1991). Others have noted the important factors involved in the assessment of families of trauma victims (Carroll, Foy, Cannon, & Zwier, 1991; Figley, 1989). Trepper and Sprenkle (1988), for example, suggested the use of the Circumplex Model for assessing and treating intrafamily child sexual abuse.

The findings by Davidson, Swartz, Storck, Krishnan, and Hammett (1985) also suggest that family variables are important in studying PTSD. They interviewed 36 patients with chronic PTSD regarding a history of familial psychopathology. Two-thirds of the patients had some psychopathology in their family. The most common were alcoholism, depression, and anxiety disorders, including a higher prevalence of alcoholic siblings than among a retrospectively derived control group of depressed and anxious male patients.

With regard to treating traumatized families, Carroll et al. (1991) promote a form of Kendall's (1987) "multiple-gating" for assessing different aspects of trauma-related family dysfunction. They suggest that the sequential utilization of family assessment data is vital to developing effective treatment plans that are targeted to specific problems, such as family abuse behavior, substance abuse, and poor communication. The first "gate" is a positive indication of PTSD through some global measure. The next gate would involve administration of a more comprehensive PTSD scale. If this is positive, one would administer an assessment of the marital dyad and then, if required, a measure of the entire family and then an assessment of the children, as indicated until the various presenting problems are measured.

Crisis Intervention

This approach predated the infamous Coconut Grove fire, which led to Lindemann's (1944) classic paper focusing on acute grief reactions, and existed long before Caplan (1964) invented the field of crisis theory and intervention. In a definitive discussion of crisis intervention as a method of preventing mental health disorders, Swanson and Carbon (1989), as part of an American Psychiatric Association task force report, suggest that the goal of crisis intervention is stabilization, immediate reduction in unwanted symptoms and by so doing, helping the individual more effectively deal with future crises on their own. The treatment tends to be brief, intensive, and goal oriented, building on the strengths of the client including her or his support systems. The same standards can be applied to systemic crisis intervention.

Fraser (1989) adopts a more systemic approach in his strategic rapid intervention (SRI) model. He views crises in the lives of families as "windows of opportunity" to effect family system change. He uses his SRI model to help families adopt more mutually supportive coping patterns in a six-phase approach. The first three help develop a therapeutic alliance with the clients, formulate goals for treatment, and establish the family's response patterns vis-à-vis the crisis, as well as identify any dysfunctional solutions generated by the family. The fourth phase is a recess from therapy during which the family and therapist review the problems and develop a tailor-made treatment plan (often with the help of a therapy team). The final two phases involve implementing the plan and bringing closure to the intervention program.

Very recently Harris (1995), drawing on the work of Slaikeu (1984) and others, has described a crisis intervention program for individuals, but especially for working with the family of traumatized people. This generic approach appears to be a useful framework for any type of crisis event and any theoretical orientation of the crisis intervener. He notes five stages of psychological first aid as an effort to prevent PTSD: (a) psychological contact, (b) exploring dimensions of the family problem, (c) examining possible solutions, (d) assisting in taking concrete action, and (e) follow-up.

Psychoeducation/Prevention

Some have argued that one of the most important interventions in terms of traumatic stress disorder is preventive (Brom & Kleber, 1989). Others have argued, however, that psychoeducational approaches—those that focus on didactic training and education about and the development of skills to cope with highly stressful events—are also a form of prevention (Hardley & Guerney, 1989). Wollert (1988), for example, developed a useful communications training program for members of sexually abused families. Similarly, Figley's (1988b, 1989) empowerment approach includes the development of an understanding of traumatic stress and the patterns of coping employed by the family, development of family supportiveness skills, and coaching in the development of a "healing theory" or new perspective regarding the trauma that facilitates recovery. This approach is discussed in more detail later in this chapter.

Grief Therapy

The field of grief therapy includes bereavement and death studies. Interestingly, this literature has always focused on traumatic stress, though the concept is rarely used. More importantly for this chapter, this field has always concerned itself with family and other systems. Although rarely using systems or family social science concepts, it has been concerned about the consequences of survivorship among members of a family or system that has lost a member through death. It studies the interpersonal relationships among members of a system and the stress associated with terminating such relationships through death.

Although some view "normal" bereavement as the absence of a traumatic stress reaction, little research has focused on differentiating between normal and abnormal. Glick et al. (1974), for example, found that within 8 weeks after the death of their husband, 40% of their sample of widows consulted a physician for various somatic problems. This confirmed previous studies by Parkes and Brown (1972), who found that half their widows had such complaints; also, 28% increased smoking, 28% increased alcohol consumption, and 26% increased tranquilizer usage. It is not surprising that Raphael (1983) found that such major problems as depression, neurotic disorders, phobias, obsessions, hypochondriasis, and various conversions follow the death of a loved one.

Redmon (1989) is the first grief therapist to acknowledge that PTSD is an expected outcome of death of a loved one, at least in the case of survivors of murder victims. Similar to Redmon, though not acknowledging the similarity, Cook and Dworkin (1992) suggest that PTSD should be viewed as a form of grief reaction and that therapy should be on "resolving the tasks of grieving" (p. 25).

Family Psychotherapy

Figley and his colleagues (Figley & Sprenkle, 1978; Hogancamp & Figley, 1983; Stanton & Figley, 1978) suggest that family therapy is most effective in treating PTSD for both the traumatized person and her or his family, because chronicity of the symptoms often becomes enmeshed in the family system. Similarly, Williams (1980) observed that the most common relationship problems for families, particularly those with a Vietnam veteran diagnosed with PTSD, were (a) a pattern of rage followed with remorseful behavior, (b) problems of low self-esteem and insecurity, (c) prolonged periods of crisis and confusion, and (d) mutual defensive barriers to both intimacy and support. These observations were confirmed in part by Carroll, Rueger, Foy, and Donahoe (1985) in a study of Vietnam combat veterans with PTSD. These authors found that combat veterans with PTSD had more marital problems in terms of self-disclosure and expressiveness, hostility and aggression toward their partner, and global marital maladjustment. Similarly, Rueger (1983) found that wives in this group were less communicative, more angry, and fearful of their partner than comparison groups of wives. This is consistent with the approach advocated by Levy and Neumann (1987), who found that treatment of combat reactions were more effective when they involved families.

Though not developed specifically for traumatized couples, a widely used marital therapy approach to treating spouse abuse appears appropriate for marital-violence-related PTSD. Neidgid and Friedman (1984) provide a detailed description of their approach, from the initial session and assessment to various decision points and, finally, the end of treatment. They adopt a systemic approach whereby they attempt to avoid blaming, accept the abused spouse's wish to remain in the relationship, and shift from the victim and perpetrator to the violent marital relationship and how it must change. Along the way they deal with the grief and sense of emotional violation that will take much longer to heal than the wounds of violence.

Jurich (1983), recognizing that families of Vietnam veterans often exhibit enmeshed parent-child ties between the veteran and his children, has developed a multistage family therapy treatment program. Focused primarily on the adolescent's struggle with individualization and the subsequent family turmoil, the approach deals only indirectly with PTSD. It is assumed that father's combat experiences have led to "foreclosed identity." This apparently makes it more difficult for teens to work through their own developmentally based struggles.

THE EMPOWERMENT APPROACH TO TREATING TRAUMATIZED FAMILIES

Figley (1989a) was the first to present a generic model for treating families traumatized by any one of a number of events. This empowerment model is based on his own research and former treatment innovations (Figley, 1983, 1985, 1986, 1988) and the existing literatures of traumatology, crisis intervention, and family therapy (parts of which are cited above). In contrast to existing approaches, however, the goal of this program is to *empower* the family to overcome and learn from their ordeal and, in so doing, be more prepared to handle future adversities.

Thus the focus in this program is on understanding and utilizing the client's family system and its natural efforts of recovering from highly stressful events. The approach attempts first to help the family recapitulate together the most important factors associated with these events and learn to manage the memories more effectively and satisfactorily. By managing the memories, family members not only cope effectively with the traumatic and post-traumatic stress but are able to make peace with the past and are more prepared to face current and future challenges.

Finally, the program helps to equip the family with the necessary knowledge about the recovery process and helps them develop effective family resources (e.g., communication, problem-solving, and conflict resolution skills) to enable them to avoid stressful events in the future. By doing so, the program attempts to develop family social supportiveness and family-relations skills.

Competency Enhancement

To effectively empower the family, the program develops social supportiveness among its members and thereby develop each family member's skills in relating to one another. Briefly, these competencies are as described below.

Family Social Supportiveness. As noted earlier, social support is a critical resource for human survival. Love, affection, kindness, companionship, a sense of belonging, protection, advice, favors, encouragement, and so many other factors that are often difficult to define and measure are the products of friendship and family relations. There is considerable variation in the quality of social support in all types of systems (e.g., work units, clubs, teams); this is certainly also the case in families.

The empowerment approach is to assess the degree to which family members are supportive to one another, *want* to be supportive, and *are able* to be supportive. Through modeling and training in some basic family-relation skills, social supportiveness can be increased significantly.

Family-Relations Skills. A major element of treating families, particularly families in crisis, is focusing on the development of a variety of interpersonal relationship skills. These include behaviors that appear to lead to effective and efficient (a) exchange of information between family members, (b) problem solving, and (c) conflict resolution.

By fostering family-relations skills, family members are able to exploit fully their own individual resources and those of other family members in helping to seek and resolve the current crisis. There is a wide variety of models for teaching these skills to people within a family context. An excellent example is Guerney's (1978) relationship enhancement (RE) program.

The crucial component of this facet of the empowerment treatment program is that family members learn to be each other's "therapist." They develop the skill and confidence to engage other family members in conversation in such a way that results in self-disclosure about important aspects of traumatic experiences, especially feelings. What is important at this point in the treatment program is to determine the most appropriate program of training if, indeed, interpersonal skills are lacking. In most cases, for clients who seek help in recovering from traumatic experiences, their natural methods of coping are ineffective.

Treatment Objectives

Irrespective of the presenting problem, sources of stress, and unique goals of each family, the empowerment program is designed to reach seven separate treatment objectives: establishing rapport and trust with the family, establishing the therapist's role, eliminating or reframing unwanted consequences, enhancing family social supportiveness, constructing new rules and skills of family communication, recapitulating the traumatic events, and building a family healing theory.

1. Establishing Rapport and Trust With the Family. This objective involves establishing a solid, therapeutic relationship between the therapist and the family. The first step in empowering traumatized families is establishing genuine rapport and trust between the helper and the helped. Some therapists have a special gift for establishing rapport and trust very early in the treatment program, yet even the most gifted therapist may be challenged by the special nature of traumatized families. Each psychotherapist must utilize his or her own methods. Because the method of treatment that is explicated here is one of empowerment, however, it should be pointed out to the clients that (a) in most cases the actual therapy will be relatively brief; (b) the role of the therapist is to *facilitate* recovery and self-reliance; (c) the task of the family is to refine and develop their own skills for coping with extraordinary circumstances; (d) success will not only improve current circumstances but also enable the family to cope more successfully with future ordeals; and (e) individually and as a family, they can be useful to others attempting to cope with similar circumstances.

2. Establishing the Therapist's Role. This objective involves the therapist's emphasizing her or his role as a consultant, facilitator, helper, guide, or investigator for the family. This is in contrast to the traditional role of being a psychotherapist. The most productive role for the professional in helping most traumatized families is to view the family's difficulty as evolving suddenly and being relatively easily corrected. Most of the elements for making the correction lie within the family members already; the clinician must simply enable the family to discover and utilize these resources.

3. Eliminating or Reframing Unwanted Consequences. This objective involves helping families identity and rid themselves of one or more trauma-related difficulties. Moreover, it is important to identify past efforts to cope or to overcome these difficulties, as well as the feelings and responses of the family members when these efforts failed.

4. Enhancing Family Social Supportiveness. This objective involves making the family self-sufficient as an effective source of social support, one of the most important human resources (Brownell & Shumaker, 1984; Gottlieb, 1983; Pilisuk & Parks, 1986; Shumaker & Brownell, 1985). Families are alerted to the ways in which they effectively support, encourage, advise, and are generally helpful to one another, and they learn to be even more supportive.

5. Constructing New Rules and Skills for Family Communication. This objective involves challenging (both directly and indirectly) unwritten rules in the family that prescribe the manner and content of communication among family members, depending upon the context (i.e., public, private, or semiprivate; Watzlawick, Beavin, & Jackson, 1967). Family rituals and secrets rigidify family interaction, resulting in a pattern of family behaviors that is generally functional in day-to-day activities but less functional during extraordinary times (e.g., holidays, vacations). Thus family interaction patterns are often dysfunctional during periods of high stress and crisis, such as in the wake of a traumatic event that impairs one or more members. New family rules and communication skills encourage the free exchange of ideas in a clear and efficient manner, including self-disclosure.

6. Recapitulating the Traumatic Material. This objective involves gradually reviewing all those memories of all family members that are troubling, both during and following the traumatic event. Each family member is encouraged to articulate his or her experiences and feelings associated with the traumatic event in as much detail as possible. Often this triggers new, vitally important information, insights, and conclusions associated with the event. As the individual stories are told about how each family member experienced the traumatic event and its wake, a picture of the family trauma will emerge (e.g., all were quite upset and worried and tried to cope in their own ways; these coping attempts helped or did not help; and at times these efforts did more harm than good, compounding the stress for the traumatized person as well as other family members).

Thus the objective here is to encourage a retelling of the experiences connected to both the trauma and its emotional wake. As the entire family listens to the individual stories of each member, new insights emerge that lead to important alterations in the perception of the situation. Specifically, the family begins to develop a consensus view that can answer the fundamental victim questions: What happened? Why did it happen? How did each family member react initially and subsequently? Will everyone be able to cope if something like this happens again? These perceptions inevitably lead to greater acceptance, as well as understanding, of past and present behavior and attitudes of fellow family members.

*7. **Building a Family Healing Theory.*** This involves bringing all these separate perspectives together into a single story or perspective about the traumatic event and its wake; each of the victim questions are answered for the entire family. Such a theory or view is most often a more optimistic perspective than was held prior to treatment. Every family member may not embrace this consensus view with equal enthusiasm, yet it is essential that every family member recognize the need for such a view and be willing to support it for the common welfare of the family. To achieve this consensus, the family healing theory may need to be rather general and avoid language that is controversial.

Course and Plan of the Treatment Program

The actual program of treatment consists of five phases following a systematic assessment. Phase one, building a commitment to the therapeutic objectives, involves developing a brief treatment plan that combines the needs of the family with the generic treatment objectives. This constitutes the requirements of effective recovery from the traumatic event. Typically clients at this stage need reassurance that what they are experiencing is normal, as well as some sense of hope that they will eventually recover from their traumatic and post-traumatic stress reactions.

The second phase, framing the problem, involves each family member telling their story, sources of stress, stress reactions, and method of coping as well as answering the five victim questions. It is not important that the family reach consensus at this point regarding the answers to these questions.

The third phase, reframing the problem, involves revising the answers to the victim questions to accommodate the additional information that has emerged during the therapy sessions. Here family members begin to articulate alternative views of the traumatic event and the circumstances subsequent to it. The therapist plays a strategic role in helping family members negotiate the meanings of various events that emerged during and following the traumatic occurrence. In many ways, this phase helps family members generate and assemble the many pieces of a puzzle. Together, the pieces form a picture that places their traumatic experiences in proper or satisfactory perspective.

The fourth phase, developing a healing theory, involves putting together each family member's individual perspectives and points of view into a family view or health theory that allows everyone to move on with their lives. The members are able to draw upon and even cherish certain aspects of the traumatic experiences (e.g., feeling stronger as a family unit because they were able to survive this ordeal) while looking ahead to the future.

Phase five, closure and preparedness, helps the family take credit for their successes and rehearse and plan for any future adversities by drawing upon what they have learned. This phase can last from one to five sessions. There is often the tendency for some families to "discovery" additional incentives for continuing the therapy; therapists must use their judgment in recognizing when the treatment program has reached sufficient closure. Most programs should never fully terminate but simply enter another phase of recovery. Here family members are urged to test their newfound insights and return at some later date to report their experiences and prepare further for future adversities.

CONCLUSION

Systemic traumatic stress is manifested in a wide variety of individual behavior and relationship patterns. They can evolve during or immediately following a highly stressful event, or they may not emerge for many years. Most often, families cope effectively with these trauma-induced problems. Sometimes, though, professional help is needed. This can come in many forms; the empowerment program described here is one approach that appears to be effective with a wide variety of families and traumatic stressors. The vital ingredients to this or any other program of intervention is to help families help themselves—providing them with the tools and knowledge necessary to work through their current crisis and, just as important, preparing them for future upheavals. If the therapist's efforts are effective, these traumatized families will become strong and even more resilient.

Recently, Figley (1995) has noted the special challenges of psychotherapists who work with traumatized systems. They are at special risk of developing what has been described as compassion fatigue or secondary traumatic stress reactions. This phenomenon is a form of burnout in which therapists absorb the traumatic material first experienced by their clients. Therapists may guard against this by carefully monitoring their own reactions for signs of PTSD and, if it is detected, seeking out the help of another therapist who specializes in treating traumatized clients. One effective method of preventing such problems is to establish a supportive network of therapists who can help process the traumatic material that emerges within clinical sessions. To ignore these signs of secondary traumatization is to ignore the power and influence of traumatized systems.

REFERENCES

Boehlein, J. K. (1987). Culture and society in posttraumatic stress disorder: Implications for psychotherapy. *American Journal of Psychotherapy, 41*(4), 519–530.

Brom, D., and Kleber, R. J. (1989). Prevention of PTSD. *Journal of Traumatic Stress, 2*(3), 335–352.

Brownell, A., and Shumaker, S. A. (1984). Social support: An introduction to a complex phenomenon. *Journal of Social Issues, 4,* 1–9.

Caplan, G. (1964). *Principles of preventive psychiatry.* New York: Basic Books.

Carroll, E. M., Rueger, D. B., Foy, D. W., & Donahoe, C. P. (1985). Vietnam combat veterans with PTSD: Analysis of marital and cohabiting adjustment. *Journal of Abnormal Psychology, 94,* 329–337.

Carroll, E. M., Foy, D. W., Cannon, B. J., & Zwier, G. (1991). Assessment issues involving the families of trauma victims. *Journal of Traumatic Stress, 4*(1), 25–40.

Cook, A. S., & Dworkin, D. S. (1992). Helping the bereaved: *Therapeutic interventions for children, adolescents, and adults.* New York: Basic Books.

Davidson, J., Swartz, M., Storck, M., Krishnan, R., & Hammett, E. (1985). A diagnosis and family study of PTSD. *American Journal of Psychiatry, 142*(1), 90–93.

Eldridge, G. D. (1991). Contextual issues in the assessment of PTSD. *Journal of Traumatic Stress, 4*(1), 7–24.

Figley, C. R. (1979). Combat as disaster: Treating combat veterans as survivors. Invided address to the American Psychiatric Association, Chicago.

Figley, C. R. (1983). Catastrophes: An overview of family reactions. In C. R. Figley and H. I. McCubbin (Eds.), *Stress and the family: Volume II: Coping with catastrophe.* New York: Brunner/Mazel, 3–20.

Figley, C. R. (1985a). The role of the family: Both haven and headache. In M. Lystad (Ed.), *Role stressors and supports for emergency workers.* U.S. Government Printing Office (DHH Publication No(Adm) 85-1408), 84–94.

Figley, C. R. (1985b). From victim to survivor: Social responsibility in the wade of catastrophe. In C. R. Figley (Ed.), *Trauma and its wake: The study and treatment of PTSD.* Brunner/Mazel: New York, 398–415.

Figley, C. R. (1986). Traumatic stress: The role of the family and social support system. In C. R. Figley (Ed.), *Trauma and its wake, Volume II: The study and treatment of post-traumatic stress disorder.* New York: Brunner/Mazel, 39–54.

Figley, C. R. (1988a). A five-phase treatment of PTSD in families. *Journal of Traumatic Stress,* 1:1, 127–139.

Figley, C. R. (1988b). Victimization, trauma, and traumatic stress. *Counseling Psychologist,* 1988(Oct), *16*(4), 635–641.

Figley, C. R. (1989a). *Helping traumatized families.* San Francisco: Jossey-Bass.

Figley, C. R. (1989b). Treating stress in families. New York: Brunner/Mazel.

Figley, C. R. (Ed.). (1995). *Compassion fatigue: STSD from treating the traumatized.* New York: Brunner/Mazel.

Figley, C. R., & McCubbin, H. I. (Eds.). (1983). *Stress and the family: Vol. II. Coping with catastrophe.* New York: Brunner/Mazel.

Figley, C. R., & Sprenkle, D. H. (1978). Delayed stress response syndrome: Family therapy implications. *Journal of Marriage and Family Counseling, 4,* 53–59.

Fraser, J. S. (1989). The strategic rapid intervention approach. In C. R. Figley (Ed.), *Treating traumatized families.* New York: Brunner/Mazel.

Glick, I. O., Weiss, R. S., and Parkes, C. M. (1974). *The first year of bereavement.* New York: Wiley Interscience.

Gottlieb, B. H. (Ed.). (198?). *Social support strategies: Guidelines for mental health practice.* Newbury Park, Calif.: Sage.

Guerney, B. G., Jr. (1977). *Relationship enhancement: Skills-training programs for therapy, problem prevention, and enrichment.* San Francisco: Jossey-Bass.

Hardley, G., & Guerney, Jr., B. G. (1989). A psychoeducational approach. In C. R. Figley (Ed.), *Treating traumatized families.* New York: Brunner/Mazel.

Harris, C. J. (1995). Sensory-based therapy for crisis counselors. In C. R. Figley (Ed.), *Compassion fatigue: STSD from treating the traumatized.* New York: Brunner/Mazel.

Hill, R. (1949). *Families under stress.* New York: Harper & Row.

Hill, R., and Hansen, D. (1965). The family in disaster. In G. Baker and D. S. Chapman (Eds.), *Man and society in disaster,* pp. 37–51. New York: Basic Books.

Hogancamp, V. E., & Figley, C. R. (1983). War: Bringing the battle home. In C. R. Figley &

H. I. McCubbin (Eds.), *Stress and the family: Vol. 2. Coping with catastrophe* (pp. 148–165). New York: Brunner/Mazel.

Hyer, L., Woods, M. G., and Boulewyns, P. A. (1991). A three-tier evaluation of PTSD among Vietnam combat veterans. *Journal of Traumatic Stress, 4*(2), 165–194.

Jurich, A. (1983). The Saigon of the family's mind: Family therapy with families of Vietnam veterans. *Journal of Marital and Family Therapy, 9*(4), 355–363.

Keane, T. M., Caddell, J. M., and Taylor, K. L. (1988). Mississippi Scale for Combat-Related Posttraumatic Stress Disorder: Three studies in reliability and validity. *Journal of Consulting & Clinical Psychology, 56*(1), 85–90.

Kendall, P. C. (1987). Ahead to basics; Assessments with children and families. *Behavioral Assessment, 9,* 321–332.

Kleber, R. J., and Brom, D. (1992). *Coping with trauma: Theory, prevention, and treatment.* Amsterdam: Swets and Zeitlinger.

Kulka, R. A., Schlenger, W. E., Fairbank, J. A., Hough, R. L., Jordan, B. K., Marmar, C. R., & Weiss, D. S. (1990). *Trauma and the Vietnam War generation.* New York: Brunner/Mazel.

Lavee, Y., McCubbin, H. I., & Olson, D. H. (1987). The effect of stressful life events and transitions on family functioning and well-being. *Journal of Marriage and the Family, 49*(4), 857–873.

Levy, A., & Neuman, M. (1987). Involving families in the treatment of combat reactions. *Journal of Family Therapy, 9*(2), 177–188.

Lewis, J. M. (1986). Family structure and stress. *Family Process, 25*(2), 235–247.

Lindemann, E. (1944). Symptomatology and management of acute grief. *American Journal of Psychiatry,* 101: 141–148.

Lyons, J. A. (1991). Issues to consider in assessing the effects of trauma: Introduction. *Journal of Traumatic Stress, 4*(1), 3–6.

Lyons, J. A., Gerardi, R. J., Wolfe, J., and Keane, T. M. (1988). Multidimensional assessment of combat-related PTSD: Phenomenological, psychometric, and psychophysiological considerations. *Journal of Traumatic Stress 1*(3), 373–394.

Mallory, P. F., Fairbank, J. A., and Keane, T. M. (1983). Validation of a multi-method assessment of PTSD in Vietnam veterans. *Journal of Consulting and Clinical Psychology, 51,* 488–494.

Maloney, L. J. (1988). Post traumatic stresses on women partners of Vietnam veterans. *Smith College Studies in Social Work, 58*(2), 122–143.

McCubbin, H. I., and Patterson, J. (1983). Family transitions: Adaptation to stress. In H. I. McCubbin and C. R. Figley (Eds.), *Stress and the family: Volume 1: Coping with normative transition* (pp. 5–25). New York: Brunner/Mazel.

McFall, M. E., Murburg, M. M., Smith, D. E., and Jensen, C. F. (1991). An analysis of criteria used by VA clinicians to diagnose combat-related PTSD. *Journal of Traumatic Stress, 4*(2), 123–136.

McFarlane, A. C. (1989). The longitudinal course of posttraumatic stress disorders following a natural disaster. *Journal of Nervous and Mental Disease, 176,* 22–29.

Montgomery, B. (1982). *Family crisis as process: Persistence and change.* Washington, D.C.: University Press of America.

Neidgid, P. H., & Friedman, D. H. (1984). *Spouse abuse: A treatment program for couples.* Champaign, IL: Research Press.

Parkes, C. M., and Brown, R. J. (1972). Health after bereavement. *Psychosomatic Medicine,* 34:5, 449–461.

Pilisuk, M., and Parks, S. H. (1986). *The healing web: Social networks and human survival.* Hanover, N.H.: University Press of New England.

Raphael, B. (1983). *The anatomy of bereavement.* New York: Basic Books.

Redmond, L. M. (1989). *Surviving: When someone you love was murdered.* Clearwater, Florida: Psychological Consultation and Education Services.

Rosenbeck, R., & Thomson, J. (1986). "Detoxification" of Vietnam War trauma: A combined family-individual approach. *Family Process, 25*(4), 559–570.

Rueger, D. B. (1983). *PTSD: Analysis of female partners' relationship perception.* Paper presented at the annual meeting of the American Psychological Association, Anaheim, CA.

Schlenger, W. E., Kulka, R. A., Fairbank, J. A., Hough, R. L., Jordan, B. K., Marmar, C. R., and Weiss, D. S. (1992). The prevalence of PTSD in the Vietnam generation: A multimethod, multisource assessment of psychiatric disorder. *Journal of Traumatic Stress, 5*(3), 333–363.

Shumaker, S. A., and Bronell, A. (1985). Introduction: Social support intervention. *Journal of Social Issues, 1,* 1–4.

Slaikeu, K. A. (1984). *Crisis intervention: A handbook for practice and research.* Boston, Allyn and Bacon.

Solomon, Z. (1988). Somatic complaints, stress reaction, and PTSD: A three year follow-up study. *Behavioral Medicine, 14*(4), 179–185.

Solomon, A., Mikulincer, M., Freid, B., & Wosner, Y. (1987). Family characteristics and PTSD: A follow-up of Israeli combat stress reaction casualties. *Family Process, 26,* 383–394.

Solomon, Z., Waysman, M., Avitzur, E., & Enoch, D. (1991). Psychiatric symptomatology among wives of soldiers following combat stress reaction: The role of the social network and marital relations. *Anxiety Research, 4,* 213–223.

Solomon, Z., Waysman, M., Belkin, R., Levy, G., Mikulincer, M., & Enoch, D. (1992). Marital relations and combat stress reaction: The wives' perspective. *Journal of Marriage and the Family, 54*(2), 316–326.

Solomon, Z., Waysman, M., Levy, G., Fried, B., Mikulincer, M., Benbenishty, R., Florian, V., & Bliech, A. (1992). From front line to home front: A study of secondary traumatization. *Family Process, 31*(3), 289–302.

Solomon, Z., Waysman, M., & Mikulincer, M. (1990). Family functioning, societal support and combat-related psychopathology: The moderating of loneliness. *Journal of Social and Clinical Psychology, 9,* 456–472.

Stanton, M. D., & Figley, C. R. (1978). Treating the Vietnam veteran within the family system. In C. R. Figley (Ed.), *Stress disorders among Vietnam veterans: Theory, research, and treatment* (pp. 281–290). New York: Brunner/Mazel.

Swanson, W. C., & Carbon, J. B. (1989). Crisis intervention: Theory and technique. In *Treatment of Psychiatric Disorders: A Task Force Report of the American Psychiatric Association* (Volume 3, 2520–2531).

Trepper, T. S., and Sprenkle, D. H. (1988). The clinical use of the Circumplex Model in the assessment and treatment of intrafamily child sexual abuse. *Journal of Psychotherapy and the Family, 4*(1–2), 93–111.

Verbosky, S. J., & Ryan, D. A. (1988). Female partners of Vietnam veterans: Stress by proximity. *Issues in Mental Health Nursing, 9*(1), 95–104.

Watzlawick, P., Beavin, J., and Jackson, D. D. (1967). *Pragmatics of human communication.* New York: Norton.

Williams, C. M. (1980). The veteran system with a focus on women partners: Theoretical considerations, problems, and treatment strategies. In T. Williams (Ed.), *Post-traumatic stress disorder of the Vietnam veteran.* Cincinnati, OH: Disabled American Veterans.

Wolfe, J., Keane, T. M., Lyons, J. A., and Gerardi, R. J. (1987). Current trends and issues in the assessment of combat-related posttraumatic stress disorder. *Behavior Therapist, 10*(2), 27–32.

Wollert, R. (1988). An evaluation of a communications training program within a self-help group for sexually abusive families. *Community Mental Health Journal, 24*(3), 229–235.

21

Theoretical and Empirical Issues in the Treatment of PTSD in Vietnam Veterans

JOHN A. FAIRBANK and ROBERT A. NICHOLSON

Controlled group studies on the effectiveness of psychological and pharmacological approaches to treating post-traumatic stress disorder (PTSD) in Vietnam combat veterans have not yet appeared in the literature. However, numerous articles in recent years have provided theoretical rationales and descriptive summaries of various treatment approaches, primarily based upon psychodynamic (Horowitz, 1973, 1974; Horowitz & Kaltreider, 1980), behavioral (Keane, Fairbank, Caddell, Zimering, & Bender, 1985; Keane, Zimering, & Caddell, 1985), and psychobiological (van der Kolk, Greenberg, Boyd, & Krystal, 1985) models for conceptualizing the treatment of combat-related PTSD. The present chapter will review these theoretical approaches and the treatment techniques that have evolved from each. In addition, this review will examine some of the current trends in PTSD treatment research and speculate on the future direction of research on treatment of combat-related PTSD in Vietnam veterans.

JOHN A. FAIRBANK • Research Triangle Institute, Research Park, North Carolina 27709. **ROBERT A. NICHOLSON** • Department of Veterans Affairs Medical Center and University of Mississippi Medical Center, Jackson, Mississippi 39216. The authors wish to thank Sandra E. Gramling for her helpful comments on an earlier version of this manuscript. Reprinted from *Journal of Clinical Psychology*, Vol. 43, pp. 44–55.

Psychotraumatology, edited by George S. Everly, Jr. and Jeffrey M. Lating. Plenum Press, New York, 1995.

PSYCHODYNAMIC METHODS

There is no single "psychodynamic" approach to understanding the development and treatment of PTSD. Rather, there are a number of complementary approaches that can be subsumed within a broadly conceived psychodynamic tradition. Early psychodynamic formulations of trauma were constructed around the concept of energy overload: An event became traumatic when external stimuli exceeded the ego's "stimulus barrier." It was postulated that when trauma occurred, the ego attempted to restore homeostasis by "binding," "discharging," or "abreacting" the excess energy (Horowitz, 1974). In some of the more recent psychodynamic formulations, however, this concept of energy overload has been supplanted by that of information overload. The task that confronts the traumatized individual is seen as one of reconciling the occurrence of the traumatic event, including the various meanings associated with it, with the individual's enduring schemata, such as his concept of himself and the world around him. Within this framework, emotions are viewed as reactions to discrepancies between external and internal information and also serve as motives for defense and control (e.g., Horowitz, 1974; Horowitz & Kaltreider, 1980).

Various phases of PTSD have been identified as a function of the kinds of defensive operations engaged in by the individual and the degree of success of these defenses. Periods of intrusive repetition of the stressful event (e.g., intrusive thoughts, nightmares, flashback experiences) are seen as the result of defensive undercontrol or failure, whereas states of denial and emotional numbness are thought to be the product of defensive overcontrol (Horowitz, 1973; Horowitz & Kaltreider, 1980). These phases may alternate with one another or even coexist. Thus a veteran may be in a state of denial about one aspect of a traumatic event, but in a state of intrusive repetition about another aspect of the same event.

Characterological and identity disturbances often observed in veterans with PTSD have been described from a psychodynamic perspective. For example, Brende and McCann (1984) have suggested that character symptoms, such as chronic dependency, withdrawal, and aggressive outbursts, emerge when the individual's usual methods of coping fail; this induces a pathological regression to more primitive levels of behavior and psychological functioning. In addition, Blackburn, O'Connell, and Richman (1984) have emphasized the problems of identity in veterans with PTSD and have noted in particular that many veterans were not able to resolve the late adolescent struggle of identity versus role confusion because traumatic war experiences disrupted normal passage through this stage of psychosocial and personality development.

Whether the fundamental problem of veterans with PTSD is described as ideational incongruity (Horowitz, 1974), "split-off experience" (Brende & McCann, 1984), emotional blocking and "unfinished business" (Crump,

1984), or disruption of the normal course of psychosocial and personality development (Blackburn et al., 1984), the optimal goal of any psychodynamic treatment of PTSD is integration of the traumatic experience, usually by means of therapeutic "revivification" (Brende, 1981). However, the particular techniques used to accomplish this end result will vary as a function of the phase of PTSD (Horowitz, 1973; Horowitz & Kaltreider, 1980), the stage of therapy (Brende & McCann, 1984), and the personality style of the patient (Horowitz, 1974). In addition, "revivification" may not always be possible, depending at least in part on the level of motivation and strength of self-concept of the patient (Horowitz, Marmar, Weiss, Dewitt, & Rosenbaum, 1984).

Horowitz (1973, 1974) has classified treatment techniques according to whether they are more appropriate for addressing states of intrusive repetition of the trauma or states of denial and numbness. During a state of severe intrusive repetition, supportive or "covering" interventions may be used to alleviate painful affects, to manage regressive symptoms, and to aid repression. On the other hand, during a phase of extreme denial, "uncovering" techniques are used both to reduce controls (e.g., through interpretation of defenses, hypnosis, suggestion) and to encourage abreaction and catharsis (e.g., through psychodrama, use of imagery). Brende and McCann (1984) further suggest that management and supportive techniques may predominate in the early stages of psychotherapy, whereas later stages may involve induction of regression to facilitate integration of the traumatic experience and emotions associated with it.

Two studies have investigated systematically the efficacy of psychodynamically oriented psychotherapy for stress response syndromes (Horowitz et al., 1984; Lindy, Green, Grace, & Titchener, 1983). These studies are similar in that they were uncontrolled investigations and did not deal exclusively with PTSD. In the study by Horowitz et al. (1984), 52 patients who were experiencing bereavement reactions after death of a loved one were treated by brief (12-session) dynamic psychotherapy. Only 14 of the patients actually met DSM-III criteria for PTSD; the majority were diagnosed as having adjustment disorder. Outcome was assessed by a variety of measures, which included measures of symptoms severity, work and interpersonal functioning, and capacity for intimacy. Horowitz et al. (1984) reported before–after effect sizes for these different types of measures that ranged from .4 for work and interpersonal functioning to 1.21 for one of the symptom measures. In the study by Lindy et al. (1983), 30 survivors of the Beverly Hills Supper Club fire received brief (6- to 12-session) dynamic psychotherapy. Only 10 of the patients completed treatment and achieved symptom reduction.

Although these studies represent an important first step in programmatic evaluation of dynamic psychotherapy in the treatment of stress response syndromes, the diagnostic heterogeneity of the treated groups and the absence of untreated control groups are serious limitations. The impact of the latter shortcoming can be seen in the discussion and interpretation of effect sizes obtained by Horowitz et al. (1984). They compared their results with the findings from a meta-analysis of psychotherapy outcome (Nicholson & Berman, 1983), in which a mean before–after effect size of .57 was reported for dynamic therapies. Thus the Horowitz et al. (1984) findings appeared to compare favorably with the results of previous research. However, it should be noted that Nicholson and Berman (1983) also reported effect sizes for comparisons between treatment and control groups. The mean effect size for such comparisons that involved dynamic therapies was −.05, which indicates that there was no difference between treated and untreated groups. Thus groups who were receiving dynamic therapy improved over time, as indicated by the before–after effect size, but this improvement did not differ from that of untreated controls, as indicated by the between-groups effect size. These considerations urge caution in interpreting the finding of significant before–after change in the study by Horowitz et al. (1984) and also underscore the need for controlled outcome research in the area.

BEHAVIORAL METHODS

Researchers at the Jackson Veterans Administration Medical Center (Keane, Fairbank, Caddell, Zimering, & Bender, 1985; Keane, Zimering, & Caddell, 1985) have offered a behavioral learning model for conceptualizing the etiology and treatment of combat-related PTSD in Vietnam veterans. Based primarily on Mowrer's (1960) two-factor learning theory, this model emphasizes the importance of both classical conditioning and instrumental conditioning in the development of psychopathology. In this formulation, the development of PTSD symptoms in humans is thought to parallel the acquisition of classically conditioned physiological and behavioral fear responses in animals (Keane, Fairbank, Caddell, Zimering, & Bender, 1985; Kilpatrick, Veronen, & Resick, 1982; Kolb, 1984). Specifically, Keane, Fairbank, Caddell, Zimering, and Bender (1985) have proposed that a traumatic combat event (e.g., helplessly witnessing the death of a fellow combatant) acts as an unconditioned aversive stimulus (UCS) that reflexively elicits extreme levels of autonomic distress in the surviving individual. Accordingly, previously neutral external stimuli (e.g., nonthreatening aspects of the physical environment) and internal stimuli (e.g., physiological and cognitive responses) that accompanied the occurrence of the traumatic UCS now may serve as conditioned stimuli (CS) capable of eliciting high levels of psychological and physiological distress.

The second factor of Mowrer's (1960) two-factor learning theory, instrumental conditioning, predicts that subjects will engage in whatever behavior is necessary to avoid or escape exposure to conditioned and unconditioned aversive stimuli. Indeed, numerous studies have demonstrated that animals exposed to a strong UCS will continue to avoid exposure to conditioned stimuli during numerous extinction trials when presentations of the CS no longer are paired with the UCS (e.g., Solomon & Wynne, 1954). Escape and avoidance of the CS are reinforced by arousal reduction; hence, as a function of instrumental conditioning, the subject is likely to attempt to avoid exposure to conditioned cues in the future. Although instrumental avoidance of the CS may produce a temporary reduction in arousal, avoidance during extinction (i.e., when the CS no longer is paired with the UCS) prevents deconditioning of aversive emotional arousal through exposure to the now "harmless" CS complex (cf. Keane, Fairbank, Caddell, Zimering, & Bender, 1985; Kolb, 1984).

The relevance and applicability of animal analog conditioning models to PTSD in humans have not been without their critics (cf. Rachman, 1985; Saigh, 1984, 1985). For example, Rachman (1985) has voiced concern that few studies of fear acquisition in humans have supported a straightforward classical conditioning model. However, as both Keane (1985) and Kolb (1984) have observed, several recent controlled investigations of Vietnam veterans' psychophysiological, cognitive, and behavioral responses to cues associated with combat experiences (e.g., Blanchard, Kolb, Pallmayer, & Gerardi, 1982; Malloy, Fairbank, & Keane, 1983) have provided indirect empirical support for a conditioning model of avoidance and arousal in combat-related PTSD.

In addition, the principles of higher-order conditioning (Kamil, 1969) and stimulus generalization (e.g., Watson & Raynor, 1920) would predict that subjects will learn to avoid an increasingly extensive array of conditioned cues that elicit memories of the traumatic event. Learning theory models for PTSD thus would predict that interventions that focus on deconditioning negative arousal to cues of the traumatic conditioning experience should be therapeutically beneficial. As such, a primary goal of behavior therapy for combat-related PTSD is reduction of the veteran's dysfunctional arousal to traumatically conditioned cues.

Two general behavioral approaches to treating PTSD have been described in the literature. The first approach is composed of exposure-based therapies, such as systematic desensitization and flooding in imagination, that primarily target memories of traumatic events and focus on reduction of arousal to cues of the traumatic conditioning experience (Fairbank & Keane, 1982; Keane & Kaloupek, 1982; Schindler, 1980). The second approach consists of a variety of stress management procedures that focus on the acquisition and maintenance of skills for coping with symptoms of PTSD and trauma-related problems (Keane, Fairbank, Caddell, Zimering, and Bender, 1985; Kilpatrick et al., 1982).

Although published reports of group outcome studies have yet to appear in the literature, there have been several encouraging data-based single-case studies on the efficacy of behavior therapy for combat-related PTSD in Vietnam veterans (Fairbank, Gross, & Keane, 1983; Fairbank & Keane, 1982; Johnson, Gilmore, & Shenoy, 1982; Keane & Kaloupek, 1982; Miller & Buchbinder, 1979; Schindler, 1980; Scrignar, 1983). Each of these studies has included as a component of treatment a deconditioning procedure, such as systematic desensitization with graduated hierarchial exposure to anxiety-eliciting cues (Schindler, 1980), flooding in vivo to stimuli associated with traumatic combat events (Johnson et al., 1982), or flooding in imagination (i.e., implosive therapy; Fairbank et al., 1983; Fairbank & Keane, 1982; Keane, Fairbank, Caddell, Zimering, & Bender, 1985; Keane & Kaloupek, 1982), and a stress management procedure, such as progressive muscle relaxation training (Fairbank et al., 1983; Fairbank & Keane, 1982; Keane & Kaloupek, 1982), anger control training (Keane, Fairbank, Caddell, Zimering, & Bender, 1985), and distraction techniques (Johnson et al., 1982). For example, Fairbank et al. (1983) treated a Vietnam veteran with chronic and severe symptoms of PTSD and depression with a behavior therapy package that consisted primarily of flooding in imagination (implosive therapy) and relaxation training. These investigators successfully used behavior therapy to treat dramatic behavioral and psychophysiological arousal associated with the memory of surviving an ambush in which the patient was severely wounded and all other members of his patrol team were killed. Once dysfunctional levels of arousal to this specific memory were reduced, a number of adaptive behavioral and interpersonal changes were reported.

Although the results obtained in data-based single case studies are encouraging and provide at least some preliminary support for the learning theory approach, the efficacy of behavior therapy for combat-related PTSD is still a long way from being firmly established. Several controlled investigations of behavior therapy for combat-related PTSD are currently in progress, and publication of these findings should clarify further the clinical utility of behavioral approaches.

BIOCHEMICAL APPLICATIONS

Numerous studies (e.g., Anisman, 1978; Christie & Chesher, 1982) have shown that exposure to stress produces central nervous system (CNS) biochemical alterations. Anisman's (1978) extensive review of the literature on stress-induced neurochemical changes indicates that neurotransmitter activity varies as a function of (1) frequency, duration, and intensity of the stressor; and (2) the subject's level of control over stress onset or termination. For example, profound norepinephrine (NE) depletion has been found under conditions of acute stress, such as occurs when laboratory animals are exposed to severe and inescapable electric shock (Maynert &

Levi, 1964). Stress also is known to precipitate peripheral endorphin release as well as to induce a centrally mediated analgesia response (Krieger, 1983).

Recently, van der Kolk et al. (1985) proposed that the neurochemical changes (i.e., adrenergic and endorphin) that occur in animals exposed to inescapable shock (IS) procedures provide the best available biological model for the development of PTSD symptoms in man. Accordingly, the behavioral sequelae of these neurochemical changes in the PTSD patient are thought to parallel the behavioral effects of IS procedures observed in animals (i.e., "learned helplessness"). This biochemical model of PTSD suggests that life-threatening traumatic events and associated stimuli may act as stressors capable of producing profound catecholamine depletion similar to the depletion of NE after acute IS in animals. Thus, some symptoms of PTSD (e.g., decreased motivation, decline in occupational functioning) are viewed as correlates of NE depletion analogous to the learned-helplessness behavior exhibited by animals exposed to IS. Moreover, trauma-induced NE depletion may lead to adrenergic hypersensitivity, which would account for PTSD symptomatology of hyperactivity (i.e., startle responses, explosive and impulsive behavior, nightmares, and intrusive recollections). Thus the model suggests that PTSD symptomatology reflects a tonic underactivity of NE-mediated behavior, with aphasic overactivation of NE-driven behavior after transitory stimulation.

The tendency for some PTSD veterans to reexpose themselves to stressful trauma-simulating events and their reports of a paradoxical sense of calm also may be attributed to the neurochemical effects of stress. Specifically, reexposure to a stressor after a traumatic event may cause an endorphin response analogous to the stress-induced analgesia observed in animals reexposed to a stressor subsequent to IS procedures. Furthermore, as van der Kolk et al. (1985) point out, there are striking similarities between the PTSD symptoms of hyperalertness, anxiety, uncontrollable anger, insomnia, and emotional lability, and the opiate withdrawal syndrome, a syndrome thought to be mediated by noradrenergic hyperactivity.

van der Kolk et al.'s (1985) proposed treatment based on this biochemical model parallels the procedures used to reverse the effects of IS in animals. Thus therapy for PTSD would include the human analog of forced exposure to escapable shock procedures in animals. However, in contrast to van der Kolk et al.'s (1985) model, most biochemically oriented interventions for PTSD appear to have evolved from the perspective of symptomatic pharmacotherapy (i.e., antidepressants for depression, anxiolytics for anxiety, neuroleptics for flashback episodes and extreme agitation; Walker, 1982).

Recently, the drug phenelzine (a monoamine oxidase inhibitor [MAOI]) has been advanced as a pharmacological treatment with therapeutic effects specific to the symptom cluster presented by the PTSD patient (Demers, McDonagh, & Moore, 1984; Hogben & Cornfield, 1981; Levenson, Lanman, & Rankin, 1982; Milanes, Mack, Dennison, & Slater, 1984; Shen & Park, 1983). Though these studies generally report that phenelzine is efficacious in the treatment of PTSD, most have tested phenelzine in combination with other forms of therapy in uncontrolled designs. For example, Hogben and Cornfield (1982) used a regimen of phenelzine and psychotherapy to treat five veterans with chronic PTSD associated with exposure to traumatic events that occurred during varying eras of military service. Subjects were a former World War II–era prisoner of war, a Korean combat veteran, two Vietnam combat veterans, and a noncombat Vietnam-era veteran. These investigators reported that a combined regimen of phenelzine and trauma-focused psychotherapy produced clinically significant symptom reduction in patients who had shown little response to earlier regimens of pharmacotherapy (including tricyclic antidepressants and neuroleptics) or psychotherapy alone or with other medications.

To date, there have been no published reports of controlled studies of pharmacotherapy in the treatment of combat-related PTSD. Studies are needed that employ accepted standards of design for research on drug therapy, including the use of relevant comparison groups (e.g., placebo control groups) and blind outcome evaluation procedures. Important research questions include the following: (a) What is the comparative utility of different pharmacological therapies (e.g., MAOIs vs. tricyclic antidepressants) in the treatment of PTSD? (b) What are the consequences of combining drug therapies with various psychotherapies? and (c) Can drug therapy be said to be more or less effective than specific psychotherapy interventions? The answers to these empirical questions await the findings of controlled studies of the separate and interactive effects of drug therapies and psychological interventions on combat-related PTSD.

SOME ISSUES, TRENDS, AND DIRECTIONS IN RESEARCH ON THE TREATMENT OF PTSD IN VIETNAM VETERANS

Although research on the treatment of combat-related PTSD is still in its infancy, clinicians and researchers interested in this disorder have considerable reason for optimism. First, research on the treatment of combat-related PTSD has a strong theoretical foundation on which to build, as indicated in the previous overview of the psychodynamic, behavioral, and psychobiological treatment models. Second, case studies and clinical replications of psychological and pharmacological interventions for PTSD have produced some encouraging findings that have provided guidelines for both researchers and clinicians.

The clear need for controlled studies of the efficacy of the various treatment approaches to combat-related PTSD has been addressed in the preceding paragraphs. Recognizing this necessity, the Veterans Administration (VA) has funded several controlled research studies that are in progress in VA medical centers around the nation. In the following paragraphs, several additional issues of importance to the study of PTSD treatment will be considered, including (a) the apparent emergence of components common to all methods of treating combat-related PTSD, (b) the analysis of untrained coping in nonclinical and clinical samples of Vietnam veterans and implications for developing treatment programs, (c) the issue of heterogeneity of subject samples, and (d) measurement of treatment outcome. The comments offered here are intended to provide direction for future research endeavors.

EVIDENCE FOR COMMON TREATMENT COMPONENTS

Although the various psychodynamic, behavioral, and psychopharmacological treatments described above are built upon quite different theoretical foundations, the treatments themselves share important components. Identification of the mechanisms responsible for therapeutic efficacy will be facilitated by focusing on those treatment components held in common by the three theoretical approaches. As noted previously, the ultimate goal of psychodynamic interventions is to facilitate integration of the traumatic event, including the various meanings and emotions associated with it. The reexperiencing of the trauma in the context of therapy has been termed "therapeutic revivification" (Brende, 1981), and it is considered crucial for the healing and integration of split-off traumatic experiences. Similarly, the deconditioning procedures most often used in behavioral treatment approaches, flooding and desensitization, involve imaginal exposure to the traumatic event (e.g., Fairbank et al., 1983; Fairbank & Keane, 1982; Keane & Kaloupek, 1982; Schindler, 1980) or in vivo exposure to stimuli associated with the trauma (Johnson et al., 1982). Finally, although most psychopharmacological treatments have been directed primarily toward amelioration of PTSD symptomatology, the biobehavioral model recently proposed by van der Kolk et al. (1985) predicts that exposure to the traumatic event would be the most efficacious approach to treatment. Furthermore, most of the uncontrolled clinical trials that have examined the efficacy of pharmacotherapy have included some form of trauma-focused psychological therapy (e.g., Hogben & Cornfield, 1981). Thus, regardless of the underlying theoretical rationale, each of the foregoing treatments has involved directly exposing the patient, in the context of a stable therapeutic relationship, to the feared traumatic memories.

From the preceding discussion, it appears that direct therapeutic exposure to the trauma has emerged as the single most important factor in the treatment of PTSD (cf. Boudewyns & Shipley, 1983). Whether exposure is a necessary component of treatment, however, remains to be established empirically. For example, the treatments described above generally have included supportive, "covering," or stress management techniques along with an exposure component. Further, Horowitz (Horowitz, 1973, 1974; Horowitz & Kaltreider, 1980) has argued that the effectiveness of these two general strategies may vary with the phase of PTSD and certain patient characteristics. In particular, Horowitz has suggested that "uncovering" techniques—which would include behavioral treatments, such as flooding in imagination, and dynamically oriented treatments, such as psychodrama—are more appropriate during states of extreme denial and numbness, whereas "covering" techniques, such as relaxation training and supportive psychotherapy, are more appropriate during states of defensive failure and excessive intrusion of the traumatic event. In addition, Horowitz et al. (1984) also have suggested that exploratory (uncovering) actions by the therapist are more effective for patients with greater motivation and more stable, coherent self-concepts, whereas supportive actions are more beneficial to patients deficient on these dimensions.

In the absence of any controlled outcome studies that compared direct therapeutic exposure and "covering" techniques under the various conditions delineated above, the validity of these assertions cannot be assessed. These questions about the relative efficacy of the two strategies for different types of patients and different phases of PTSD seem to be appropriate starting points for controlled outcome research. Comparison of these strategies should be informed by research on treatment of phobic and other anxiety-based disorders. Such research has suggested that the timing of the various components may be crucial. For example, initial research indicated that exposure treatments were superior to cognitive coping strategies in treatment of agoraphobia (e.g., Emmelkamp, Kuipers, & Eggeraat, 1978) and that a combination of the two approaches was no more effective than exposure alone (Emmelkamp & Mersch, 1982). However, recent investigation indicates that an appropriate combination of the two treatments may yield greater improvement by the time of a follow-up assessment than exposure alone (Marshall, 1985).

COPING IN CLINICAL AND NONCLINICAL SAMPLES

In recent years, behavioral scientists have attempted to identify and measure the cognitive and behavioral strategies that individuals use to adapt to a variety of adverse conditions (e.g., Lazarus, 1981; Moos & Billings, 1982; Pearlin & Schooler, 1978). Recent significant advances in the measurement of cognitive coping (e.g., Billings & Moos, 1981; Folkman & Lazarus, 1980, 1985; Stone & Neale, 1984) have given rise to controlled investigations of the effects of specific coping strategies on adaptation to extreme stress. For example, Fairbank, Hensen, and Fitterling (1985) studied cognitive coping in 30 veterans of World War II: 10 former prisoners of war (POWs) with a diagnosis of PTSD; 10 former POWs who were well adjusted and did not meet DSM-III criteria for a diagnosis of PTSD; and 10 well-adjusted non-combat veterans who were not exposed to traumatic wartime stressors.

Subjects completed a standardized inventory of coping strategies (Ways of Coping Checklist-Revised; Lazarus & Folkman, 1984) under two experimental conditions: (1) induction of a distressing memory of military service during World War II; and (2) induction of thoughts about a recent stressor (e.g., financial difficulties associated with recent retirement). These investigators found that under both experimental conditions, former POWs with PTSD reported using a wider repertoire of coping responses than the two comparison groups, including more maladaptive coping strategies (e.g., wishful thinking). Conversely, well-adjusted former POWs more often implemented adaptive cognitive coping strategies (e.g., emphasizing positive aspects of the experience) than the veterans with PTSD. The data from this preliminary investigation suggest that well-adjusted and symptomatic former POWs differ markedly in the ways in which they cope with memories of extreme stress and current problems.

Although no studies have assessed directly coping and psychological adjustment in Vietnam veterans, information derived from such investigations could have important applications to the assessment and treatment of PTSD. For example, identification of empirically derived differences in coping between Vietnam veterans with PTSD and combat veterans who are well adjusted could have implications for the development of intervention strategies. These data could reduce the risk that clinicians might implement treatment programs that are no more effective than what veterans with PTSD do on their own (cf. Kaloupek & Stoupakis, 1985).

The seeking of social support in times of distress long has been recognized as a prevalent and adaptive coping strategy (Sarason, Sarason, Potter, & Antoni, 1985). Indeed, numerous studies have documented a direct relationship between variables, such as social network size and psychological adjustment (Escobar et al., 1983). Recent empirical studies (Carroll, Rueger, Foy, & Donahue, 1985; Escobar et al., 1983; Keane, Scott, Chavoya, Lamparski, & Fairbank, 1985) have described low levels of social support and dysfunctional patterns of social interaction in Vietnam veterans with PTSD. For example, Keane, Scott, Chavoya, Lamparski, and Fairbank (1985) interviewed three groups of Vietnam veterans to obtain their ratings of the social support resources that they perceived as available to them over three different time periods: (1) the 3-month period that immediately preceded military service; (2) the 3-month period immediately after service in the military; and (3) the 3 months immediately prior to the interview. Results indicated that across the three time periods, combat veterans with PTSD perceived themselves as having progressively fewer social support resources on which to rely than did the subjects in either of the two comparison groups. Data such as these strongly suggest that there is a need for controlled investigations of the interventive effects of mobilizing social support systems of Vietnam veterans with PTSD.

HETEROGENEITY OF SUBJECT SAMPLES

Lettieri (1985) has made the observation that researchers and clinicians in the area of substance abuse treatment frequently combine heterogeneous groups of alcohol-dependent persons into a single "alcoholic" category. He argues that the use of heterogeneous or "omnibus" groups of subjects has tended to impede the detection of efficacious treatments for alcohol abuse by masking the therapeutic changes that may have occurred for some individuals within the heterogeneous groups. In point of fact, Lettieri's (1985) concerns about the negative impact of heterogeneous samples on treatment outcome research are relevant to research on PTSD. Even the most cursory review of the PTSD literature quickly reveals that selection criteria for PTSD research subjects have varied greatly across studies. All too often, subjects in PTSD studies are recruited by use of subject selection procedures fraught with questionable reliability and validity, such as assigning subjects to diagnostic groups based on retrospective review of medical charts or the use of self-report inventories for PTSD that have unknown psychometric properties. Although the publication, acceptance, and use of DSM-III criteria for PTSD has done much to increase the homogeneity of subject samples, progress in this area needs to continue. In particular, clinicians and researchers must arrive at a clear consensus on some issues basic to the diagnosis of PTSD, such as the definition of traumatic stress. The controversial nature of this issue has been demonstrated by recent spirited debate over the conditions necessary and sufficient for defining an event as a traumatic stressor (Heimberg, 1985; Keane, 1985; Rachman, 1985; Saigh, 1985). Until issues such as these are resolved empirically, the use of heterogeneous samples of subjects in PTSD research will continue, which potentially will decrease the probability of detecting efficacious treatments.

MEASUREMENT OF TREATMENT OUTCOME

PTSD is a multifaceted disorder that may include sensory, motor, neuroendocrine, cognitive, characterological, and identity disturbances (Brende & McCann, 1984). Existing research reflects this complexity in the variety of measures that have been used to assess outcome. Behavioral studies have relied upon daily self-monitoring of such symptoms as nightmares and flashbacks (Fairbank et al., 1983; Keane & Kaloupek, 1982). In one investigation, the patient's self-report of nightmare occurrence was corroborated by the patient's spouse (Schindler, 1980). In addition, during presentation of traumatic scenes during implosive therapy, SUDS anxiety ratings (Fairbank & Keane, 1982; Keane & Kaloupek, 1982), physiological indices of anxiety, such as heart rate (Fairbank & Keane, 1982; Keane & Kaloupek, 1982) and electrodermal activity (Fairbank & Keane, 1982), and motoric indices of anxiety recorded by independent observers (Fairbank et al., 1983) have been obtained. Finally, results based on standard self-report (e.g., Spielberger State-Trait Anxiety Inventory; Keane & Kaloupek, 1982) or clinician-rated psychometric instruments (e.g., Hamilton Depression Rating Scale; Fairbank et al., 1983) also have been reported. One systematic study of psychodynamically oriented psychotherapy (Horowitz et al., 1984) similarly used a variety of both self-report (e.g., intrusion and avoidance subscales on the Impact of Event Scale; Symptom Checklist-90) and clinician-rated (e.g., Stress Response Rating Scale) measures.

Though the studies as a whole have made use of a variety of outcome measures, as is fitting for a multidimensional disorder such as PTSD, there is in fact little consistency from one study to another with regard to the specific measures employed, which reduces the comparability of the findings across studies. As research on treatment of PTSD continues, the proliferation of measures unique to various research programs could impair integration of findings and impede progress. The development of a standard assessment battery (or at least some common assessment instruments) that could be used across settings would prevent this problem. In this regard, it is clear that data from multiple response systems (cognitive, behavioral, and psychophysiological) would provide the most comprehensive assessment of treatment efficacy. For example, the multimethod assessment package developed at the Jackson VA Medical Center (Malloy et al., 1983) could be used to provide behavioral, subjective/cognitive, and psychophysiological indices of anxiety in response to visual and auditory stimuli associated with the traumatic event (cf. McCaffrey & Fairbank, 1985). This multimethod assessment package, accompanied by daily self-monitoring of the hallmark symptom of PTSD, reexperiencing of the trauma (nightmares, flashbacks, intrusive thoughts), could provide the core of such a standard assessment battery. Of course, the self-report of symptoms should be verified, whenever possible, by data obtained from significant others.

SUMMARY

The long overdue acceptance of PTSD as a diagnostic entity, as reflected by its inclusion in the *Diagnostic and Statistical Manual of Mental Disorders* (American Psychiatric Association, 1980) has been followed by a proliferation of research on the etiology, assessment, and treatment of this disorder. Research in each of these areas is inextricably linked. The development and evaluation of effective treatment procedures depends in no small measure on progress in elucidating the etiology and natural history of the disorder and in developing reliable and valid methods of diagnosis. Fortunately, considerable progress in each of these areas has been made during the past 5 years. Such research, along with the theoretical formulations and initial treatment outcome research described in this paper, has provided a strong foundation for the development and refinement of efficacious treatments for post-traumatic stress disorder. As such, the next 5 years promise even greater returns.

REFERENCES

American Psychiatric Association. (1980). *Diagnostic and statistical manual of mental disorders* (3rd ed.). Washington: Author.

Anisman, H. (1978). Neurochemical changes elicited by stress. In H. Anisman & G. Bignami (Eds.), *Psychopharmacology of aversively motivated behavior* (pp. 119–172). New York: Plenum.

Billings, A. G., & Moos, R. H. (1981). The role of coping responses and social resources in attenuating the stress of life events. *Journal of Behavioral Medicine, 4,* 139–157.

Blackburn, A. B., O'Connell, W. E., & Richman, B. W. (1984). PTSD, the Vietnam veteran, and Adlerian natural high therapy. *Individual Psychology: Journal of Adlerian Theory, Research and Practice, 40,* 317–332.

Blanchard, E. B., Kolb, L. C., Pallmayer, T. P., & Gerardi, R. J. (1982). The development of a psychophysiological assessment procedure for post-traumatic stress disorder in Vietnam veterans. *Psychiatric Quarterly, 54,* 220–228.

Boudewyns, P. A., & Shipley, R. H. (1983). *Flooding and implosive therapy: Direct therapeutic exposure in clinical practice.* New York: Plenum.

Brende, J. O. (1981). Combined individual and group therapy for Vietnam veterans. *International Journal of Group Psychotherapy, 31,* 367–378.

Brende, J. O., & McCann, I. L. (1984). Regressive experiences in Vietnam veterans: Their relationship to war, post-traumatic symptoms and recovery. *Journal of Contemporary Psychotherapy, 14,* 57–75.

Carroll, E. M., Rueger, D. B., Foy, D. W., & Donohoe, C. P. (1985). Vietnam combat veterans with post-traumatic stress disorder: Analysis of marital and cohabitating adjustment. *Journal of Abnormal Psychology, 95,* 329–337.

Christie, M. J., & Chesher, G. B. (1982). Physical dependence on physiologically released endogenous opiates. *Life Sciences, 30,* 1173–1177.

Crump, L. E. (1984). Gestalt therapy in the treatment of Vietnam veterans experiencing PTSD symptomatology. *Journal of Contemporary Psychotherapy, 14,* 90–98.

Demers, R. G., McDonagh, P. H., & Moore, R. J. (1984). Pyridoxine deficiency with phenelzine. *Southern Medical Journal, 77,* 641–642.

Emmelkamp, P. M. G., Kuipers, C. M., & Eggeraat, J. B. (1978). Cognitive modification versus prolonged exposure in vivo. *Behaviour Research and Therapy, 16,* 33–41.

Emmelkamp, P. M. G., & Mersch, P. P. (1982). Cognition and exposure in vivo in the treatment of agoraphobia: Short-term and delayed effects. *Cognitive Therapy and Research, 6,* 77–88.

Escobar, J. I., Randolph, E. T., Puente, G., Spiwak, F., Asamen, J. K., Hill, M., & Hough, R. L. (1983). Post-traumatic stress disorder in Hispanic Vietnam veterans. *Journal of Nervous and Mental Disease, 171,* 585–596.

Fairbank, J. A., Gross, R. T., & Keane, T. M. (1983). Treatment of post-traumatic stress disorder: Evaluating outcome with a behavioral code. *Behavior Modification, 7,* 557–568.

Fairbank, J. A., Hansen, D., & Fitterling, J. (1985, August). *Psychological stress and coping in aging former prisoners of war.* Paper presented at the annual meeting of the American Psychological Association, Los Angeles.

Fairbank, J. A., & Keane, T. M. (1982). Flooding for combat-related stress disorders: Assessment of anxiety reduction across traumatic memories. *Behavior Therapy, 13,* 499–510.

Folkman, S., & Lazarus, R. S. (1980). An analysis of coping in a middle-aged community sample. *Journal of Health and Social Behavior, 21,* 219–239.

Folkman, S., & Lazarus, R. S. (1985). If it changes it must be a process: Study of emotion and coping during three stages of a college examination. *Journal of Personality and Social Psychology, 48,* 150–170.

Heimberg, R. G. (1985). What makes traumatic stress traumatic? *Behavior Therapy, 16,* 417–428.

Hogben, G. L., & Cornfield, R. B. (1981). Treatment of traumatic war neurosis with phenelzine. *Archives of General Psychiatry, 38,* 440–445.

Horowitz, M. J. (1973). Phase oriented treatment of stress response syndromes. *American Journal of Psychotherapy, 27,* 506–515.

Horowitz, M. J. (1974). Stress response syndromes, character style, and dynamic psychotherapy. *Archives of General Psychiatry, 31,* 768–781.

Horowitz, M. J., & Kaltreider, N. B. (1980). Brief psychotherapy of stress response syndromes. In T. B. Karasu and L. Bellak (Eds.), *Specialized techniques in individual psychotherapy.* New York: Brunner/Mazel.

Horowitz, M. J., Marmar, C., Weiss, D. S., Dewitt, K. N., & Rosenbaum, R. (1984). Brief psychotherapy of bereavement reactions: The relationship of process to outcome. *Archives of General Psychiatry, 41,* 438–448.

Johnson, C. H., Gilmore, J. D., & Shenoy, R. S. (1982). Use of a feeding procedure in the treatment of a stress-related anxiety disorder. *Journal of Behavior Therapy and Experimental Psychiatry, 13,* 235–237.

Kaloupek, D. G., & Stoupakis, T. (1985). Coping with a stressful medical procedure: Further investigation of volunteer blood donors. *Journal of Behavioral Medicine, 8,* 131–149.

Kamil, A. C. (1969). Some parameters of the second-order conditioning of fear in rats. *Journal of Comparative and Physiological Psychology, 67,* 364–369.

Keane, T. M. (1985). Defining traumatic stress: Some comments on the current terminological confusion. *Behavior Therapy, 16,* 419–423.

Keane, T. M., Fairbank, J. A., Caddell, J. M., Zimering, R. T., & Bender, M. E. (1985). A behavioral approach to assessing and treating post-traumatic stress disorder in Vietnam veterans. In C. R. Figley (Ed.), *Trauma and its wake: The assessment and treatment of post-traumatic stress disorder.* New York: Brunner/Mazel.

Keane, T. M., & Kaloupek, D. G. (1982). Imaginal flooding in the treatment of a post-traumatic stress disorder. *Journal of Consulting and Clinical Psychology, 50,* 138–140.

Keane, T. M., Scott, W. O., Chavoya, G. A., Lamparski, D. M., & Fairbank, J. A. (1985). Social support in Vietnam veterans with post-traumatic stress disorder: A comparative analysis. *Journal of Consulting and Clinical Psychology, 53,* 95–102.

Keane, T. M., Zimering, R. T., & Caddell, J. M. (1985). A behavioral formulation of post-traumatic stress disorder in Vietnam veterans. *Behavior Therapist, 8,* 9–12.

Kilpatrick, D. G., Veronen, L. J., & Resick, P. A. (1982). Psychological sequelae to rape: Assessment and treatment strategies. In D. M. Doleys, R. L. Meredith, & A. R. Ciminero (Eds.), *Behavioral medicine: Assessment and treatment strategies.* New York: Plenum.

Kolb, L. C. (1984). The post-traumatic stress disorders of combat: A subgroup with a conditioned emotional response. *Military Medicine, 149,* 237–243.

Krieger, D. (1983). Brain peptides, what, where, and why. *Science, 222,* 975–985.

Lazarus, R. S. (1981). The stress and coping paradigm. In S. Eisdorfer, D. Cohen, A. Kleinman, & P. Maxim (Eds.), *Theoretical bases for psychopathology.* New York: Spectrum.

Lazarus, R. S., & Folkman, S. (1984). *Stress, appraisal, and coping.* New York: Springer.

Lettieri, D. J. (1985, August). *Recovery from alcoholism: Patient, treatment, and environmental factors.* Paper presented at the annual meeting of the American Psychological Association, Los Angeles.

Levenson, H., Lanman, R., & Rankin, M. (1982). Traumatic war neurosis and phenelzine [letter]. *Archives of General Psychiatry, 38,* 1345.

Lindy, J. D., Green, B. L., Grace, M., & Titchener, J. (1983). Psychotherapy with survivors of the Beverly Hills Supper Club fire. *American Journal of Psychotherapy, 37,* 593–610.

Malloy, P. F., Fairbank, J. A., & Keane, T. M. (1983). Validation of a multimethod assessment of post-traumatic stress disorders in Vietnam veterans. *Journal of Consulting and Clinical Psychology, 51,* 488–494.

Marshall, W. L. (1985). The effects of variable exposure in flooding therapy. *Behavior Therapy, 16,* 117–135.

Maynert, E. W., & Levi, R. (1964). Stress-induced release of brain norepinephrine and its inhibition by drugs. *Journal of Pharmacological Experimental Therapy, 143,* 90–95.

McCaffrey, R. J., & Fairbank, J. A. (1985). Post-traumatic stress disorder associated with transportation accidents: Two case studies. *Behavior Therapy, 16,* 406–416.

Milanes, F. J., Mack, C. N., Dennison, J., & Slater, V. L. (1984). Phenelzine treatment of post-Vietnam stress syndrome. *VA Practitioner, 1,* 40–49.

Miller, T. W., & Buchbinder, J. T. (1979, December). *Clinical effects of cognitive-behavior therapy with a post-traumatic war neurosis Vietnam veteran.* Paper presented at the meeting of the Association for Advancement of Behavior Therapy, San Francisco.

Moos, R., & Billings, A. (1982). Conceptualizing and measuring coping resolves and processes. In L. Goldberger & S. S. Brenitz (Eds.), *Handbook of stress: Theoretical and clinical aspects.* New York: Macmillan.

Mowrer, O. H. (1960). *Learning theory and behavior.* New York: Wiley.

Nicholson, R. A., & Berman, J. S. (1983). Is follow-up necessary in evaluating psychotherapy? *Psychological Bulletin, 93,* 261–278.

Pearlin, L. I., & Schooler, C. (1978). The structure of coping. *Journal of Health and Social Behavior, 19,* 2–21.

Rachman, S. (1985). A note on the conditioning theory of fear acquisition. *Behavior Therapy, 16,* 426–428.

Saigh, P. A. (1984). Pre- and postinvasion anxiety in Lebanon. *Behavior Therapy, 15,* 185–190.

Saigh, P. A. (1985). On the nature and etiology of traumatic stress. *Behavior Therapy, 16,* 423–426.

Sarason, I. G., Sarason, B. R., Potter, E. H., & Antoni, M. H. (1985). Life events, social support, and illness. *Psychosomatic Medicine, 47,* 156–163.

Schindler, F. E. (1980). Treatment by systematic desensitization of a recurring nightmare of a real life trauma. *Journal of Behavior Therapy and Experimental Psychiatry, 11,* 53–54.

Scrignar, C. B. (1983). *Stress strategies: The treatment of the anxiety disorders.* New York: Karger.

Shen, W. W., & Park, S. (1983). The use of monoamine oxidase inhibitors in the treatment of traumatic war neurosis: Case report. *Military Medicine, 148,* 430–431.

Solomon, R. L., & Wynne, L. C. (1954). Traumatic avoidance learning: The principles of anxiety conservation and partial irreversibility. *Psychological Review, 61,* 353–385.

Stone, A. A., & Neale, J. M. (1984). New measure of daily coping: Development and preliminary results. *Journal of Personality and Social Psychology, 46,* 892–906.

van der Kolk, B., Greenberg, M., Boyd, H., & Krystal, J. (1985). Inescapable shock, neurotransmitters, and addition to trauma: Toward a psychobiology of post-traumatic stress. *Biological Psychiatry, 20,* 314–325.

Walker, J. I. (1982). Chemotherapy of traumatic war stress. *Military Medicine, 147,* 1029–1033.

Watson, J. B., & Raynor, R. (1920). Conditioned emotional reactions. *Journal of Experimental Psychology, 3,* 1–14.

22

Cross-Cultural Care for PTSD

Research, Training, and Service Needs for the Future

JOSEPH WESTERMEYER

Have post-traumatic stress reactions and their related disorders already been adequately addressed? Have we gone through the worst of disastrous Third World wars, refugee hoards, hostage taking, drunk-driving victims, rape victims, and other victims of violence? I think not—and for several reasons.

First, we cannot assume that tribal or Third World violence is abating. On the contrary, an argument can be made that it is just getting started. Colonialism, neocolonialism, and socioeconomic hegemony—despite their many moral and cultural evils—did establish the conditions for a *pax Romana,* largely because war undermines markets. Tribal warfare, revolution, civil wars, national expansionism, and even some regional imperialism are currently in progress in Latin America, Africa, and Asia. Their victims have been coming to the United States by the hundreds of thousands in the last decade and will likely continue to arrive, legally and illegally. It should also be borne in mind that these conflicts do not go by the international conventions of war that have largely prevailed in recent European wars. Torture, rape, mutilation, terror, mass executions, "no prisoner" battlefield policies,

---

JOSEPH WESTERMEYER • Department of Psychiatry, University of Minnesota Hospitals and Clinics, Minneapolis, Minnesota 55455; and Department of Psychiatry, Department of Veterans Affairs Medical Center, Minneapolis, Minnesota 55417. Reprinted from *Journal of Traumatic Stress*, Vol. 2, No. 4, 1989.

Psychotraumatology, edited by George S. Everly, Jr. and Jeffrey M. Lating. Plenum Press, New York, 1995.

forced work and concentration camps, violence against unarmed civilian populations, purposeful starvation of minorities and rebellious subgroups, abuse of children, and use of bacterial and gas weapons are occurring and will probably continue (Zarjenvski, 1985).

Second, substance abuse shows little sign of abating among those subgroups who perpetuate violence while intoxicated (Dezelsky et al., 1985). Though there may be some decline of alcohol-related events in older men, it is continuing or perhaps even increasing in younger men—the group responsible for most alcohol- and drug-related vehicular accidents, assault, rape, child abuse, homicide, and other violence (Westermeyer, 1975, 1986a). The driving-while-intoxicated (DWI) subpopulation shows no signs of responding optimally to education, treatment, or other intervention; they are a different subgroup from other subgroups of substance abusers. The increasingly younger substance abusers of today are less stable socially than the older alcoholic of past generations: Rape, assault, robbery, and careless driving are more common in this group, who are more apt to be single, unemployed, untrained and unskilled, and socially alienated.

A third factor involves the increase of cross-cultural work in facilities serving mental health needs. These range from counseling offices to community mental health clinics to psychiatric clinics and hospital units. Until recent years these services, largely purveyed in a fee-for-service context, were available primarily to better-educated, wealthier, English-speaking patients. Nowadays all groups have greater access to mental health services. Not only are the services more readily available, but also the number of cross-cultural contacts are increasing. One factor is the increase of refugees and economic migrants coming to the United States from Asia, the Soviet Union, Africa, and Latin America. A second factor is the rural-to-urban migration of many ethnic minorities in the United States: American Indians, southwestern Hispanics, Scots-Irish-English from the Appalachians, and southern blacks.

A fourth factor involves the high rate of psychiatric disorder and disability among virtually all migrants. These rates are especially high among refugees, with the involuntary loss of country, occupation, and status that usually attends these moves, along with the high incidence of torture, other violence, and terror in this group. Thus the mental health needs of these incoming populations are greater than those of our indigenous populations. If these needs are not effectively met, the national costs in disability and unemployment escalate (Westermeyer 1985c, d, e; Williams & Westermeyer, 1986).

A fifth reason involves methodological research issues. Most victims of post-traumatic stress disorder (PTSD) do not realize financial gains from their disorder, while some may. These latter include some veterans and vehicular accident victims. This can dramatically alter the clinical picture (Sparr and Pankratz, 1983). Hostages, refugees, and torture victims do not ordinarily realize secondary economic gains from PTSD. Thus research into these groups can aid in testing out etiological or perpetuating factors. Until the etiology of PTSD is better understood, many clinicians will continue to doubt the validity of this disorder. Because all PTSD victim groups are biased populations in one way or another, there is also an advantage in sampling from many different demographic, clinical, and cultural groups in order to distinguish core elements of PTSD.

TRAINING NEEDS

Current Status

Over the last 50 years an extensive literature has developed on both cross-cultural psychiatry and PTSD. However, few training programs in the mental health disciplines include explicit course work or training in either area. This is probably attributable to numerous factors: the scarcity of academicians and clinical supervisors experienced in these areas, the sparse distribution of research findings in an extensive multidisciplinary literature, the unevenness in the quality of the PTSD and cross-cultural work (some of which is more polemic than research), the sometimes political nature of the work (which confuses or alienates many professionals), the need to examine one's own ethnocentrism and racial prejudices, an unwillingness to consider both fascination with and revulsion toward violence, the personal horror at explicitly discussing the violent events experienced by patients and their sequelae, and the existential turmoil in dealing with the randomness, unpredictability, and senselessness of much violence and victimization.

Cross-Cultural Assessment and Treatment

Many mental health professionals shy away from assessing or treating patients of different cultural or linguistic backgrounds, even averring at times that it is impossible. It is indeed more difficult and more time-consuming than intracultural work, but it is not impossible (Westermeyer, 1976a; 1985d; Westermeyer et al., 1984; Westermeyer & Sines, 1979; Westermeyer & Walker, 1982). For it to become feasible, however, mental health professionals must acquire knowledge, skills, and experience (preferably supervised) in conducting this type of work.

The tasks of cross-cultural assessment must first be broken down into its subcomponents. When, where, and how to work with translators is a critical first step (Westermeyer, 1986a). Methods for establishing rapport across cultures (and often across language and race) require special training and supervision. Clinical approaches fundamental to establishing the presence or absence of psychopathological signs and symptoms must be known. Is a certain idea expressed by the patient a culturally consistent belief or is it a delusion? Has the patient been hallucinating or merely experiencing a socially approved trance event? Does a particular behavior fit a normal cultural pattern, or is it culturally strange and unexpected? Means for answering these questions are available and should be known by today's clinicians (Westermeyer, 1985d).

Cross-cultural treatment also involves certain special aspects. Transference as well as countertransference can have cultural, racial, historical, and political dimensions that should be addressed during training. Individual therapy can be influenced by culture in various ways: For example, a female patient may not be permitted to see a male therapist without a family chaperone being present. Racial identity must be distinguished from ethnic identity (Westermeyer, 1979). Couples and family therapy may also be affected by culture: In many traditional groups, any direct confrontation or negative report about an extended family matriarch or patriarch may be impossible in that person's presence. Group therapy especially can be remarkably different among various cultures: Some groups expound on their symptoms and personal "sins," whereas others prefer to relate their adventures, accomplishments, and coping despite adversity. Even pharmacotherapy depends heavily upon cultural expectations regarding duration of treatment, changes in dosage, control over regimens (i.e., by the patient, family, or clinician), and tolerance of side effects. Psychiatric hospitalization conveys markedly differing symbolism from one group to another: Some see it as a desirable endorsement of illness, whereas others view it as a shame on the family. Compliance with treatment plans depends strongly on the clinician's ability to recognize the principles of treatment, to set treatment priorities, and to negotiate treatment across cultural boundaries.

Assessment and Treatment of PTSD Across Cultural Boundaries

Many clinicians in the United States are unfamiliar with taking a PTSD history. The principles for such diagnostic and therapeutic interviewing are well known, having been developed during and after World War II at a time when PTSD was known as "shell shock." Research following the Boston Coconut Grove disaster contributed greatly to this body of knowledge and skill (Adler, 1943; Lindemann, 1944). Unfortunately, this accumulated wisdom was gradually abandoned, with the result that an entire generation of clinicians have minimal familiarity with it. The resurgence of interest in Vietnam veterans has resulted in some rediscovery, but with much political conflict marring this effort.

My own experience with students, residents in training, and many colleagues trained in the last decade or two is that they do not take a relevant PTSD history in cases where it is warranted. Victims of accidents and American war veterans sometimes receive such attention (Van Putten & Emory, 1973). Rape victims, battered spouses, and victims of child abuse may or may not. Refugees, veterans of other armies, and torture victims almost never do. Even when a history of the violent event is obtained, there is a tendency to ignore the premigration and/or pretrauma life experience, although these are known to play an important role in the genesis of PTSD, treatment approaches, and outcome. The relevance of the traumatic event to the patient and the particular clinical problem at hand is sometimes overlooked. A common notion is that PTSD victims will report their symptoms if merely invited to report their problem, when in fact shame, guilt, suppression, and displacement typically make the PTSD diagnosis unavailable unless the clinician asks specific questions.

A general method for eliciting PTSD symptoms and evaluating the relevance of these symptoms to the particular individual does exist. This includes the following:

1. Pretraumatic losses (e.g., parental loss), coping, achievements, roles, and psychiatric disorders
2. Nature, extent and duration of the traumatic event(s)
3. Patient's thoughts and feelings about these events at the time, during the interim, and now
4. Directed history regarding PTSD symptoms (see Horowitz et al., 1980)
5. Life changes concurrent with onset of PTSD symptoms, such as arrival in new culture, discharge from service, divorce, loss of job, assault, theft or vandalism (Christenson et al., 1981)
6. Thorough psychiatric evaluation, with special reference to conditions commonly associated with PTSD (i.e., depression, substance abuse, panic attacks, generalized anxiety, phobia, paranoia, psychophysiological disorders, dissociative reactions)

In addition to this generic history, special history taking and therapeutic interviewing are warranted depending on the nature of the traumatic events. This has been well described for veterans of military service (Haley, 1974; Sonnenberg et al., 1985). Special topical areas must also be covered for children, torture victims, concentration camp survivors, hostages, rape victims, and others. With refugees the following topics should be discussed in detail:

1. Preflight occupation, social status, coping mechanisms, psychiatric disorders
2. Reasons for initiating the flight from the mother country
3. Patient's willingness to leave, along with the amount of care and deliberation given to the decision (i.e., many leave unwillingly because family members or fellow villagers are leaving; decisions may be careful and balanced after due deliberation, or precipitously made in a moment of fear)
4. Nature and duration of the flight, with losses, traumatic events, injuries, and other experiences during the flight
5. Experiences (positive and negative) in countries of refuge

6. Losses as a result of the flight (e.g., relationships, social roles and status, property, vocation and avocations, daily activities)
7. Elements of continuity from preflight to postflight life (e.g., language, household members, religion, occupation, sports, hobbies)
8. Problems in the new country (e.g., language, finances, marital or family disruption, affiliation with expatriate community, security from assault and theft)
9. Behaviors and affiliations vis-à-vis the country of origin (e.g., food, cultural celebrations, contacts with those still in the country)
10. Behaviors and affiliations in the country of refuge (e.g., number of indigenous friends, citizenship, use of indigenous resources and institutions such as banks or political parties)
11. Feelings about the country of refuge, its culture and people, and prospects of living out one's life in the new country (e.g., clarification about wanting to return to country of origin, location and content of any dreams)

The professional in training, as well as clinicians unfamiliar with this work, will benefit from role modeling by an experienced clinician actually conducting this type of therapeutic work. Didactic presentations and one-to-one supervisions are also important. Those new to this type of work share certain problems in achieving the requisite skills, including the following:

1. Fascination with "the story" of the events, to the exclusion of considering how the events interacted with the individual and his or her previous life, as well as how the past events have psychological and social relevance for the patient in the here and now
2. Horror, revulsion, or remorse at the patient's story, so that the patient is led away from it into other more pleasant topics
3. Unwillingness to pursue the traumatic events in detail for fear of adding additional suffering to the patient, who is often distraught while recalling the events (like questions about suicide, asking about traumatic life events does not create distress, but only elicits it if it already exists)
4. Unwillingness to question the patient about his or her premigration life, as though the patient's life began only after arrival in the clinician's community
5. Inability to obtain, or perhaps to tolerate negative reports and feelings about the clinician's own country-of-origin, citizenry, and culture

Once clinicians are trained to assess PTSD in the cross-cultural context, the next learning task is treatment of PTSD in the cross-cultural context. This, too, involves a number of adaptations of standard therapeutic practice. It may be necessary to work through a translator—a complex, but learnable skill. More facilitation and clarification are needed in earlier stages, as compared to intracultural therapy. Psychodynamic interpretations and patient education must be phrased in concepts, symbols, analogies, or proverbs familiar to the patient. Confrontation must be gently attempted, ideally within a social network approach involving the family, because cross-cultural patients are often especially sensitive to poor self-image and feelings of rejection and alienation. As with assessment, skill in this kind of therapy is most rapidly achieved during supervision with a number of different cases.

Trainees must learn to recognize and deal with special problems which often attend the treatment of PTSD across cultures. One of these involves translators who have had crises and traumas similar to those of the patient. Translators may avoid inducing stress in themselves by not translating accurately, avoiding the topic, changing the subject, informing the clinician that the interview is too stressful for the patient, and so forth. Those translators who persist despite their own discomfort should have the opportunity to discuss their own feelings privately after the interview. Household members usually realize something is amiss (because of prominent symptoms, such as night terrors), but they may not appreciate the existence of PTSD. At times they may not even know about the traumatic event(s). The patient may be protecting the family by not telling them about their disorder, or previous traumatic events. This lack of family awareness must be addressed in therapy.

SERVICE NEEDS

Problem in the Treatment System

Ideally all mental health clinicians should be able to recognize, assess, and treat PTSD in cross-cultural contexts, but this is not likely to happen in the foreseeable future. Since the ideal is not feasible, what is possible?

There is a problem with outreach or bilingual workers, inexperienced clinicians, clinics, and programs holding onto cross-cultural cases of PTSD even when the patient is severely disturbed or not responding to treatment. Any clinician encountering cross-cultural patients should be able at least to conduct skillful evaluations. If they cannot do so, they should be able to refer to facilities that can accomplish this. Because many cross-cultural patients receive their care in public clinics or health maintenance organizations (HMOs), there are economic forces that inveigh against referrals to outside facilities. Substandard care results; cases of negligence or malpractice are now in the courts. Legal redress may change this situation for indigenous patients who know how to use the American court system, but it may not be so available for cross-cultural patients. Public defenders do not readily confront the system that is paying them, nor do they usually understand the nuances of cross-cultural care. Expatriate or other ethnic organizations may be able to remedy this by initiating class action suits.

Another approach is the training of professionals in cross-cultural assessment and treatment. In psychiatry and psychology, there are only a few hundred persons with expertise in this field. Many of them hold academic positions. Training funds for G-4 residency positions, G-5 fellowship positions, and postdoctoral fellowships could greatly increase the cadre of national expertise in this field. The cost would be relatively small, and impact on services could occur within a few to several years (i.e., a relatively short time).

Facilities serving cross-cultural patients should be able to demonstrate training, skill, experience, and expertise in cross-cultural evaluation and treatment. Without such abilities, clinicians, clinics, and programs should not receive service funds. Currently no such policies or procedures exist. Given minimal resources, many facilities provide service workers with minimal training and experience for cross-cultural work when extra training and experience are required. Bilingual workers without professional training or licensure may be falsely identified as "counselors" or "therapists" when they are not.

Another dilemma involves delay in treatment for PTSD and its associated conditions. Timely and effective interventions are needed for populations at risk. Social and primary health care workers untrained in psychiatric assessment, as well as those professionals in the mental health field unable to diagnose and assess psychiatric conditions across cultural boundaries, contribute to this problem (Westermeyer & Williams, 1986).

Problems with the Professionals

Psychiatrists and psychologists providing cross-cultural services especially need cross-cultural training. Most practicing psychologists do not have skills in selecting "culture fair" psychometrics and administering them across cultural and language boundaries. Most practicing psychiatrists do not know how to distinguish delusions from culture-bound beliefs, or to conduct a mental status exam that is cross-culturally sensitive. Misdiagnosis, "overdiagnosis" (i.e., perceiving more pathology than exists), and "underdiagnosis" (i.e., eliciting less pathology than exists) lead to therapeutic failures, as treatment plans are built on a false foundation.

Another problem (among psychiatrists as well as psychologists) is the failure to consider, test for, and recognize organic factors. Head injuries are especially common in torture victims, concentration camp internees, and refugees from war and political strife. In my own clinical experience, these patients have often not been even asked about head injuries, periods of unconsciousness, seizures, and other manifestations of head injury. Prolonged periods of malnutrition and epidemic infectious disease in refugee camps in children have also been associated with learning disabilities, impulsiveness, developmental problems, and mental retardation. Prolonged periods of untreated psychiatric disorder can precipitate or exacerbate physical illness, from allergies to migraine to tuberculosis and lung flukes. Conversely, physical illness in refugees and other trauma victims struggling to adapt to new circumstances can serve as the "last straw" and precipitate psychiatric disorders. We have seen a number of potentially life-threatening problems present with psychiatric symptoms (e.g., extrauterine pregnancy, hemoglobinopathies, gallbladder stones, hepatoma, uterus perforated by an IUD, fungal meningitis, respiratory and gastrointestinal cancer, and chronic infection); three of these patients have died as a result of delayed diagnosis. Neuropsychological and neuropsychiatric assessment are regularly indicated in refugees and other post-traumatic patients. Professionals with expertise in neuropsychology and neuropsychiatry should be on the full-time staff of any facility serving as a referral center for cross-cultural patients. Part-time professional consultants or supervisors who do not themselves examine, assess, and treat these patients may be worse than no psychiatrists at all.

Consultation for associated medical conditions should be readily available to mental health facilities serving cross-cultural patients. A nearby team of surgeons, internists, family practitioners, radiologists, and laboratory medical and other specialists should have familiarity in working with cross-cultural patients and their particular maladies. For example, those working with Indochinese refugees must know about the common infectious disorders, the high rates of trauma, the special congenital problems (e.g., hemoglobinopathies) and the special cancers (e.g., hepatoma, craniopharyngioma, choriocarcinoma) that occur in these groups. Because many physicians are unskilled or uninterested in cross-cultural work, referrals must be carefully established and monitored. In many countries, physicians or other white-coated persons attend at torture sessions, contributing to patients' fear of physicians and nurses.

Access to culturally sensitive social resources in the community is also vital. Regular working relationships should be established with local vocational rehabilitation services, social agencies, rape services, and expatriate organizations, depending on the type of patient being served. As in mental health and other clinical settings, many social service agency workers have no skill or interest in providing cross-cultural services, and skill at cross-cultural psychiatric assessment may not be available. Liaison and follow-up are therefore critical.

Strategic Approaches to Organizing Services

Agencies serving particular groups (e.g., refugees, rape victims) can feel threatened by mental health involvement with one of their clients. They may perceive this as a failure on their part, as though they should be able to provide a complete spectrum of services for every single client. Or they may feel that their limitations will be exposed, their funding will be removed, or some other unnamed catastrophe may ensue. This feeling of being threatened can lead to behaviors that augur against the patient's care, such as holding onto seriously disturbed or disturbing clients who need psychiatric attention, withholding information, or withdrawing from the case.

Another common obstacle is a certain possessiveness, so that the particular group is perceived as "ours"—"our" refugees, or "our" rape victims. This viewpoint is almost inevitable when one type of victim alone is served. Unfortunately, this attitude stems from and further contributes to the type of social isolation that victims experience. It can also lead to primary and lifelong identity as a victim, rather than integrating the fact of victimization into other, more stable and healthy identities (e.g., worker, parent, man or woman).

At times special agencies are created to meet a particular need (i.e., refugees, rape or torture victims). This has the advantage that a particular service can be rapidly developed and implemented. Working through established institutions and facilities can be time-consuming, and the priority on the particular service can be readily undermined in the face of many other needs. There are also certain problems from this approach. Perhaps most importantly, funding for special agencies is fragile. Isolated services tend to disappear once the political emphasis shifts. The isolated facility also does not have access to generic services provided in larger institutions, so that major problems are missed, or recognized but ignored, or totally mismanaged when the isolated facility does not have the full range of resources to address the problem. Because special populations tend to be relatively small (e.g., several dozen to several thousand people), a full range of social, medical, and mental health services cannot be created to serve the special population alone. Victims in these groups must at times obtain services in nonspecial resources, which creates problems if those in the general facilities are unaware or insensitive to the individual's special needs. Another difficulty is the isolation of both staff and clientele from the societal mainstream. The staff does not grow professionally by learning to address a variety of persons as well as clinical problems; consequences include burnout, professional isolation, vulnerability in the job market, and a self-image of being in constant struggle with the outside world. Clients or patients may emulate the staff by remaining isolated instead of entering and participating in the mainstream of society. Clients in this type of agency or clinic are especially apt to become immobilized with an ongoing self-label as "refugee" or "rape victim," instead of integrating the violent event into their lives and then moving on. Thus, in the long run, isolated services can become counterproductive.

Development of special services involves certain logistical problems. This involves both a geographic and chronological dimension. Refugee moves, prisoner-of-war releases, and hostage taking are episodic events, with large numbers appearing at infrequent times. Rapes, child abuse, amok-type homicides, and other victimizations occur more consistently but may be too infrequent or sparsely distributed (say, in a rural area or small town) to warrant a special program. Again, there is the issue of general skills versus special programs: to what extent should generalists have these more esoteric skills, versus how many special programs can be supported. Some compromise between the two must be struck. For episodic problems, such as isolated mass public violence or hostages or released prisoners of war, a national cadre of experts may be necessary. The latter might then educate, train, consult with, and guide local caregivers in providing useful services. Another strategy involves a regional or national center, such as the torture victim program in Canada or the several refugee centers scattered about Europe. These centers have several advantages, including a cadre of experts, consultation to outside professionals and facilities, triage, referral for assessment and sometimes treatment, and rehabilitation services. Some of these centers are freestanding, but those with greater longevity tend to have a stable institutional base (Westermeyer, 1986b, c).

Placement of programs in nonspecialized or general agencies, departments, clinics, hospitals, or other institutions also has advantages and disadvantages. Access to a wide range of resources is a major advantage, because some victims do need highly expert help that cannot be provided in a small program. Placement in a general institution also avoids isolation by providing daily interaction on both staff levels and client-patient levels with other staff and clients/patients who do not belong to the victims' special group. Special program staff can gradually be assimilated into the general staff on firm funding as they acquire training, certification, or skills with generic application. On the negative side, most staff at general facilities do not have the skill or experience to deal with special victim populations. There is also the risk that funds for special populations (as well as special knowledge, skill, and experience) will be lost into the general staff activities if care is not taken to prevent it.

Experience with refugee populations in Europe after World War II demonstrated the superiority of a combined special-but-general approach. This involved establishing a special program within a generic institution, including psychiatric facilities, general hospital units, and social agencies. Funding was more stable, patients/clients had ready access to generic services, and staff worked with other people and problems besides the refugee group.

In the United States the cross-cultural care and PTSD of American Indians and other native peoples are not adequately addressed. This particular population has an extensive rural-to-urban migration, high rates of violence, and high mortality of family members (Westermeyer, 1976b, c; Westermeyer & Brantner, 1972; Westermeyer & Peake, 1983). Besides high prevalence of PTSD, sensitive cross-cultural services are minimal from the standpoint of quality, quantity, access, and timeliness. If centers can be established for refugees and others, why not for the original Americans?

Treatment of PTSD and Associated Conditions

Services must take into account the fact that PTSD rarely occurs by itself. It often accompanies other major disorders that require attention (Escobar et al., 1983; Sierles et al., 1983). These include major depression (Silver & Iacono, 1984; Westermeyer, 1986b, d), substance abuse (Keehn, 1980; Lacoursiere et al., 1981; Peak et al., 1981; Westermeyer, 1985b, c), panic disorder, generalized anxiety, phobias, antisocial and other personality disorders (Kolb and Mutalipassi, 1982), behavioral and learning problems in children and adolescents, psychophysiological disorders, psychosis (Yesavage, 1983), childhood developmental problems, organic brain syndrome (especially in victims of violence), and associated medical and social problems (Corcoran, 1982). Treatment of PTSD alone may occasionally relieve these conditions, but often does not. Conversely, attention to these associated problems alone may or may not relieve the PTSD.

Treatment modalities for PTSD include grief work, counseling about social network development, education about self-help methods for dealing with PTSD symptoms, hypnotherapy, desensitization including imaginal flooding, behavioral therapies, narcosynthesis, various pharmacotherapies, existential approaches, and other psychotherapeutic individual/family/group interventions, self-help groups, and the value of sublimation in dealing with PTSD (Hamburg & Adams, 1967; Hogben & Cornfield, 1981; Keane & Kaloupek, 1982; Sledge et al., 1980; Westermeyer et al., 1983a). A variety of culturally sensitive psychotherapies must be available, including individual, group, and family/marital approaches. Therapists working with PTSD patients must be highly skilled and experienced, as they will have to be able to deal with remorse, survival guilt, delayed grief, childhood traumas reawakened by the traumas experienced in adult life, sexual violence, sexual dysfunction, impacted anger, abreaction, hysteria, conversion symptoms, fugue and other dissociative reactions, regression, brief psychosis, displaced violence, and substance abuse. Staff should be aware of common posttraumatic symptoms that occur in patients short of full PTSD, because these can exacerbate other psychopathology or produce embarrassment of self-doubt. Common concomitants of severe stress should be understood, such as spontaneous ejaculation during severe anxiety or terror (Redmond et al., 1983). Many victims of severe traumatic events may not have a full PTSD syndrome but still suffer from existential crises regarding the value of life, startle reactions at noises or circumstances simulating the original trauma, identification with the aggressor, overresponsibility for untoward consequences of war and other random violence (Smith, 1982), "missed" or absent or "impacted" grief (Shatan, 1974), recurrent dreams or intrusive thoughts regarding trauma from long ago (Cavenar & Nash, 1976; Wilkinson, 1983), and chronic dysthymia (Westermeyer, 1985d, e). Prestress coping methods and character should be known before undertaking a particular psychotherapeutic approach (Horowitz, 1974). Family relationships can also be seriously disrupted as a result of catastrophe or violence (Titchener & Kapp, 1976), so that family assessment and—as needed—family therapy should be available. Another factor in family assessment may be higher-than-expected rates of psychopathology, including depression and anxiety, in the other family members of PTSD patients (Davidson et al., 1985). Legal problems may be more apt to occur among certain PTSD subgroups (Walker, 1981), so that access to culturally sensitive attorneys may be required.

RESEARCH NEEDS

Priorities and Methods

As in any research endeavor, research questions must be assigned priorities. Priority research efforts should address major issues of prevention, reducing morbidity, and enhancing treatment effectiveness and cost efficacy. Lower priority should be assigned to factors that are merely historical or cannot be effectively altered in the here and now. Research should be applicable and properly scientific. Pitfalls of being overly scientistic should be avoided (as in the alcoholism field, where hundreds of millions of dollars have gone into rat and liver studies with minimal clinical application, whereas actual clinical studies have been largely ignored because strict experimental conditions cannot be applied).

One area to which I would assign high priority in cross-cultural PTSD research involves here-and-now social-environmental factors. From a clinical perspective PTSD in refugees, migrating minorities, concentration camp survivors, and American veterans of war appears to be precipitated and/or perpetuated by factors such as the following: unemployment, marital discord, geographic relocation with diminution of the intimate social network, theft/robbery/vandalism of one's property, and other current events and stresses. Comparison groups could consist of subjects from the same population who are not experiencing PTSD. The principal advantage of this work is that it would focus on here-and-now factors correlated with pathology. Correlations do not prove causality, of course. Further complicating the matter is the fact that even demonstrating causality does not necessarily imply that reversing causal factors (e.g., unemployment) will necessarily reverse pathological processes once they are present. This would lead to the next generation of research projects, detailed in the next few paragraphs.

Potential sources of bias must be recognized and protected against. For example, several Hmong associates and I recently undertook a study of traumatic events (premigration, migration, and postmigration) and post-traumatic symptoms among Hmong refugees. Complicating this study was the fact that all of us, including myself, had undergone significant stressors similar to our subjects—including exposure to attack or combat, death of close friends or family members, mortal danger to self and family, and so forth. We had also experienced a range of post-traumatic symptoms and associated conditions. In order to control for our own potential sources of bias we adopted the following data collection techniques:

1. The Hmong research associates collected data on the traumatic events or stressors.
2. I obtained clinical data regarding post-traumatic symptoms and associated conditions while blind to the above data.
3. The subjects completed self-rating scales to which we as researchers remained blind prior to other data collecting.

This care is particularly important in undertaking PTSD research because of the strong countertransference apt to occur toward victims. In addition, many clinicians and researchers interested in PTSD have had personal or family histories that involve extraordinary stress (e.g., offspring of refugees, former combat stressors, refugee workers).

Associated Conditions

It is well known that PTSD in some populations (e.g., refugees) commonly accompanies other psychiatric disorders, such as depression and substance abuse (Williams & Westermeyer, 1986). We do not, however, know whether this is also true in other populations of victims. For example, the high rates of alcoholism in certain American Indian groups could be related to the high rates of violence and subsequent unresolved PTSD. However, these crucial questions are not easily operationalized into research projects. This is not so much caused by a lack of research instruments, because these are available or can be developed. A more serious problem involves sampling, because violence rarely affects victims who are not a biased sample. One can readily consider the numerous biases that can and do influence who becomes a victim of a drunken driver, a torture victim, a concentration camp survivor, a hostage, or a refugee. It seems likely that associated conditions will vary among these subgroups. It is also not clear that stress alone may precipitate other conditions besides PTSD alone. For example, marijuana use by Vietnam era veterans does not appear specifically related to service stress (Ritter et al., 1985). These associated conditions may greatly affect the result of any treatment and rehabilitation approaches.

Another methodological problem involves the persistence of vulnerability to PTSD over a long period. Individuals may experience PTSD decades later, especially around retirement, the death of a spouse, or a major illness. This creates both theoretical and methodological problems. For example, those surviving into later ages (say, after the Holocaust in Europe during World War II) may be a highly atypical group. Studies into such subgroups of victims must take care in not generalizing the results to all victims.

Treatment of PTSD

The research literature does not tell us how to treat PTSD effectively. Most of us employ a shotgun approach, employing whatever resources are at hand coupled with some clinical intuition (often a valuable, but sometimes a misleading determinant of action) and some out-and-out guessing. Numerous potential research questions come to mind here. Does treatment of the associated condition by itself (e.g., depression or substance abuse) relieve the PTSD symptoms? This certainly occurs, but with unknown regularity. Is it most useful to treat PTSD victims in groups or as individuals or within families? If in groups, should the groups be related to past events (e.g., having been beaten or tortured), to current events (e.g., unemployed, divorced, widowed), to current diagnosis (e.g., depressed, alcoholic), or to some combination of these and other factors? Are self-help groups (see Shatan, 1973) of value, or do they reaffirm social isolation? Should professionals try to promulgate them (e.g., hostage groups, rape victim groups, refugee veterans groups)? Should these groups be social, mutually supportive, or (like Alcoholics Anonymous or Recovery) quasi-therapeutic groups? To what extent should family members or significant others be involved in the therapeutic process? Is social network therapy cost-efficient? Which social interventions and milieu modifications are effective and cost-efficient? What is the role of pharmacotherapy (such as imipramine or clonidine), especially for persistent PTSD symptoms or dysthymia in the absence of major depression, anxiety, or panic?

Secondary Prevention of PTSD

Another issue involves preventive measures. Hostages, refugees, prisoners of war, rape victims, and torture victims are at extremely high risk for psychiatric morbidity (Eitinger, 1961; Norris & Feltman-Summers, 1981; Thyysen et al., 1970; Westermeyer, 1986d; Westermeyer et al., 1983a, b, c). Consequently, some early intervention, screening, or ongoing psychiatric monitoring is being implemented in these groups, such as veterans and hostages (Corcoran, 1982). How effective and cost-efficient are these secondary preventive efforts? Should they be employed with other groups at high risk, such as concentration camp survivors, robbery victims, or refugees? Are there certain subgroups within these victims who are at particular risk to PTSD and/or associated conditions (Worthington, 1978)?

Previous psychiatric disorder may be a risk factor in subsequently developing PTSD. Other factors that generally predict psychiatric disorder may also predict PTSD, such as parental loss during childhood, a family history of substance abuse or other psychiatric disorder, certain personality types (Ursano, 1981), legal problems, never being married (over a certain age), and being divorced or widowed (Westermeyer et al., 1983a, b).

Comparison groups of individuals from the same populations without PTSD are required to answer these questions. Selecting these comparison groups involves the same problems of sampling referred to above.

Secondary Gain in PTSD

Further research into PTSD among these populations might help to clarify the issue of secondary gain in PTSD. Certain PTSD populations can stand to gain as a result of their PTSD symptoms: veterans (Atkinson et al., 1982), vehicular accident victims, and certain hostages. At this time the issue of secondary gain is a complex and uncertain one in PTSD. One study indicates that secondary gain does not greatly affect certain descriptive aspects of the therapeutic process itself (Burstein, 1983). Another study documents the existence of fictitious PTSD (Sparr & Pankrantz, 1983)—a problem that appears to have increased with the popularization and politicalization of PTSD. Many PTSD patients in the cross-cultural context have little or no element of financial remuneration for their symptoms. They thus compose a group in which PTSD can be studied independent of this complicating factor. Comparison can then be made back to PTSD patients among whom the possibility of economic gain exists. This is an important issue to the acceptance of PTSD among mental health clinicians, because many view it simply as an induced disorder solely related to secondary gain.

Course of PTSD

The treated and untreated course of PTSD has been relatively little studied (Archibald & Tuddenham, 1965; Ursano et al., 1981; Westermeyer, 1985a; Westermeyer et al., 1984a, b). Is this a relatively benign disorder with good outcome when not accompanied by other psychiatric disorders? Is self-help as effective as professional intervention in the eventual course? In the event of no treatment, among which groups does PTSD persist? If persistent, does it lead to social disability or psychiatric conditions? Or is it a sequela of social disability or psychiatric conditions? One epidemiological study of refugees suggests that treatment for major depression can have long-lasting benefit in reducing post-traumatic symptoms (Westermeyer, 1984b). Even with successful treatment, how often does the PTSD recur? And among whom? (And it does recur in some cases, at times with recurrence of an associated psychiatric disorder, or at times precipitated by a medical or social stressor, such as a major illness or retirement.)

Special Issues in Cross-Cultural Research

Any research in cross-cultural context involves special methodological, political, and ethical questions. Trust is a major issue: Cross-cultural patients are especially apt to feel like guinea pigs. This dynamic is further accentuated in PTSD victims. Researchers must be sensitive to the "gook syndrome," in which those of different race or ethnicity are seen as less human or civilized than oneself. Anthropology and cultural psychiatry provide an extensive fund of knowledge, experience, and skill for dealing with these issues.

One effective method is to involve the group to be studied in the research itself. This requires that they be involved from early on in setting the goals, designing the protocol, collecting the data, and analyzing and publishing the results. I have found this to be a valuable strategy in undertaking sensitive and difficult research among Native Americans and Hmong peoples (Westermeyer et al., 1982–1984; Westermeyer & Peake, 1983).

From the Computer to the Clinic

Dissemination of research findings to the professional community is a key element in any research undertaking. In fact, considerable literature exists on PTSD (Edwards, 1946) and cross-cultural psychiatric care as well as on cross-cultural populations at risk to PTSD, but it is not read by many involved in services. This is attributable to several factors: the inevitable delay between research and application, the generally low educational level of service providers in this area (who do not read the research literature and are not concerned with recertification), and the span of the literature across several decades and many journals and fields. Several recent books will help in filling this gap. Even an updated bibliography would help to advance the field. Some bibliographies are available for particular areas, such as culture and psychiatry, Native Americans and mental health, and refugees, social readjustment, and mental health.

Primary Prevention of PTSD

Like substance abuse, central nervous system syphilis, and mental retardation from fetal alcohol syndrome, PTSD need not be an inherent feature of the human condition. If it cannot be entirely eliminated, it can be reduced—at least in theory. Efforts to reduce loss, violence, and social disruption are under way in many corners of the world (e.g., Amnesty International, various refugee organizations). Research evaluation of these efforts would permit their effectiveness and cost efficacy to be evaluated.

Handgun legislation is being attempted in several metropolitan areas and states. Epidemiological comparisons could be made using two controls.

One would be a "before versus after legislation" in the regions. Another would be comparisons with adjacent areas not having such regulations. The U.S. Centers for Disease Control (CDC) in Atlanta could undertake this work.

Refugees fleeing Indochina have high mortality rates during flight, as well as high psychiatric morbidity after flight (Westermeyer et al., 1984a; Westermeyer et al., 1983). Australia, in an attempt to reduce this high morbidity and mortality, is now accepting "orderly departure" refugees only. PTSD among these "orderly departure" refugees could be compared with rates among other refugees. Comparisons could also be undertaken in the United States, where both kinds of refugees are accepted.

Mothers Against Drunk Drivers (MADD) groups are spreading nationally as well as internationally. Their methods are diverse and include legislative changes, pressures on lax court policies, and public education and attitude change via the mass media. How effective are these groups in reducing victimization via drunken driving? Comparisons within one population over time and of two populations (one with MADD and one without MADD) could be undertaken. Again, the CDC in Atlanta might perform this work.

Refugee placement in the United States has often been designed to produce PTSD rather than to ameliorate it. These policies are adapted and implemented by the U.S. State Department—an organization not known for its humanitarian expertise or concerns. Firm data on refugee placement policies and their financial consequences may lead to alteration in certain policies, which include placement of "unaccompanied adolescents" away from their own cultural groups, disruption of extended families that exceed eight persons, "broadcasting" of refugee groups thinly across the nation rather than multicentric distribution, and abandonment of special services after 1 year (Williams & Westermeyer, 1983; Westermeyer et al., 1985b, c).

Certain groups accepted in the United States as refugees have an extremely high risk to mental disorder. These include unaccompanied children and adolescent refugees, Amerasian children and their solo mothers, solo mothers with young children, solo young males, torture victims, former opium addicts (e.g., from Laos), and other former mentally ill persons. The national government has brought them to the United States but then does not provide services for them. Likewise, county and state governments ignore their special needs. Consequently their misery is exacerbated rather than ameliorated by bringing them to the United States. Responsibility is not and likely will not be borne by state and local governments. Philanthropic funds focus on the unmet needs of indigenous citizens, as well as short-lived projects. If funding is not provided on a national level, needs will not be served. And if needs are not served, it is at least unethical and perhaps illegal to admit such persons to the United States merely for political or public relations reasons.

We know that subsequent environmental factors can precipitate, maintain, or exacerbate PTSD months, years, or even decades after the original event. These environmental factors include hostile rejection of returning veterans, inability to speak the local language among refugees, and unemployment among migrants (Keane & Fairbank, 1983; Westermeyer, 1985d, e, f; Westermeyer et al., 1984a, b). Policies, procedures, and interventions to reduce or eliminate these factors known to be associated with psychopathology should be identified and implemented (Westermeyer & Williams, 1986).

REFERENCES

Adler, A. (1943). Neuropsychiatric complications in victims of Boston's Coconut Grove fire. *J. Amer. Med. Assoc, 123,* 1098–1101.

Archibald, H. E., & Tuddenham, R. D. (1965). Persistent stress reaction following combat: A 20 year follow up. *Arch. Gen. Psychiatry, 12,* 475–481.

Atkinson, R. M., Henderson, R. G., Sparr, L. F., et al. (1982). Assessment of Viet Nam veterans for post-traumatic stress disorder in Vietnam Administration disability claims. *Am. J. Psychiatry, 139,* 1118–1121.

Burstein, A. (1983). Treatment of post-traumatic stress disorder with imipramine. *Psychosomatics, 25,* 681–687.

Cavenar, J. O., & Nash, J. L. (1976). The effects of combat on the normal personality: War neuroses in Viet Nam returnees. *Comp. Psychiatry, 17,* 647–653.

Christenson, R. M., Walker, J. I., Ross, D. R., et al. (1981). Reactivation of traumatic conflicts. *Am. J. Psychiatry, 138,* 984–985.

Corcoran, J. D. T. (1982). The concentration camp syndrome and USAF Vietnam prisoners of war. *Psychiatr. Ann, 10,* 991–994.

Davidson, J., Swartz, M., Storck, M., et al. (1985). A diagnostic and family study of post-traumatic stress disorder. *Am. J. Psychiatry, 142,* 90–93.

Dezelsky, T. L., Toohey, J. V., & Shaw, R. S. (1985). Non-medical drug use behaviour at five United States universities: A 15-year study. *Bull. Narc, 37,* 49–53.

Edwards, J. G. (1946). Psychiatric aspects of civilian disasters. *Brit. Med. J, 1,* 944–947.

Eitinger, L. (1961). Pathology of the concentration camp syndrome. *Arch. Gen. Psychiatry, 5,* 79–87.

Escobar, J. I., Randolph, E. T., Puente, G., et al. (1983). Post-traumatic stress disorder in Hispanic Vietnam veterans: Clinical phenomenology and sociocultural characteristics. *J. Nerv. Ment. Dis, 171,* 585–596.

Haley, S. (1974). When the patient reports atrocities: Specific treatment considerations for the Vietnam veteran. *Arch. Gen. Psychiatry, 30,* 191–196.

Hamburg, D. A., & Adams, J. E. (1967). A perspective on coping behavior: Seeking and utilizing information in major transitions. *Arch. Gen. Psychiatry, 17,* 277–284.

Hogben, G. I., & Cornfield, R. B. (1981). Treatment of traumatic war neurosis with phenelzine. *Arch. Gen. Psychiatry, 38,* 440–445.

Horowitz, M. (1974). Stress response syndromes, character style and dynamic psychotherapy. *Arch. Gen. Psychiatry, 31,* 768–781.

Horowitz, M. J., Wilner, K., Kaltreider, N., et al. (1980). Signs and symptoms of post-traumatic stress disorder. *Arch. Gen. Psychiatry, 37,* 85–92.

Keane, R. M., & Fairbank, J. A. (1983). Survey analysis of combat-related stress disorders in Viet Nam veterans. *Am. J. Psychiatry, 140,* 348–350.

Keane, R. M., & Kaloupek, D. G. (1982). Imaginal flooding in the treatment of a post-traumatic stress disorder. *J. Consult. Clin. Psychol, 50,* 138–140.

Keehn, R. J. (1980). Follow-up studies of World War II and Korean conflict prisoners. *Am. J. Epidemiol, 111,* 194–211.

Kolb, L. C., & Mutalipassi, L. R. (1982). The conditional emotional response: A sub-class of the chronic and delayed post-traumatic stress disorder. *Psychiatric Ann, 12,* 979–987.

Lacoursiere, R. B., Godfrey, K. E., & Ruby, L. M. (1980). Traumatic neurosis in the etiology of alcoholism: Viet Nam combat and other trauma. *Am. J. Psychiatry, 137,* 966–968.

Lindemann, E. (1944). Symptomatology and management of acute grief. *Am. J. Psychiatry, 101,* 141–148.

Norris, J., & Feldman-Summers, S. (1981). Factors related to psychological impacts of rape on the victim. *J. Abnorm. Psychol, 90,* 562–567.

Peak, W. E., Robinowitz, R., Roberts, W. R., et al. (1981). Adjustment differences among male substance abusers varying in degree of combat experience in Vietnam. *J. Consult. Clin. Psychol, 49,* 426–437.

Redmond, D. E., Kosten, T. R., & Reiser, M. F. (1981). Spontaneous ejaculation association with anxiety: Psychophysiological considerations. *Am. J. Psychiatry, 140,* 1163–1166.

Ritter, C., Clayton, R. R., & Voss, H. L. (1985). Vietnam military service and marijuana use. *Am. J. Drug Alcohol Abuse, 11,* 119–130.

Shatan, C. F. (1973). The grief of soldiers: Vietnam combat veterans' self-help movement. *Am. J. Orthopsychiatry, 43,* 640–653.

Shatan, C. F. (1974). Through the membrane of reality: "Impacted grief" and perceptual dissonance in Viet Nam combat veterans. *Psychiatr. Opin, 11,* 6–15.

Sierles, F. S., Chen, J. J., McFarland, R. E., et al. (1983). Post-traumatic stress disorder and concurrent psychiatric illness: A preliminary report. *Am. J. Psychiatry, 140,* 1177–1179.

Silver, S. M., & Iacono, C. U. (1984). Factor-analytic support for DSM-III's post-traumatic stress disorder for Vietnam veterans. *J. Clin. Psychol, 40,* 5–14.

Sledge, W. H., Boydstun, J. A., & Rahe, J. A. (1980). Self-concept changes related to war captivity. *Arch. Gen. Psychiatry, 37,* 430–443.

Smith, J. R. (1982). Personal responsibility in traumatic stress reactions. *Psychiatr. Ann, 10,* 1021–1030.

Sonnenberg, S. J., Blank, A. S., & Talbott, J. A. (1985). *The trauma of war: Stress and recovery in Vietnam veterans.* Washington, DC: American Psychiatric Association.

Sparr, L., & Pankratz, L. D. (1983). Factitious post-traumatic stress disorder. *Amer. J. Psychiatry, 140,* 1016–1019.

Thyysen, P., Hermann, K., & Willanger, R. (1970). Concentration camp survivors in Denmark: Persecution, disease, disability, compensation. *Dan. Med. Bull, 17,* 65–108.

Titchener, J. L., & Kapp, F. T. (1976). Family and character change at Buffalo Creek. *Am. J. Psychiatry, 133,* 295–299.

Ursano, R. J. (1981). The Vietnam era prisoners of war: Precaptivity personality and the development. *Am. J. Psychiatry, 138,* 315–318.

Ursano, R. J., Boydstun, J. A., & Wheatley, R. D. (1981). Psychiatric illness in U.S. Air Force Vietnam prisoners of war: A five-year follow-up. *Amer. J. Psychiatry, 138,* 310–314.

Van Putten, T., & Emory, W. H. (1973). Traumatic neuroses in Viet Nam returnees: A forgotten diagnosis? *Arch. Gen. Psychiatry, 29,* 695–698.

Walker, J. I. (1981). Viet Nam combat veterans with legal difficulties: A psychiatric problem? *Am. J. Psychiatry, 138,* 1384–1385.

Westermeyer, J. (1975). Social aspects of violence. In J. Lieberman (Ed.), *Mental health: The public health challenge* (pp. 213–217). Washington, DC: American Public Health Association.

Westermeyer, J. (1976a). Clinical guidelines for cross-cultural treatment of chemical dependence. *Am. J. Drug Alc. Abuse, 3,* 315–322.

Westermeyer, J. (1976b). The average of Indian families in crisis. In S. Unger (Ed.), *The destruction of Indian family life* (pp. 47–56). New York: Association for American Indian Affairs.

Westermeyer, J. (1976c). Use of a social indicator system to assess alcoholism among American Indian people in Minnesota. *Am. J. Drug Alcohol Abuse, 3,* 447–456.

Westermeyer, J. (1979). The "apple" syndrome: The effects of racial-ethnic discontinuity. *J. Operat. Psychiatry, 10,* 134–140.

Westermeyer, J. (1985a). The course of depression and depressive symptoms: A review and analysis. *Integr. Psychiatry, 3,* 144-154.

Westermeyer, J. (1985b). *A clinical guide to alcohol and drug problems.* Philadelphia: Praeger.

Westermeyer, J. (1985c). Among drinking practices in the United States: The influence of migration. In L. Bennett & G. Ames (Eds.), *The American experience with alcohol* (pp. 373–391). New York: Plenum.

Westermeyer, J. (1985d). Mental health of Southeast Asian refugees: Observations over two decades from Laos and the United States. In T. C. Cowan (Ed.), *Southeast Asian mental health: Treatment, prevention, services, training and research* (pp. 65–89). Washington, DC: National Institute for Mental Health.

Westermeyer, J. (1985e). Psychiatric epidemiology among Indochinese refugees: Methods and findings. *Asian Refugee Mental Health* (NIMH report).

Westermeyer, J. (1985f). Psychiatric diagnosis across cultural boundaries. *Amer. J. Psychiatry, 142,* 798–805.

Westermeyer, J. (1986a). Clinical considerations in cross cultural diagnosis. *Hospital and Community Psychiatry.*

Westermeyer, J. (1986b). Migration and psychopathology. In C. Williams & J. Westermeyer (Eds.), *Refugee mental health issues in resettlement countries.* New York: Hemisphere.

Westermeyer, J. (1986c). Psychiatric care of refugees. In R. H. Sandler (Ed.), *Medical care of refugees.* New York: Oxford University Press.

Westermeyer, J. (1986d). Two self rating scales for depression in Hmong refugees: Assessment in clinical and nonclinical samples. *J. Psychiatric Res.*

Westermeyer, J., & Brantner, J. (1972). Violent death and alcohol use among the Chippewa of Minnesota. *Minnesota Med, 55,* 749–752.

Westermeyer, J., Neider, J., & Vang, T. F. (1984a). Acculturation and mental health: A study of Hmong refugees at 1.5 and 3.5 years postmigration. *Social Sci. Med, 18,* 87–93.

Westermeyer, J., & Peake, E. (1983). A ten year follow up of alcoholic Native Americans in Minnesota. *Am. J. Psychiatry, 140,* 189–194.

Westermeyer, J., & Sines, L. (1979). Reliability of cross-cultural psychiatric diagnosis with an assessment of two rating contexts. *J. Psychiatric Res, 15,* 199–213.

Westermeyer, J., Vang, T. F., & Lyfong, G. (1983). Hmong refugees in Minnesota: Characteristics and self-perceptions. *Minnesota Med, 66,* 431–439.

Westermeyer, J., Vang, T. F., & Neider, J. (1983a). A comparison of refugees using and not using a psychiatric service: An analysis of DSM-III criteria and self-rating scales in cross-cultural context. *J. Opera. Psychiat, 14,* 36–41.

Westermeyer, J., Vang, T. F., & Neider, J. (1983b). Migration and mental health: Association of pre- and post-migration factors with self-rating scales. *J. Nerv. Ment. Dis, 171,* 92–96.

Westermeyer, J., Vang, T. F., & Neider, J. (1983c). Refugees who do and do not seek psychiatric care: An analysis of premigratory and postmigratory characteristics. *J. Nerv. Ment. Dis, 171,* 86–91.

Westermeyer, J., Vang, T. F., & Neider, J. (1984). Symptom change over time among Hmong refugees: Psychiatric patients versus nonpatients. *Psychopathology, 17,* 168–177.

Westermeyer, J., & Walker, D. (1982). Approaches to treatment of alcoholism across cultural boundaries. *Psychiatry Ann, 12,* 434–439.

Westermeyer, J., & Williams, C. (1986). Planning mental health services for refugees. In C. Williams & J. Westermeyer (Eds.), *Refugee mental health issues in resettlement countries.* New York: Hemisphere.

Wilkinson, C. B. (1983). Aftermath of a disaster: The collapse of the Hyatt Regency Hotel skywalks. *Am. J. Psychiatry, 140,* 1134–1139.

Williams, C., & Westermeyer, J. (1983). Psychiatric problems among adolescent Southeast Asian refugees: A descriptive study. *J. Nerv. Ment. Dis, 171,* 79–85.

Williams, C., & Westermeyer, J. (1986). *Mental health of refugees in resettlement countries.* New York: Hemisphere.

Worthington, E. R. (1978). Demographic and preservice variables as predictors of post-military service adjustment. In C. R. Figley, *Stress disorders among Vietnam veterans.* New York: Brunner/Mazel.

Yesavage, J. A. (1983). Dangerous behavior by Viet Nam veterans with schizophrenia. *Am. J. Psychiatry, 140,* 1180–1183.

Zarjenski, Y. (1985). Forty years in the service of refugees. *Refugees, 22,* 20–21.

About the Editors

George S. Everly, Jr., Ph.D., F.A.P.M. is Chairman of the Board and Chief Executive Officer of the International Critical Incident Stress Foundation, a nonprofit organization that provides education, training, and consultative support services to emergency services, disaster response, and humanitarian aid organizations worldwide. A Fellow of the Academy of Psychosomatic Medicine and of the American Institute of Stress, Dr. Everly is the author, coauthor, or editor of 10 textbooks and over 100 scientific and professional papers, including *A Clinical Guide to the Treatment of the Human Stress Response* (Plenum, 1989) and *Critical Incident Stress Debriefing* (1993). As one of the first psychologists trained in disaster mental health by the American Red Cross, he led the efforts to establish the disaster mental health network for the Maryland Psychological Association and for the Central Maryland Chapter of the American Red Cross, where he serves as mental health coordinator. A former Harvard Scholar, Dr. Everly has held appointments on the faculties of Harvard University, Harvard Medical School, and Johns Hopkins University. He is currently adjunct professor of psychology at Loyola College in Maryland.

Jeffrey M. Lating, Ph.D. is currently director of clinical training at Union Memorial Hospital, Baltimore. A graduate of Swarthmore College and the University of Georgia, Dr. Lating interned at Homewood Hospital Center of the Johns Hopkins Health System. He was a postdoctoral fellow in medical psychology at the Johns Hopkins Hospital.

Index